New Approaches and Technologies in Orthodontics

New Approaches and Technologies in Orthodontics

Editors

Letizia Perillo
Vincenzo Grassia
Fabrizia d'Apuzzo

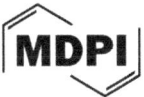

Basel • Beijing • Wuhan • Barcelona • Belgrade • Novi Sad • Cluj • Manchester

Editors

Letizia Perillo
Multidisciplinary Department
of Medical-Surgical and
Dental Specialties, University
of Campania Luigi Vanvitelli
Naples
Italy

Vincenzo Grassia
Multidisciplinary Department
of Medical-Surgical and
Dental Specialties, University
of Campania Luigi Vanvitelli
Naples
Italy

Fabrizia d'Apuzzo
Multidisciplinary Department
of Medical-Surgical and
Dental Specialties, University
of Campania Luigi Vanvitelli
Naples
Italy

Editorial Office
MDPI
St. Alban-Anlage 66
4052 Basel, Switzerland

This is a reprint of articles from the Special Issue published online in the open access journal *Journal of Clinical Medicine* (ISSN 2077-0383) (available at: https://www.mdpi.com/journal/jcm/special_issues/dentofacial_orthodontics).

For citation purposes, cite each article independently as indicated on the article page online and as indicated below:

Lastname, A.A.; Lastname, B.B. Article Title. *Journal Name* **Year**, *Volume Number*, Page Range.

ISBN 978-3-7258-1221-9 (Hbk)
ISBN 978-3-7258-1222-6 (PDF)
doi.org/10.3390/books978-3-7258-1222-6

© 2024 by the authors. Articles in this book are Open Access and distributed under the Creative Commons Attribution (CC BY) license. The book as a whole is distributed by MDPI under the terms and conditions of the Creative Commons Attribution-NonCommercial-NoDerivs (CC BY-NC-ND) license.

Contents

Letizia Perillo, Fabrizia d'Apuzzo and Vincenzo Grassia
New Approaches and Technologies in Orthodontics
Reprinted from: *J. Clin. Med.* **2024**, *13*, 2470, doi:10.3390/jcm13092470 1

Ludger Keilig, Lena Brieskorn, Jörg Schwarze, Werner Schupp, Christoph Bourauel and Anna Konermann
Treatment Efficiency of Maxillary and Mandibular Orovestibular Tooth Expansion and Compression Movements with the Invisalign® System in Adolescents and Adults
Reprinted from: *J. Clin. Med.* **2024**, *13*, 1267, doi:10.3390/jcm13051267 6

Mirei Keitoku, Ikuo Yonemitsu, Yuhei Ikeda, Huan Tang and Takashi Ono
Differential Recovery Patterns of the Maxilla and Mandible after Eliminating Nasal Obstruction in Growing Rats
Reprinted from: *J. Clin. Med.* **2022**, *11*, 7359, doi:10.3390/jcm11247359 22

Olivia Griswold, Chenshuang Li, Justin C. Orr, Normand S. Boucher, Shalin R. Shah and Chun-Hsi Chung
Lip Bumper Therapy Does Not Influence the Sagittal Mandibular Incisor Position in a Retrospective CBCT Study
Reprinted from: *J. Clin. Med.* **2022**, *11*, 6032, doi:10.3390/jcm11206032 38

Teodora Consuela Bungău, Luminița Ligia Vaida, Abel Emanuel Moca, Gabriela Ciavoi, Raluca Iurcov, Ioana Mihaela Romanul and Camelia Liana Buhaș
Mini-Implant Rejection Rate in Teenage Patients Depending on Insertion Site: A Retrospective Study
Reprinted from: *J. Clin. Med.* **2022**, *11*, 5331, doi:10.3390/jcm11185331 48

Patricia Solano Mendoza, Paula Aceytuno Poch, Enrique Solano Reina and Beatriz Solano Mendoza
Skeletal, Dentoalveolar and Dental Changes after "Mini-Screw Assisted Rapid Palatal Expansion" Evaluated with Cone Beam Computed Tomography
Reprinted from: *J. Clin. Med.* **2022**, *11*, 4652, doi:10.3390/jcm11164652 59

Arwa Gera, Shadi Gera, Michel Dalstra, Paolo M. Cattaneo and Marie A. Cornelis
Validity and Reproducibility of the Peer Assessment Rating Index Scored on Digital Models Using a Software Compared with Traditional Manual Scoring
Reprinted from: *J. Clin. Med.* **2021**, *10*, 1646, doi:10.3390/jcm10081646 79

Georgios Kanavakis, Anna-Sofia Silvola, Demetrios Halazonetis, Raija Lähdesmäki and Pertti Pirttiniemi
Incisor Occlusion Affects Profile Shape Variation in Middle-Aged Adults
Reprinted from: *J. Clin. Med.* **2021**, *10*, 800, doi:10.3390/jcm10040800 90

Ralph M. Steegman, Annemarlien Faye Klein Meulekamp, Arjan Dieters, Johan Jansma, Wicher J. van der Meer and Yijin Ren
Skeletal Changes in Growing Cleft Patients with Class III Malocclusion Treated with Bone Anchored Maxillary Protraction—A 3.5-Year Follow-Up
Reprinted from: *J. Clin. Med.* **2021**, *10*, 750, doi:10.3390/jcm10040750 100

Anuraj Singh Kochhar, Ludovica Nucci, Maninder Singh Sidhu, Mona Prabhakar, Vincenzo Grassia, Letizia Perillo, Gulsheen Kaur Kochhar, et al.
Reliability and Reproducibility of Landmark Identification in Unilateral Cleft Lip and Palate Patients: Digital Lateral Vis-A-Vis CBCT-Derived 3D Cephalograms
Reprinted from: *J. Clin. Med.* **2021**, *10*, 535, doi:10.3390/jcm10030535 . . . . **112**

Ionut Luchian, Mihaela Moscalu, Ancuta Goriuc, Ludovica Nucci, Monica Tatarciuc, Ioana Martu and Mihai Covasa
Using Salivary MMP-9 to Successfully Quantify Periodontal Inflammation during Orthodontic Treatment
Reprinted from: *J. Clin. Med.* **2021**, *10*, 379, doi:10.3390/jcm10030379 . . . . **123**

Chenshuang Li, Leanne Lin, Zhong Zheng and Chun-Hsi Chung
A User-Friendly Protocol for Mandibular Segmentation of CBCT Images for Superimposition and Internal Structure Analysis
Reprinted from: *J. Clin. Med.* **2021**, *10*, 127, doi:10.3390/jcm10010127 . . . . **132**

Nikolaos Gkantidis, Konstantinos Dritsas, Christos Katsaros, Demetrios Halazonetis and Yijin Ren
3D Method for Occlusal Tooth Wear Assessment in Presence of Substantial Changes on Other Tooth Surfaces
Reprinted from: *J. Clin. Med.* **2020**, *9*, 3937, doi:10.3390/jcm9123937 . . . . **145**

Leixuri de Frutos-Valle, Conchita Martín, José Antonio Alarcón, Juan Carlos Palma-Fernández, Ricardo Ortega and Alejandro Iglesias-Linares
Novel Sub-Clustering of Class III Skeletal Malocclusion Phenotypes in a Southern European Population Based on Proportional Measurements
Reprinted from: *J. Clin. Med.* **2020**, *9*, 3048, doi:10.3390/jcm9093048 . . . . **158**

Seo-Hyun Park, Soo-Hwan Byun, So-Hee Oh, Hye-Lim Lee, Ju-Won Kim, Byoung-Eun Yang and In-Young Park
Evaluation of the Reliability, Reproducibility and Validity of Digital Orthodontic Measurements Based on Various Digital Models among Young Patients
Reprinted from: *J. Clin. Med.* **2020**, *9*, 2728, doi:10.3390/jcm9092728 . . . . **171**

Hyeran Helen Jeon, Hellen Teixeira and Andrew Tsai
Mechanistic Insight into Orthodontic Tooth Movement Based on Animal Studies: A Critical Review
Reprinted from: *J. Clin. Med.* **2021**, *10*, 1733, doi:10.3390/jcm10081733 . . . . **182**

Fabrizia d'Apuzzo, Ludovica Nucci, Ines Delfino, Marianna Portaccio, Giuseppe Minervini, Gaetano Isola, Ismene Serino, et al.
Application of Vibrational Spectroscopies in the Qualitative Analysis of Gingival Crevicular Fluid and Periodontal Ligament during Orthodontic Tooth Movement
Reprinted from: *J. Clin. Med.* **2021**, *10*, 1405, doi:10.3390/jcm10071405 . . . . **197**

Maria Contaldo, Alberta Lucchese, Carlo Lajolo, Cosimo Rupe, Dario Di Stasio, Antonio Romano, Massimo Petruzzi, et al.
The Oral Microbiota Changes in Orthodontic Patients and Effects on Oral Health: An Overview
Reprinted from: *J. Clin. Med.* **2021**, *10*, 780, doi:10.3390/jcm10040780 . . . . **217**

Darius Bidjan, Rahel Sallmann, Theodore Eliades and Spyridon N. Papageorgiou
Orthopedic Treatment for Class II Malocclusion with Functional Appliances and Its Effect on Upper Airways: A Systematic Review with Meta-Analysis
Reprinted from: *J. Clin. Med.* **2020**, *9*, 3806, doi:10.3390/jcm9123806 . . . . **230**

Laura Templier, Cecilia Rossi, Manuel Miguez, Javier De la Cruz Pérez, Adrián Curto, Alberto Albaladejo and Manuel Lagravère Vich
Combined Surgical and Orthodontic Treatments in Children with OSA: A Systematic Review
Reprinted from: *J. Clin. Med.* **2020**, *9*, 2387, doi:10.3390/jcm9082387 . . . . **248**

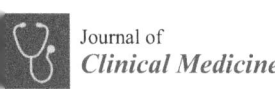

Editorial

New Approaches and Technologies in Orthodontics

Letizia Perillo, Fabrizia d'Apuzzo and Vincenzo Grassia *

Multidisciplinary Department of Medical-Surgical and Dental Specialties, University of Campania Luigi Vanvitelli, 80138 Naples, Italy; letizia.perillo@unicampania.it (L.P.); fabrizia.dapuzzo@unicampania.it (F.d.)
* Correspondence: vincenzo.grassia@unicampania.it

1. Introduction

In recent years, new diagnostic and treatment approaches in orthodontics have arisen, and there is thus a need for researchers and practitioners to stay up to date with these innovations [1–3].

In recent years, artificial intelligence (AI) development has advanced, allowing each expert to provide better alternatives to patients, to make more precise diagnoses, and to reduce treatment costs and timeframes [4,5].

New technologies and procedures, such as intraoral scanners, digital models, and measurements, along with increasing use of CBCT [6], have slowly expanded, enhancing overall patient care, treatment plan management, and prevention, particularly in the early stages [7,8].

The everyday use of AI technology has increased the potential of each treatment step in real time, including examining the outcome, evaluating all feasible options, and staging the state of oral hygiene.

Currently, impacted teeth, facial deformities [9], OSA [10], and other oral disorders or pathologies [11] may be detected more quickly, allowing for more direct and timely communication while also enhancing patient compliance [12]. Furthermore, technology has enabled the accurate timing and positioning of many types of orthodontic devices, such as functional appliances and mini-screws, as well as the ability to determine which factors are connected to the orthodontic treatment movement (OTM) [13,14].

The literature is regularly updated with fresh research, allowing doctors to provide more effective and less onerous therapies to each patient [15]. As a result, the goal of this Special Issue was to encourage research in all areas of orthodontics, with an emphasis on diagnostic and therapeutic advances to widen our knowledge and support scientific and clinical discoveries.

2. An Overview of Published Articles

Kanavakis G. et al. [16] evaluated the effects of overjet (OVJ) and overbite (OVB) on the profile of middle-aged patients. They concluded that OVJ significantly leads to changes to upper lips, while OVB has minor consequences for the general shape of the profile. However, considering the variety of genetic and environmental factors that affect the soft tissues of the face, these outcomes could become more significant.

A younger sample size, from 12 to 17 years, was analyzed by Bungău T.C. et al. [17], who examined the rejection rate of mini-implants in orthodontics. The application of these devices can be helpful in several approaches according to the severity of the malocclusion. The authors investigated the rejection rate up to three months after positioning. In conclusion, mini-implants showed the highest percentage of rejection (25%) in the buccal mandibular bone during the first month, while in the second month, it was recorded in the lingual region. Thus, mini-implants are useful devices during orthodontic treatment (OT), but their stability must be improved.

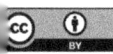

Malocclusions have also been studied by other authors. Frutos-Valle L. and colleagues [18] established a Class III skeletal malocclusion sub-phenotype characterization based on proportional cranial measurements using principal component and cluster analyses. They recognized four phenotypic subgroups, from C1 to C4, according to the severity of the malocclusion. Therefore, the authors provided a new subset of Class III skeletal malocclusions, improving diagnostic and therapeutic approaches to this malocclusion.

Similarly, Class III malocclusion was analyzed by Steegman R.M. et al. [19]. This group presented a prospective controlled study to assess the skeletal effect of anchored bone extension (BAMP) in Class III patients with a cleft using CBCT. Their results, with a follow-up of about 3.5 years, provide the first evidence to support BAMP as an effective and reliable treatment option for growing subjects with mild-to-moderate Class III malocclusion up to an average age of 15 years.

The potential use of CBCT was also considered by Griswold O. et al. [20], who conducted a longitudinal retrospective study to compare patients treated only with rapid maxillary expansion (RME) and patients treated with RME and LB using CBCT. Pre- and post-treatment CBCTs were superimposed to determine changes in anterior lower teeth. Both study groups showed no significant changes in the proclination of the lower incisors. Hence, the use of LB would seem not to affect the position of the mandibular incisors significantly.

CBCT was used by other researchers for their studies as well, including Solano Mendoza P. et al. [21], who assessed skeletal and dental changes after mini-screw-assisted rapid palatal expansion (MARPE) in adolescent patients. They conducted an uncontrolled prospective study on 17-year-old subjects with transverse maxillary deficiency. Pre- (T1) and post-expansion (T2) CBCT and digital casts were taken to evaluate changes to the premolar and first molar areas. Therefore, they concluded that MARPE is a successful means of obtaining skeletal maxillary expansion in adolescents, observing only small dentoalveolar changes that are not clinically detectable.

Similarly, Li C. et al. [22] created an efficient and accurate orthodontist-friendly protocol to segment the mandible while maintaining access to internal structures based on CBCT images. At the end of the measurements, it was seen that the mandibular bones of all tested DICOM files were successfully segmented. In addition, all anatomical structures were found in voxel-based overlap, demonstrating the ability of CBCTs to conduct precise internal structure analysis.

Finally, also Kochhar A.S. et al. [23] conducted a retrospective study to compare the accuracy of the identification of reference points and their reproducibility using 3D cephalograms derived from CBCT and digital lateral–lateral radiographs in patients with cleft lip and cleft palate. The identification of the points and their reproducibility on CBCT were found to be statistically significant compared to the lateral–lateral radiographs.

Several digital tools have been employed by Park S.H. et al. [24]. They evaluated the reliability, reproducibility, and validity of orthodontic measurements, such as tooth width, arch length, and arch length discrepancy, on plaster models (P), digital scanning models (MSD), and intraoral scanned digital models (ISD). Most orthodontic measurements have shown high validity. Measurements based on the digital program appeared highly reliable, reproducible, and accurate compared to conventional measurements. Despite this, clinicians should be aware of the errors induced by the distortion caused by using digital models.

Moreover, Gkantidis N. and colleagues [25] developed a 3D overlay technique to evaluate morphological changes in dental surfaces other than occlusal ones. It has been seen that this new technique offers a convenient, accurate, and risk-free assessment of tooth wear. Similarly, Keilig et al. [26] evaluated the efficiency of teeth alignment with clear aligners (CAs) using the 3D overlap, considering the different variability. They deduced that CAs can implement tooth movements effectively through the inclination of clinical crowns. However, digital planning needs to take individual patient parameters into account to make OT more predictable and efficient.

The use of digital instruments and manual techniques was compared by Gera A. et al. [27], who evaluated the validity and reproducibility of the peer assessment rating (PAR) index and its components using software versus a manual method. There were no significant differences in average PAR scores between both methods, but statistical tests confirmed the excellent validity and reproducibility of the PAR index on digital models compared to manual scoring on equivalent printed models through a gauge digital model.

Another field of research was addressed by Templier L. and coworkers [28], who conducted literature research to evaluate and summarize current scientific data on the effectiveness of both adenotonsillectomy (AT) and OT with rapid maxillary expansion (RME) and/or mandibular advancement (MA) in children with obstructive sleep apnea (OSA). They concluded that AT, together with RME and/or MA, is an efficient treatment in pediatric patients with OSA. AT, RME, and/or MA, when performed together, lead to a decrease in the hypopnea apnea index (AHI) and respiratory disorders index (RDI) and an increase in oxygen saturation and the oxygen desaturation index (ODI). However, the risk of relapse may occur even after proper treatment, so myofunctional therapy (MT) should also be implemented during follow-up.

The effects of functional appliances (FA) on upper airway dimensions were analyzed by Bidjan D. et al. [29] through a systematic review and meta-analysis. They gathered 20 non-randomized clinical trials, according to which orthopedic treatment with FA, both fixed and removable, is associated with an increased volume of the oropharynx and nasopharynx compared to natural growth. Removable FAs showed noticeably greater effects compared to fixed ones. In addition, the patient's age and treatment duration also significantly affected the outcome of FAs on the respiratory tract. Although nasal obstruction (NO) during growth causes the suppression of maxillofacial growth, it is unclear whether the elimination of NO differentially affects maxillary and mandibular growth.

The NO was also investigated by Keitoku M. and colleagues [30]. They performed a study on male mice, removing the sutures for resume nasal breathing to assess if elimination of the NO could allow for normal maxillofacial growth, determining, at the same time, the right timing of intervention. They have, therefore, evaluated immunohistochemical changes in the hypoxia-inducible factor (HIF)-1α, osteoprotegerin (OPG), and nuclear factor receptor activator kappa-B ligand (RANKL) of condylar cartilage. Their study suggests that the elimination of NO is effective in recovering maxillofacial growth. In addition, the optimal timing of surgery differed between the jaw and the jaw.

Other studies have focused on biomarkers. In particular, Luchian I. and collaborators [31] have evaluated the effects of periodontal treatment (PT) alone or in combination with OT on the levels of MMP-9. The results showed that both PT and OT significantly improved clinical parameters and lowered MMP-9 levels compared to the control group. However, the combination of PT and OT improved both clinical parameters and the reduction in MMP-9 levels. It was also shown that the degree of malocclusion also significantly affects MPP-9 levels.

d'Apuzzo F. et al. [32] studied the composition, structure, and molecular interaction of gingival crevicular fluid (GCF) and periodontal ligament (PDL) during orthodontic tooth movement (OTM) with optical vibrational techniques to put in place more personalized treatments, reducing any side effects. At the same time, Jeon H. H. and colleagues [33] examined alveolar bone remodeling during the OTM and the involved mechanisms, such as mechanosensing, sterile inflammation-mediated osteoclastogenesis, and tensile force-induced osteogenesis. They found that the cells most involved in the OTM response are periodontal fibroblasts, mesenchymal stem cells, osteoblasts, osteocytes, and osteoclasts. At the same time, intercellular signals that stimulate the OTM include RANKL, TNF-α, DKK1, sclerostin, TGF-β, and BPM.

Finally, Contaldo M. et al. [34] focused on the biological and microbiological changes related to the OT to highlight further correlations between orthodontic devices and qualitative and quantitative changes in the oral microbiota. Orthodontic patients reported significant differences in supragingival and subgingival plaque during the entire OT. Some fixed appliances, such as bonded molar brackets or elastomeric ligatures, showed high risks of periodontal disease and tooth decay for patients.

3. Conclusions

To summarize, these data provide the foundation for establishing the best possible diagnosis and serve as a reference point for future scientific study in orthodontics. Analyses and surveys conducted using new analysis equipment and cutting-edge technology demonstrated great repeatability and validity when compared to manual approaches, which had previously been regarded as the gold standard. In reality, the findings of this research provide a trustworthy foundation for treatment planning and can assist doctors in implementing therapy for all types of patients. Further study is needed to corroborate these assumptions, which should be chosen based on varied individual scenarios while constantly taking biological variety into account. Nonetheless, while AI is certainly useful to orthodontists and other health professionals, doctors will always be responsible for making ultimate health choices.

Conflicts of Interest: The authors declare no conflict of interest.

References

1. Liu, J.; Zhang, C.; Shan, Z. Application of Artificial Intelligence in Orthodontics: Current State and Future Perspectives. *Healthcare* **2023**, *11*, 2760. [CrossRef] [PubMed]
2. Bichu, Y.M.; Hansa, I.; Bichu, A.Y.; Premjani, P.; Flores-Mir, C.; Vaid, N.R. Applications of Artificial Intelligence and Machine Learning in Orthodontics: A Scoping Review. *Prog. Orthod.* **2021**, *22*, 18. [CrossRef] [PubMed]
3. Kazimierczak, N.; Kazimierczak, W.; Serafin, Z.; Nowicki, P.; Nożewski, J.; Janiszewska-Olszowska, J. AI in Orthodontics Revolutionizing Diagnostics and Treatment Planning—A Comprehensive Review. *J. Clin. Med.* **2024**, *13*, 344. [CrossRef] [PubMed]
4. Ahmed, N.; Abbasi, M.S.; Zuberi, F.; Qamar, W.; Halim, M.S.B.; Maqsood, A.; Alam, M.K. Artificial Intelligence Techniques Analysis, Application, and Outcome in Dentistry—A Systematic Review. *BioMed Res. Int.* **2021**, *2021*, 9751564. [CrossRef] [PubMed]
5. Gianfreda, F.; Pesce, P.; Marcano, E.; Pistilli, V.; Bollero, P.; Canullo, L. Clinical Outcome of Fully Digital Workflow for Single-Implant-Supported Crowns: A Retrospective Clinical Study. *Dent. J.* **2022**, *10*, 139. [CrossRef] [PubMed]
6. Kim, S.-H.; Kim, K.B.; Choo, H. New Frontier in Advanced Dentistry: CBCT, Intraoral Scanner, Sensors, and Artificial Intelligence in Dentistry. *Sensors* **2022**, *22*, 2942. [CrossRef] [PubMed]
7. Nucci, L.; d'Apuzzo, F.; Nastri, L.; Femiano, F.; Perillo, L.; Grassia, V. Enamel Interproximal Reduction and Periodontal Health. *Semin. Orthod.* **2023**, *30*, 146–149. [CrossRef]
8. Lam, M.; Dekel, E.; Nucci, L.; Grassia, V.; Naoumova, J.; Pacheco-Pereira, C.; Perillo, L.; Chaushu, S.; Flores-Mir, C. The Effect of the Dental Follicle Volume of Palatally Impacted Canines on the Relative Position of the Adjacent Teeth. *Eur. J. Orthod.* **2024**, *46*, cjad071. [CrossRef] [PubMed]
9. Bharti, P.; Gupta, H.; Kumar, A. Treatment of Post-Traumatic Facial Deformities. *J. Maxillofac. Oral Surg.* **2023**, *22*, 972–978. [CrossRef] [PubMed]
10. Shi, Y.; Zhang, Y.; Cao, Z.; Ma, L.; Yuan, Y.; Niu, X.; Su, Y.; Xie, Y.; Chen, X.; Xing, L.; et al. Application and Interpretation of Machine Learning Models in Predicting the Risk of Severe Obstructive Sleep Apnea in Adults. *BMC Med. Inform. Decis. Mak.* **2023**, *23*, 230. [CrossRef]
11. Patil, S.; Albogami, S.; Hosmani, J.; Mujoo, S.; Kamil, M.A.; Mansour, M.A.; Abdul, H.N.; Bhandi, S.; Ahmed, S.S.S.J. Artificial Intelligence in the Diagnosis of Oral Diseases: Applications and Pitfalls. *Diagnostics* **2022**, *12*, 1029. [CrossRef] [PubMed]
12. Perillo, L.; d'Apuzzo, F.; De Gregorio, F.; Grassia, V.; Barbetti, M.; Cugliari, G.; Nucci, L.; Castroflorio, T. Factors Affecting Patient Compliance during Orthodontic Treatment with Aligners: Motivational Protocol and Psychological Well-Being. *Turk. J. Orthod.* **2023**, *36*, 87–93. [CrossRef] [PubMed]
13. Laganà, G.; Malara, A.; Lione, R.; Danesi, C.; Meuli, S.; Cozza, P. Enamel Interproximal Reduction during Treatment with Clear Aligners: Digital Planning versus OrthoCAD Analysis. *BMC Oral Health* **2021**, *21*, 199. [CrossRef] [PubMed]
14. Akbari, A.; Gandhi, V.; Chen, J.; Turkkahraman, H.; Yadav, S. Vibrational Force on Accelerating Orthodontic Tooth Movement: A Systematic Review and Meta-Analysis. *Eur. J. Dent.* **2023**, *17*, 951–963. [CrossRef] [PubMed]
15. Bessadet, M.; Drancourt, N.; El Osta, N. Time Efficiency and Cost Analysis between Digital and Conventional Workflows for the Fabrication of Fixed Dental Prostheses: A Systematic Review. *J. Prosthet. Dent.* **2024**, *in press*. [CrossRef] [PubMed]
16. Kanavakis, G.; Silvola, A.-S.; Halazonetis, D.; Lähdesmäki, R.; Pirttiniemi, P. Incisor Occlusion Affects Profile Shape Variation in Middle-Aged Adults. *J. Clin. Med.* **2021**, *10*, 800. [CrossRef] [PubMed]
17. Bungău, T.C.; Vaida, L.L.; Moca, A.E.; Ciavoi, G.; Iurcov, R.; Romanul, I.M.; Buhaș, C.L. Mini-Implant Rejection Rate in Teenage Patients Depending on Insertion Site: A Retrospective Study. *J. Clin. Med.* **2022**, *11*, 5331. [CrossRef] [PubMed]
18. Frutos-Valle, L.D.; Martín, C.; Alarcón, J.A.; Palma-Fernández, J.C.; Ortega, R.; Iglesias-Linares, A. Novel Sub-Clustering of Class III Skeletal Malocclusion Phenotypes in a Southern European Population Based on Proportional Measurements. *J. Clin. Med.* **2020**, *9*, 3048. [CrossRef]

19. Steegman, R.M.; Klein Meulekamp, A.F.; Dieters, A.; Jansma, J.; Van Der Meer, W.J.; Ren, Y. Skeletal Changes in Growing Cleft Patients with Class III Malocclusion Treated with Bone Anchored Maxillary Protraction—A 3.5-Year Follow-Up. *J. Clin. Med.* **2021**, *10*, 750. [CrossRef]
20. Griswold, O.; Li, C.; Orr, J.C.; Boucher, N.S.; Shah, S.R.; Chung, C.-H. Lip Bumper Therapy Does Not Influence the Sagittal Mandibular Incisor Position in a Retrospective CBCT Study. *J. Clin. Med.* **2022**, *11*, 6032. [CrossRef]
21. Solano Mendoza, P.; Aceytuno Poch, P.; Solano Reina, E.; Solano Mendoza, B. Skeletal, Dentoalveolar and Dental Changes after "Mini-Screw Assisted Rapid Palatal Expansion" Evaluated with Cone Beam Computed Tomography. *J. Clin. Med.* **2022**, *11*, 4652. [CrossRef] [PubMed]
22. Li, C.; Lin, L.; Zheng, Z.; Chung, C.-H. A User-Friendly Protocol for Mandibular Segmentation of CBCT Images for Superimposition and Internal Structure Analysis. *J. Clin. Med.* **2021**, *10*, 127. [CrossRef] [PubMed]
23. Kochhar, A.S.; Nucci, L.; Sidhu, M.S.; Prabhakar, M.; Grassia, V.; Perillo, L.; Kochhar, G.K.; Bhasin, R.; Dadlani, H.; d'Apuzzo, F. Reliability and Reproducibility of Landmark Identification in Unilateral Cleft Lip and Palate Patients: Digital Lateral Vis-A-Vis CBCT-Derived 3D Cephalograms. *J. Clin. Med.* **2021**, *10*, 535. [CrossRef]
24. Park, S.-H.; Byun, S.-H.; Oh, S.-H.; Lee, H.-L.; Kim, J.-W.; Yang, B.-E.; Park, I.-Y. Evaluation of the Reliability, Reproducibility and Validity of Digital Orthodontic Measurements Based on Various Digital Models among Young Patients. *J. Clin. Med.* **2020**, *9*, 2728. [CrossRef]
25. Gkantidis, N.; Dritsas, K.; Katsaros, C.; Halazonetis, D.; Ren, Y. 3D Method for Occlusal Tooth Wear Assessment in Presence of Substantial Changes on Other Tooth Surfaces. *J. Clin. Med.* **2020**, *9*, 3937. [CrossRef] [PubMed]
26. Keilig, L.; Brieskorn, L.; Schwarze, J.; Schupp, W.; Bourauel, C.; Konermann, A. Treatment Efficiency of Maxillary and Mandibular Orovestibular Tooth Expansion and Compression Movements with the Invisalign® System in Adolescents and Adults. *J. Clin. Med.* **2024**, *13*, 1267. [CrossRef]
27. Gera, A.; Gera, S.; Dalstra, M.; Cattaneo, P.M.; Cornelis, M.A. Validity and Reproducibility of the Peer Assessment Rating Index Scored on Digital Models Using a Software Compared with Traditional Manual Scoring. *J. Clin. Med.* **2021**, *10*, 1646. [CrossRef] [PubMed]
28. Templier, L.; Rossi, C.; Miguez, M.; Pérez, J.D.L.C.; Curto, A.; Albaladejo, A.; Vich, M.L. Combined Surgical and Orthodontic Treatments in Children with OSA: A Systematic Review. *J. Clin. Med.* **2020**, *9*, 2387. [CrossRef]
29. Bidjan, D.; Sallmann, R.; Eliades, T.; Papageorgiou, S.N. Orthopedic Treatment for Class II Malocclusion with Functional Appliances and Its Effect on Upper Airways: A Systematic Review with Meta-Analysis. *J. Clin. Med.* **2020**, *9*, 3806. [CrossRef]
30. Keitoku, M.; Yonemitsu, I.; Ikeda, Y.; Tang, H.; Ono, T. Differential Recovery Patterns of the Maxilla and Mandible after Eliminating Nasal Obstruction in Growing Rats. *J. Clin. Med.* **2022**, *11*, 7359. [CrossRef]
31. Luchian, I.; Moscalu, M.; Goriuc, A.; Nucci, L.; Tatarciuc, M.; Martu, I.; Covasa, M. Using Salivary MMP-9 to Successfully Quantify Periodontal Inflammation during Orthodontic Treatment. *J. Clin. Med.* **2021**, *10*, 379. [CrossRef] [PubMed]
32. d'Apuzzo, F.; Nucci, L.; Delfino, I.; Portaccio, M.; Minervini, G.; Isola, G.; Serino, I.; Camerlingo, C.; Lepore, M. Application of Vibrational Spectroscopies in the Qualitative Analysis of Gingival Crevicular Fluid and Periodontal Ligament during Orthodontic Tooth Movement. *J. Clin. Med.* **2021**, *10*, 1405. [CrossRef] [PubMed]
33. Jeon, H.H.; Teixeira, H.; Tsai, A. Mechanistic Insight into Orthodontic Tooth Movement Based on Animal Studies: A Critical Review. *J. Clin. Med.* **2021**, *10*, 1733. [CrossRef] [PubMed]
34. Contaldo, M.; Lucchese, A.; Lajolo, C.; Rupe, C.; Di Stasio, D.; Romano, A.; Petruzzi, M.; Serpico, R. The Oral Microbiota Changes in Orthodontic Patients and Effects on Oral Health: An Overview. *J. Clin. Med.* **2021**, *10*, 780. [CrossRef] [PubMed]

Disclaimer/Publisher's Note: The statements, opinions and data contained in all publications are solely those of the individual author(s) and contributor(s) and not of MDPI and/or the editor(s). MDPI and/or the editor(s) disclaim responsibility for any injury to people or property resulting from any ideas, methods, instructions or products referred to in the content.

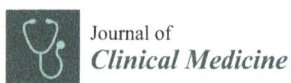 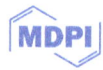

Article

Treatment Efficiency of Maxillary and Mandibular Orovestibular Tooth Expansion and Compression Movements with the Invisalign® System in Adolescents and Adults

Ludger Keilig [1,2], Lena Brieskorn [1], Jörg Schwarze [3], Werner Schupp [4], Christoph Bourauel [1,†] and Anna Konermann [5,*,†]

1. Oral Technology, University Hospital Bonn, 53111 Bonn, Germany
2. Department of Prosthodontics, University Hospital Bonn, 53127 Bonn, Germany
3. Private Practice, 50674 Cologne, Germany
4. Private Practice, 50996 Cologne, Germany
5. Department of Orthodontics, University Hospital Bonn, University of Bonn, Welschnonnenstr. 17, 53111 Bonn, Germany
* Correspondence: konermann@uni-bonn.de
† These authors contributed equally to this work.

Abstract: Objectives: Aligners are an effective and esthetic orthodontic treatment option for permanent and mixed dentition. There are only a few studies dealing with the effectiveness of orovestibular tooth movement using aligners and applying adequate examination methods. In the present retrospective study, the aligner efficiency of orovestibular movements for the entire dentition was systematically evaluated using 3D superimposition, taking into account the influence of jaw, tooth type and Invisalign® system. Methods: Group 1 (n = 18 adults, Invisalign®) and Group 2 (n = 17 adolescents, Invisalign® Teen) were treated with Invisalign® Ex30 aligner material and Invisalign® specific auxiliary means. In this non-interventional retrospective study, pre- and post-treatment maxillary and mandibular plaster cast models were scanned and superimposed with ClinChecks® via Surface–Surface Matching Algorithm on unmoved teeth providing stable references. Effectivity of planned versus clinically realized movements was evaluated for each tooth. Statistics were performed with a t-test and Bonferroni–Holm correction (α = 0.05). Results: Orovestibular movement efficiency was excellent without statistical significance regarding jaw, tooth type or Invisalign® system. Mandibular translational tooth movements were highly effective, and outstanding for premolars (91–98%). Maxillary translational tooth movements were successful for incisors and premolars, but less effective for canines and molars. Almost all teeth were moderately or very effectively corrected by crown tipping, performing better for mandibular (70–92%) than maxillary (22–31%) canines as much as for adolescent upper front teeth (81–85%) and lower canines (92%). Conclusions: Aligners are able to effectively implement translational orovestibular movements, supported by tilting the crowns for even more efficient implementation of the movements. This phenomenon was observed in our studies for all teeth in both jaws, regardless of the Invisalign® system used. Treatment planning should nevertheless take into account the individual patient parameters with regard to the movements to be performed in order to make the aligner therapy as successful as possible in terms of realizing the desired therapeutic goal.

Keywords: aligner; Invisalign®; orovestibular tooth movement; orthodontics; treatment efficiency

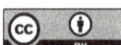

1. Introduction

Clear aligners have emerged as validated orthodontic treatment modality worldwide in the past two decades and still gain increasing popularity, particularly owing to their esthetic benefits. Generally, each aligner can affect tooth movements of 0.25 to 0.3 mm and of 2° on average [1]. In order to achieve these movements, aligner therapy requires higher patient compliance compared to multibracket therapy due to the removability of the devices, but the advantages outweigh the disadvantages, particularly from a patient perspective [2]. To mention the most relevant aspects, dental hygiene, caries control and speaking without limitations are possible and devoid of difficulty, and furthermore the high wearing comfort as much as the invisibility of the appliances make aligners attractive not only for adults but also for adolescents [3–8]. Since 2009, the option of aligner treatment is no longer restricted to adults or adolescents with full second dentition, but also available for teenagers with mixed dentition and erupting teeth due to the launch of Invisalign® Teen by Align Technology Inc. (Santa Clara, CA, USA). Investigations revealed that teenagers treated with aligners feature better compliance in oral hygiene, less plaque, and fewer gingival inflammatory reactions than the ones under fixed appliance therapy [3]. However, no data on the effectiveness of treatment with Invisalign® Teen exist to date, as such studies only focused on the compliance of adolescents wearing aligners [8,9].

Initially, aligners were considered a therapy device for correction of minor malpositioned teeth, but not for complex cases [10]. To date, the range of indications has been successively expanded through continuous advancements of the system [11–13]. In the current literature, clear aligner treatment is already estimated equivalent to the multi-bracket appliance as the gold standard in mild and moderate cases, but it is nonetheless an ongoing discussion whether aligner treatment is capable of perfectly correcting complex malocclusions as well [10,14,15]. A major point for skepticism is the assumption that the system most likely induces a tipping of moved teeth rather than a bodily translation, which represents a disadvantage compared to brackets [16,17]. In order to overcome this burden, additional tools have been developed for supporting the intended tooth movements, namely composite attachments on buccal and lingual tooth surfaces and power ridge points imprinted in the aligners that modify force projection [18–20]. When chronologically reflecting the weak data availability in the literature on aligner treatment spectrum and effectiveness, it was stated in 2000 that aligners enable correction of mild to moderate interproximal spaces and crowding, and that experts might be capable of conducting dental expansions, class II/III corrections and space closure upon extraction [21]. In the following years, investigations on the realization of specific tooth movements such as intrusion, rotation, incisor torque or molar distalization have been conducted, many of them implementing the impact of attachments and power ridges on the overall accuracy of treatment outcomes [18,19,22]. Just recently, a few studies started to focus on the feasibility and predictability of arch expansion with aligners [5,23–25]. However, these works manifested limitations regarding the methodologies applied and the overall study design. Mostly, linear measurements on digital arch models were performed, which is considerably defective due to the disregard of three-dimensionality. Other works applied the gingival margin as reference topology even though this structure is virtually designed in the ClinCheck® or did not directly correlate 3D models and ClinChecks®.

In order to overcome these burdens, superimposition techniques have to be used, which were implemented for the first time in aligner research by Kravitz et al. in 2009 [26]. By superimposing predicted tooth movements of the ClinCheck® onto achieved tooth positions of virtual models with Invisalign®'s proprietary superimposition software Tooth-Measure, potential discrepancies could be analyzed with an accuracy of 0.2 mm and 1.0° [26]. However, the major limitation of this study was the fact that only cases with corrections in the front region were incorporated and posterior tooth movements were disregarded owing to the necessity to superimpose the models on stationary teeth.

Our investigation is the first work that focuses on bridging this gap, combining both application of superimposition techniques and investigation on the whole jaws with anterior and posterior maxillary and mandibular regions. In the present retrospective study, we were able to combine both aspects with an advanced and seminal superimposition technique. The first aim of our investigation was to evaluate aligner efficiency of arch expanding and compressing tooth movements for all teeth of upper and lower jaws with this methodology. Secondly, we focused on analyzing potential differences in aligner performance with regard to upper and lower jaw and to tooth specimen for these orovestibular movements. Finally, we pursued the question whether treatment results are impacted by the aligner version, namely the conventional Invisalign® system versus Invisalign® Teen. In summary, the basic idea of our study is to evaluate the effects of the three aspects investigated, namely jaw, tooth group and aligner system, on the efficiency of orovestibular tooth movement. Our null hypothesis is that there are no statistically significant differences between these aspects. Our alternative hypothesis is that there may be statistically significant differences in treatment outcomes based on jaw, tooth group and aligner system.

2. Materials and Methods

2.1. Patient Collective

The data and clinical models were obtained from a patient collective, randomly selected without specification of the initial malocclusion or the amount of planned tooth correction in order to receive a broad spectrum of cases, subdivided into 2 groups. The study was conducted in accordance with the Declaration of Helsinki. The protocol did not need approval by the Ethics Committee of the University of Bonn since this was a non-interventional retrospective study. The patients had already finalized their treatment according to their orthodontic indication before the beginning of this study and had given their written consent to the treatment in advance.

Group 1 incorporated 18 adult patients treated with the conventional Invisalign® system, and Group 2 comprised 17 adolescent participants treated with Invisalign® Teen. A complete analysis for evaluation of the necessary number of patients was not possible, as for these concrete clinical questions no previous statistical data exist in the literature. Patient selection criteria included good general health, no medication affecting bone or soft tissue metabolism, no prosthetic restorations on the moved teeth, no premature occlusal contact on the front teeth, no radiographic signs of horizontal bone loss or vertical bony defects and no manifestations of root resorptions. All patients were treated with Invisalign® Exceed30 (EX30) aligner material and received Invisalign® specific auxiliary means such as attachments according to their individual needs. The number of aligners was prescribed by the malocclusion and varied between individuals.

2.2. Data Selection and Preparation

Data and documents for analyses comprised plaster cast models of upper and lower jaws from the initial (M.in) and the final situation after end of treatment (M.fin) for each patient. Here, only cases with at least 3 unmoved, not neighboring teeth per jaw were included in order to guarantee a stable superimposition. Plaster casts were digitized with a laser scanner (Micromeasure® 70, Micromeasure GmbH, Bischoffen, Germany). Models were fixed on an adjustable, motorized stage guided via the software 'ScanOs' (micromeasure GmbH), enabling digitization of even undercut areas. To achieve a perfect digitization, each model was scanned from four different perspectives. Resulting scatterplots were reduced to areas with teeth and gingiva and subsequently overlayed to a common surface. Achieved data were exported to an ASCII text data file. According to the manufacturer, distances between laser lines measure 100 µm on the x-axis and 53 µm on the y-axis. The data of the virtually planned treatment goals, the digital ClinChecks® (C), were provided as STL files by Align Technology Inc., consolidated for upper and lower jaws. The program ReMESH (version 2.1, Marco Attene, Istituto di Matematica Applicata e Tecnologie Informatiche Consiglio Nazionale delle Ricerche, Genova, Italy) was used to unravel the data for both jaws separately and to save them as independent files. Superimpositions of the three aforementioned digital data sets (M.in, M.fin, C) were realized by overlaying the models on the teeth that were not moved and thus served as stable references (Figure 1). After application of this selection criterion, 7 upper and 4 lower jaw models of Group 1 and 5 upper and 4 lower jaw models of Group 2 had to be excluded, as in these cases all teeth had to be moved according to the treatment plan. In addition, some models had to be eliminated due to inaccuracies or defects in the material. Thus, the overall collective used for analyses comprised 10 upper and 10 lower jaw models for Group 1 and 12 upper and 11 lower jaw models for Group 2.

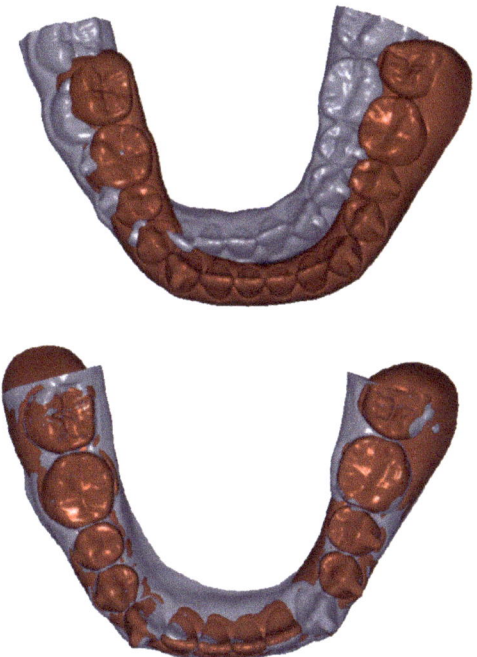

Figure 1. Representative example of a ClinCheck® (red, presented as surface) and a corresponding plaster cast model (grey, presented as surface) of the initial situation before treatment from a lower jaw. The upper picture shows the condition before matching and the lower picture represents the same situation after matching on the unmoved lower first and second premolars and the first molars in both quadrants.

2.3. Methodology of Investigations

Digitized models and ClinChecks® were visualized and edited with a specific 3D graphic software (Surfacer 10.5, Imageware/Siemens PLM Software, Plano, TX, USA), segmenting each tooth from the scatterplot surfaces before replicating it. Finally, complete model surfaces with alveolar ridges and separate tooth surfaces were available for each tooth. All teeth were investigated except the second and third molars. Superimpositions were realized with the Surface–Surface Matching Algorithm [27], overlaying the unmoved teeth of the final situation and the ClinCheck®, respectively, according to the principle of distance minimizing on the unmoved teeth of the initial situation (Figure 1). This results in a common reference system to which the rest of the alveolar ridge can be matched. It is generally known that even unmoved teeth can change their initial position and slightly move during orthodontic treatment due to interarch forces. Therefore, we verified whether the intertooth distance from the unmoved teeth differed from those of the final ClinCheck®, and excluded those unmoved teeth without a perfect fit in both categories.

After the general superimposition of the corresponding digital models in the different stages, we used the following procedure to determine the origin for the local coordinate system of each crown separately. First, we segmented the corresponding crown from the M.in model. Then we determined the minimum and maximum x and y coordinates over all points within the point set of this crown, and used $x_0 = (x_{max} + x_{min})/2$ and $y_0 = (y_{max} + y_{min})/2$ as the x and y coordinates for the local crown origin. This is basically the center of a 2D bounding box parallel to the occlusal plane. Finally, we determined the maximum z coordinate over all points within the point set of this crown, and used $z_0 = z_{max}$ as the z coordinate for the local crown origin.

Consequently, for analyses of single tooth movements, we specified a point in the center of the occlusal plane for each single tooth crown from the initial model M.in used as local coordinate origin. This local origin was then used in the subsequent superimposition of the corresponding crowns in the different models. A superimposition of individual scatterplots was conducted to calculate the clinically realized tooth movements by adjustment from M.in to C. The resulting differences in tooth positions calculated via Excel 2010 (Microsoft Corporation, Remond, WA, USA) gave information on six types of movement of the crowns: translations along the x-, y- and z-axis (Tx, Ty, Tz) and rotations around the x-, y- and z-axis (Rx, Ry, Rz). As movements of the roots were not retraceable with the given information, no differences were made between controlled and uncontrolled tipping and torque.

In order to equalize measurement results, a right-handed cartesian coordinate system with orthogonal coordinate axes was assigned to each model by which they were aligned in the Surfacer software (Surfacer 10.5, Imageware/Siemens PLM Software, Plano, TX, USA). Instead of the longitudinal axis of the tooth, which is not determinable via ClinCheck®, we used the global z-axis from this coordinate system established by means of a plane equaling the occlusal plane. As tooth-specific movements should be evaluated, the right-handed model-specific coordinate system had to be transformed into a tooth-specific coordinate system (Figure 2). For this, the x-axis was assigned to the transversal, the y-axis to the sagittal and the z-axis to the vertical direction.

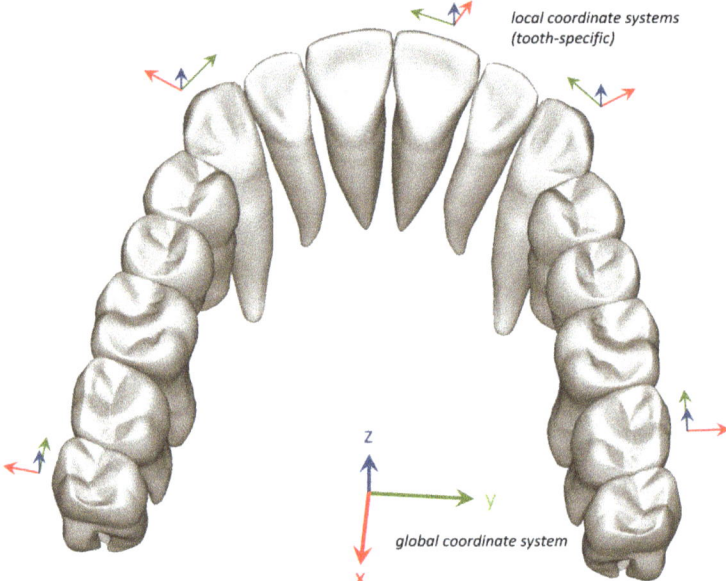

Figure 2. Illustration of an exemplary upper arch with global coordinate system (tall) and several tooth-specific coordinate systems (small). Tooth movements with course on the tooth-specific coordinate system along the x-axis correspond to mesio-distal movements, along the y-axis to orovestibular movements and along the z-axis to intrusions versus extrusions.

2.4. Data Analysis and Statistics

Effectivity of planned compared to clinically realized movements was evaluated for each tooth. Only teeth that showed planned translations above 0.2 mm and/or planned rotations above 2° were included in the following analysis. This was done as inaccuracies in the digitalization process in combination with inaccuracies of the proposed method result in high relative differences for small tooth movements. Including such small tooth movements would negatively influence the signal-to-noise ratio in the gathered data. Analyses were conducted if the sample size incorporated 3 cases or more. Tooth movements were separately calculated for each tooth from first incisor to the first molar of the upper and lower jaw, where first and second quadrant and third and fourth quadrant were taken together. In addition, we did not differentiate between expansion and compression-effecting movements and regarded them together as orovestibular movements.

The accuracy of the determined tooth movements depends on the extent of the movement. Systematic errors, either from the digitalization process or from methodical errors, influence small movements more than large movements. This holds especially when determining the efficiency as the quotient of the realized movements divided by the planned movements, i.e.,

$$e = \frac{m^{real}}{m^{plan}}$$

To compensate for this, we used the method of weighted means. Basically, this assumes that each calculated efficiency itself can be considered as a mean value over a single value, each with a separately assigned weight representing the reliability of these data. For each efficiency we used the general weighted means formula

$$\bar{e} = \frac{\sum_{i=0}^{n} w_i \cdot e_i}{\sum_{i=0}^{n} w_i}$$

to determine the mean values $\bar{e}$, and chose the weights as $w_i = \left| m_i^{plan} \right|$.

Statistics were performed for three different aspects:

1. Whether there were significant differences in the realization of expansion and compression movements with regard to the tooth type, namely incisors, canines, premolars and molars.
2. Whether the fact that bone structure differs in maxilla and mandibula was reflected by different effectivity of these orovestibular movements.
3. Whether due to either aspect 1 or 2, Group 1 and Group 2 exhibit significant variances.

Statistical analyses were done with a t-test and subsequent correction according to Bonferroni–Holm. A significance level of $\alpha = 0.05$ was considered statistically significant. A rating scale visualized in Figure 3 was used to categorize results to simplify and standardize an objective nomenclature. Values between 0 and 49% indicate a correction below the expected result, 50–69% and 131–150% a moderate effectivity, 70–89% and 111–130% a high effectivity, 91–110% a very high effectivity and 151% or higher an overcorrection.

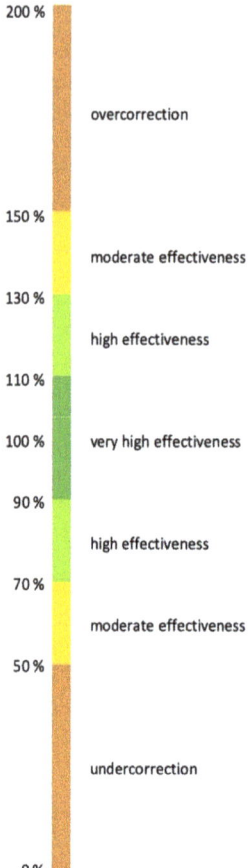

Figure 3. Rating scale for the categorization of results. Colored bars correlate with the mean relative effectivity and its corresponding interpretations. Values between 0 and 49% indicate a correction below the expected result, 50–69% and 131–150% a moderate effectivity, 70–89% and 111–130% a high effectivity, 91–110% a very high effectivity and 151% or higher an overcorrection.

3. Results

3.1. Effectiveness of Translational Movements for the Different Tooth Types of Upper and Lower Jaws

Most extent orovestibular movements were planned for upper and lower first incisors with 1.0 mm and 1.2 mm, and featured efficiencies of 80% and 82%, respectively (Figure 4A). Lower second premolars showed a very high effectivity of 96% for a similar amount of movement, and lower first premolars also presented a very high effectivity of 93% for 0.7 mm planned movement. Second incisors of both jaws, upper premolars, lower canines and lower molars manifested a high effectivity between 71 and 87% for mean planned movements of 0.5–1.0 mm. Exclusively the upper canines with 44% and upper molars with 55% could only reach a correction below the expected result or a moderate effectivity for 0.8 and 0.5 mm movement, respectively. Statistical outcomes did not significantly differ among single teeth or between upper and lower jaws.

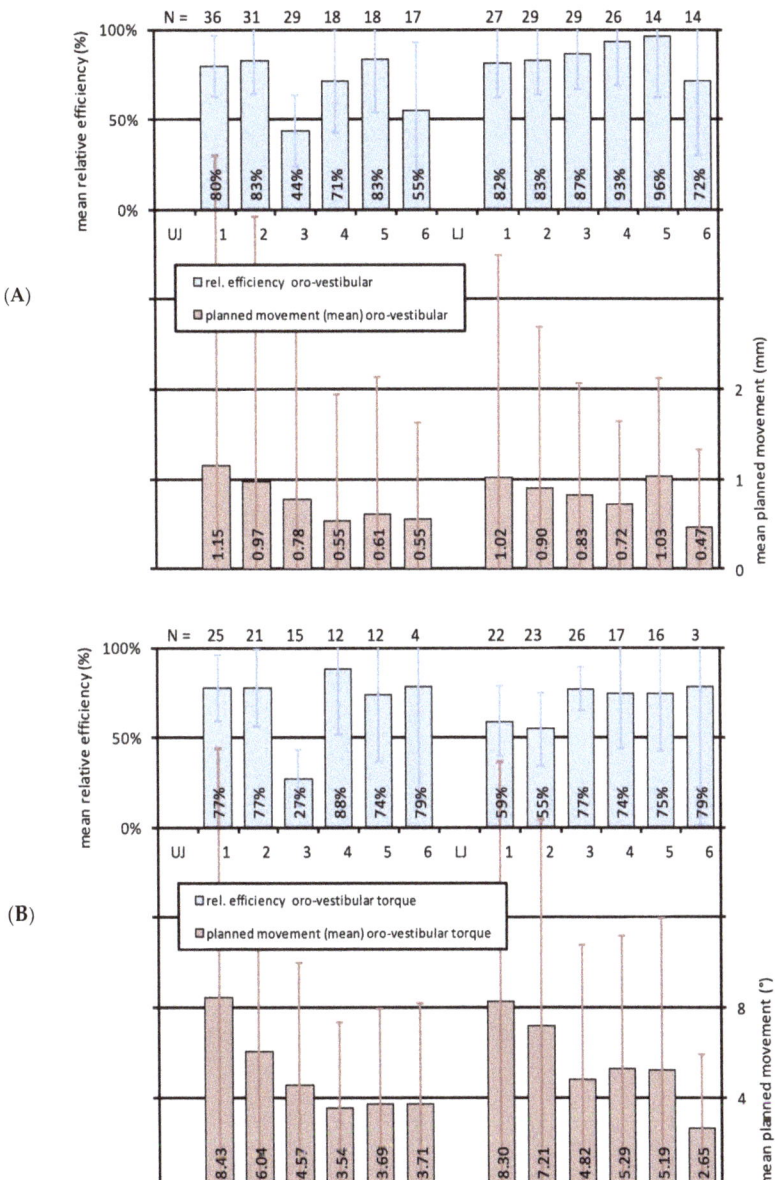

Figure 4. (**A**) Bar graph illustrating the relative effectivity of translational orovestibular tooth movements for the whole study cohort. Upper bars (blue) indicate the relative effectivity and the error in percent for each tooth of the upper (UJ, left) and the lower (LJ, right) jaw. Lower bars (red) show the mean planned movements in mm with standard deviations (SD). N-numbers of the corresponding mean values are specified on top of the illustration. (**B**) Bar graph illustrating the relative effectivity of rotations around the y-axis, equivalent to orovestibular torque, for the whole study cohort. Upper bars (blue) indicate the relative effectivity and the error in percent for each tooth of the upper (UJ, left) and the lower (LJ, right) jaw. Lower bars (red) show the mean planned movements in mm with standard deviations (SD). N-numbers of the corresponding mean values are specified on top of the illustration.

3.2. Effectiveness of Orovestibular Tipping for the Different Tooth Types of Upper and Lower Jaws

Planned orovestibular crown tipping resulted in large standard deviations for all teeth investigated except for the first molars, which is illustrated in Figure 4B. Most extent movements were again seen for upper and lower first incisors with 8.4° and 8.3°. Regarding first and second incisors together, upper front teeth seemed to superiorly implement tipping with an effectivity of 77% compared to the lower ones with 59% and 55%. A high effectivity in orovestibular crown tipping was seen for upper and lower premolars and molars and for lower canines with 74–88%. Contrarily, upper canines were corrected below the expected result with 27% for planned movements of 4.6°. Statistical analyses revealed no significant differences among single teeth or between upper and lower jaws.

3.3. Effectiveness of Translational Movements in Upper and Lower Jaws for Adolescent and Adult Patients

As seen for orovestibular movements of the whole cohort, both adult patients of Group 1 and adolescents of Group 2 displayed the same pattern of planned movement amounts for the different tooth groups when regarded separately. Interestingly, Group 2 manifested a moderate effectivity for upper first and second incisors (68%, 78%), whereas Group 1 presented a high effectivity of 90% and 87% for those teeth. Performance was reciprocal for upper canines, as they remained corrected below the expected result for Group 1 (34%), but at least featured a moderate effectivity for Group 2 (62%). For the rest of the teeth, values were approximately congruent for both groups, showing slightly better values for most of the lower teeth for Group 2. Results are displayed in Figure 5A,B. No significant differences between groups could be noted.

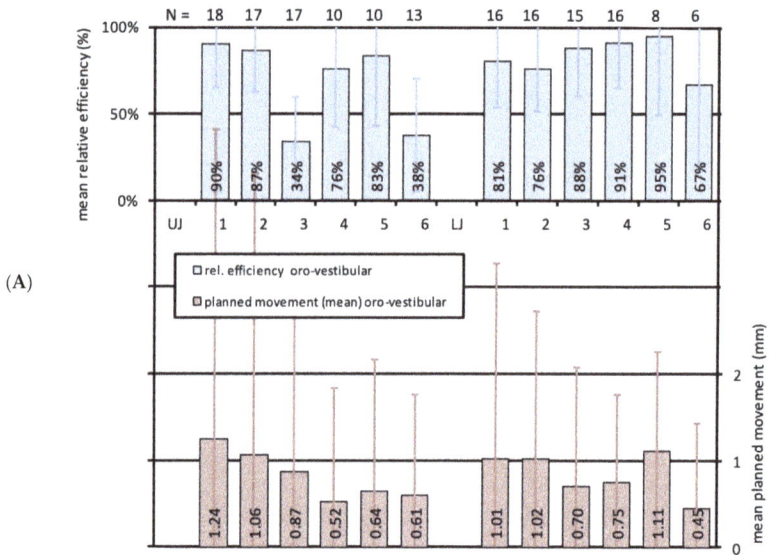

(A)

Figure 5. *Cont.*

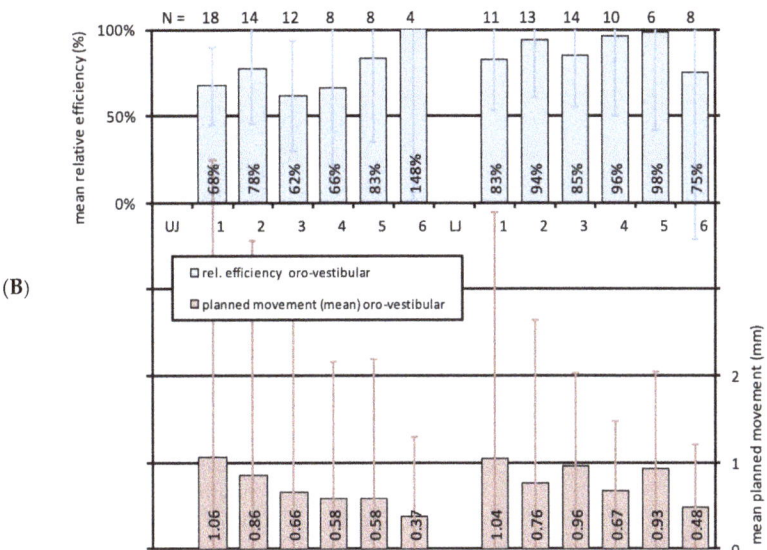

Figure 5. (**A**) Bar graph illustrating the relative effectivity of translational orovestibular tooth movements for Group 1 (adults, Invisalign®). Upper bars (blue) indicate the relative effectivity and the error in percent for each tooth of the upper (UJ, left) and the lower (LJ, right) jaw. Lower bars (red) show the mean planned movements in mm with standard deviations (SD). N-numbers of the corresponding mean values are specified on top of the illustration; (**B**) Bar graph illustrating the relative effectivity of translational orovestibular tooth movements for Group 2 (adolescents, Invisalign® Teen). Upper bars (blue) indicate the relative effectivity and the error in percent for each tooth of the upper (UJ, left) and the lower (LJ, right) jaw. Lower bars (red) show the mean planned movements in mm with standard deviations (SD). N-numbers of the corresponding mean values are specified on top of the illustration.

3.4. Effectiveness of Orovestibular Tipping in Upper and Lower Jaws for Adolescent and Adult Patients

In concordance with the results for the whole cohort, crown tipping was most pronounced for the first upper and lower incisors in both groups. Interestingly, performance was much better in Group 2 for upper and lower first incisors, upper second incisors and upper second premolars. Lower second premolars and lower canines even featured a very high effectivity of 94% and 92%, which is reflected in Figure 6B. Lower molars in Group 1 and upper plus lower molars in Group 2 could not be incorporated into analyses due to a sample size below three. In Group 2, a correction below the expected result was seen for upper canines (22%) and lower second incisors (46%), and a moderate effectivity for lower first (61%) and upper second premolars (67%) with correction values of 4.6° and 3.3°, respectively. For Group 1, the very high effectivity of 116% was striking for the upper molars, with a mean planned orovestibular tipping movement of 3.5°, which is shown in Figure 6A. However, the amount of data is moderate with a sample size of $n = 3$. Values were better for the upper incisors and second premolars compared to the lower ones, and vice versa for the lower canines and first premolars. Upper canines could only provide a correction below the expected result of 31% for a movement of 5.2°, exhibiting a small standard deviation. Analyses evidenced that statistical outcomes did not significantly differ between groups.

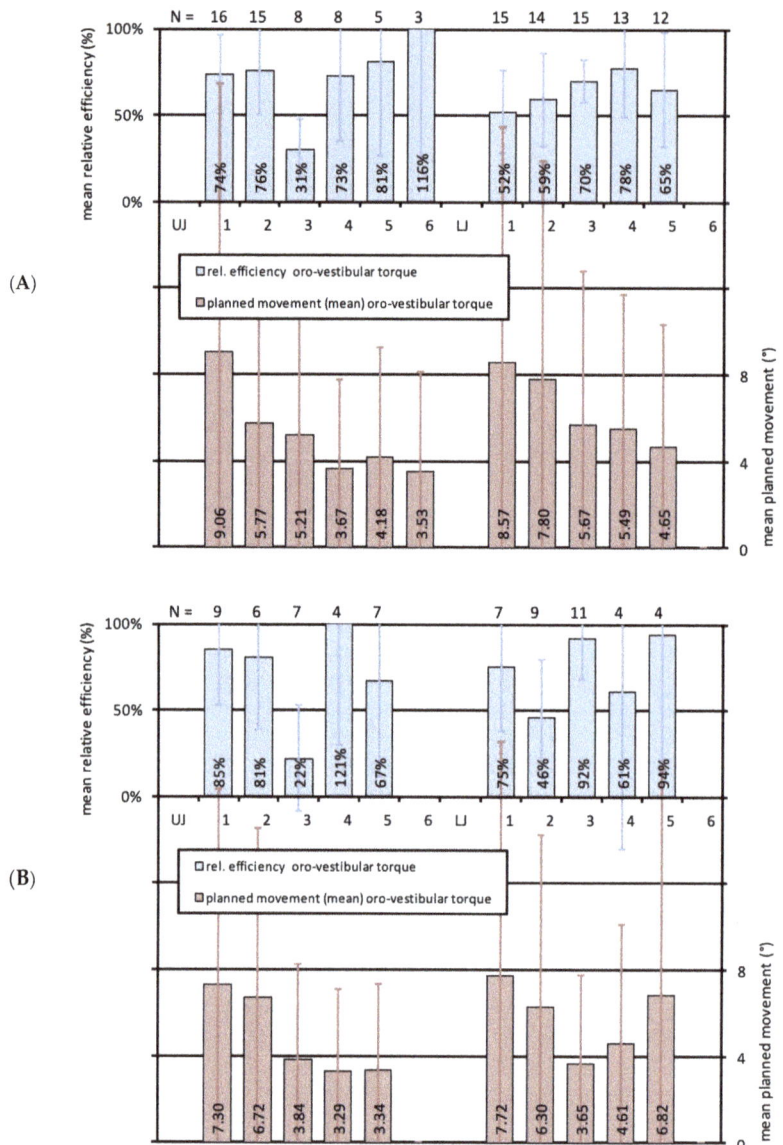

Figure 6. (**A**) Bar graph illustrating the relative effectivity of rotations around the y-axis, equivalent to orovestibular torque, for Group 1 (adults, Invisalign®). Upper bars (blue) indicate the relative effectivity and the error in percent for each tooth of the upper (UJ, left) and the lower (LJ, right) jaw. Lower bars (red) show the mean planned movements in mm with standard deviations (SD). N-numbers of the corresponding mean values are specified on top of the illustration; (**B**) Bar graph illustrating the relative effectivity of rotations around the y-axis, equivalent to orovestibular torque, for Group 2 (adolescents, Invisalign® Teen). Upper bars (blue) indicate the relative effectivity and the error in percent for each tooth of the upper (UJ, left) and the lower (LJ, right) jaw. Lower bars (red) show the mean planned movements in mm with standard deviations (SD). N-numbers of the corresponding mean values are specified on top of the illustration.

4. Discussion

Against the background of its effectivity, the spectrum of aligner orthodontic treatment indication represents a permanent and controversial discussion in the literature. Particularly with regard to the realization of arch expanding and compressing tooth movements in orovestibular direction, the data availability is insufficient. The present study aimed at surveying the conformity of planned and actually achieved orovestibular tooth movements individually for each tooth from the first incisor up to the first molar in both jaws. Consequently, this work is, to our knowledge, the first one analyzing this question comprehensively and in this complexity for the whole dentition. Our investigations revealed that the efficiency of orovestibular movements was excellent, with no statistical significance in relation to jaw, tooth type or Invisalign® system. Translational tooth movements in the mandible were highly effective and outstanding for premolars (91–98%). Translational tooth movements in the upper jaw were successful for incisors and premolars, but less effective for canines and molars. Almost all teeth were moderately or very effectively corrected by crown tipping, with better results for mandibular teeth (70–92%) than maxillary teeth (22–31%), as well as upper anterior teeth (81–85%) and lower canines (92%) in adolescents.

The underlying assumptions of our investigations were a varying performance of aligners in effecting arch expansion and compression movements, which is caused on the one hand by the different bone structure of maxilla and mandible, and on the other hand by the varying root anatomy of tooth groups. Furthermore, we gave attention to potential differences in the treatment effectivity between the conventional Invisalign® system and Invisalign® Teen, which has never been analyzed so far. Our investigations revealed that orovestibular tooth movements effecting arch expansion or compression can be differentially realized via translational movement or via crown tipping. Key parameters are the tooth specimen as much as patient age, namely teenager or adult. However, the overall performance of aligners regarding the tooth movements investigated was very good and differences were not statistically significant for the tooth types of both jaws, which confirms the aligner treatment as a very valid treatment option. Thus, our null hypothesis that there are no statistically significant differences between treatment outcomes and jaw, tooth group or aligner system could not be refuted by the results of the study.

Translations in oral and vestibular direction could be realized with high or even very high effectivity for the lower jaw of adolescents and likewise for adults, except the lower molars of the latter ones. Particularly, the performance for translational movements was outstanding for first and second lower premolars (91–98%). In the upper jaw, these translational movements could be successfully conducted in the front and premolar region as well, but are less effective for the canines and molars. These results are in concordance with the observations of Kravitz et al. [26], postulating that translational movements in orovestibular direction are best convertible with aligners. However, this study exclusively focused on the front region and additionally only reached values of 41% effectivity in the mean. At this point, it should be recalled that some authors suppose a pretense of bodily translational movement by an actual tipping [16,17]. As the focus of our study exclusively involved crown movements, this thesis can neither be supported nor neglected.

When regarding the implementation of orovestibular crown tipping in our study, almost all teeth could be moderately or very effectively corrected. Lower jaw performance was much better in the feasibility of canine movements (70–92%) compared to upper jaws (22–31%). Generally, tipping movement implementation was more effective in adolescents than in adults for selected teeth, namely upper front teeth and lower canines. Former investigations found similar results and concluded a good feasibility of protrusions and accordingly tipping in orovestibular direction, though this work also exclusively regarding the front region and not the whole dentition, as done in our study [6]. Contrarily, other investigations only found effectivity between 40–47% or reasoned an inferior performance of aligners compared to multibracket appliances for these movements [10,26].

When discussing the present data, some limitations have to be kept in mind. The superimposition works best with identical geometries, but during data processing by

Align Technology Inc., the tooth surfaces are smoothed and soft tissues are replaced by an idealized geometry. The clinical data on the other hand represent raw scan data without smoothing. This accounts for both methods of clinical recording of the actual situation, namely scanning of plaster casts and direct intraoral scanning. These differences might lead to an additional measurement noise in the determination of tooth movements. However, there is no way to avoid this methodological pitfall, as the ClinCheck® models provide the exclusive method to determine the planned tooth movements. We also aimed at achieving perfect superimposition conditions. Therefore, we exclusively included cases with at least three unmoved teeth per jaw, and additionally excluded those which regardless exhibited movement on these presumably stable teeth.

Secondly, a methodological drawback of the study is the fact that the principle of superimposition is error-prone regarding the interpretation of results. However, the chosen type of examination is the only methodology available to date for addressing questions such as those in this study. Thus, the principle of superimposition represents the most appropriate research design applicable for the analyses to perform. The susceptibility to errors is evidenced by some of our measurements featuring orovestibular efficiency ratios exceeding 100%, which is impossible and a consequence of inaccuracies in the superimposition technique. However, as stated above, these system-immanent errors cannot be prevented, but can only be consciously perceived as false values and excluded from the interpretation of the data.

As another point, it certainly has to be considered that our patients were treated with Invisalign® Exceed30 (EX30) aligner material preceding SmartTrack (LD30), which represents the next generation of aligner material [28]. As LD30 exhibits higher elasticity, better arch adaptability, greater consistency of orthodontic force application and lower warping after use than EX30, current aligners presumably perform even better in efficiency of orovestibular movements [28]. Nonetheless, our study is the first and only one that evaluated orovestibular movements to this extent, applying superimposition techniques and investigating the whole jaws with each single tooth.

We found that lower canines and premolars have more orovestibular relative efficiency than lower incisors, despite the fact that incisors have smaller roots and can therefore be moved more easily. Here, the tooth geometry will not have a decisive influence on the efficiency of the movement, as premolars in particular, but also canines, have a better grip than anterior teeth, but this is compensated for when planning the tooth movement by attachments that change the tooth geometry to allow a better force transmission. This observed phenomenon could be due to a methodological drawback of the study, which is the origin used to evaluate the rotations. As the shape of the roots cannot be determined in this study due to the technical limitations dictated by the ClinCheck®, we cannot use the center of resistance to describe tooth movements, especially the rotations. To overcome this burden, we instead used a point defined by the highest central point of each crown extracted from the initial model M.in to calculate the rotations. This can be error-prone for analytical outcomes when the tooth is tilted, as the center of the tooth crown will also move and can be misleadingly interpreted as an orovestibular displacement, even though it is a tilt of the tooth. This can influence the relationship between physical translations and compensatory rotations, but as we used the same origin for both calculations, namely planned and clinical, this systemically necessary procedure is acceptable. Nevertheless, with the future gain of further technical possibilities, such system-related limitations will be overcome in favor of higher accuracy in data calculations reflecting clinical practice even more precisely.

A recent study also investigated arch expansion with aligners and their effect on different stride and torque and found that the posterior teeth cause a certain buccal tilt when the maxillary arch is expanded [29]. Compliant with our investigations, this study also examined the effects on all tooth types, but only in the upper jaw, whereas data on the lower jaw are not available. Furthermore, the examinations were carried out using finite element analysis, which does not provide real clinical data like ours. This also accounts for a current study likewise dealing with expansion efficiency and propagating that torque compensation should be implemented in the planning to enhance torque control during arch expansion, which also applied finite element analysis and only objected the upper jaw [30]. Another very recent study evaluated aligner performance regarding the efficiency and predictability of expansion, here in a retrospective study like ours likewise comparing maxillary and mandibular pre-treatment, planned treatment and post-treatment models [31]. They found that the greatest expansion was found in both the upper and lower premolars, and that aligners are effective for simultaneous intraoral expansion in both jaws. The weakness of this study is that linear measurements of the interdental widths were recorded for the examinations, including the intercanine width between the cusp tips, the interpremolar widths between the palatal cusp tips of the first and second premolars and the intermolar width between the tips of the mesopalatine cusps of the first molars. However, this method is far less accurate and much more error-prone than our analysis of individual tooth movements, which involved superimposing individual scatter plots. Another retrospective study and systematic review focused on the efficiency of Invisalign First® regarding the quality of expansion movements in the mixed dentition [32]. However, the digital models from pre-treatment, ClinCheck® -predicted tooth positions and post-treatment were again only analyzed for the maxillary dental arch width and expansion efficiency. Furthermore, measurements were again linear with reference points on the mesiopalatal cusp tip of the temporary and permanent molars, palatal cusp tip of the premolars and cusp tip of temporary and permanent canine, lacking the necessary accuracy as described above.

In summary, this retrospective study combines the topic of aligner efficiency of orovestibular movements and systematically implements it for the entire dentition by applying the 3D superimposition methodology. The results obtained with this advanced and seminal superimposition technique have the potential for clinical contribution to improved and contemporary orthodontic treatment planning, optimized aligner performance and, thus, successful treatment outcomes and patient satisfaction. Directions for future research in this field that have emerged from our study are certainly the even more targeted use of specific auxiliary means such as attachments according to individual patient needs in order to make tooth movement even more efficient, as well as continuous optimization of the already more than sufficient, but still perfectible, material properties of the aligners.

5. Conclusions

Taken together, translational orovestibular movements can be very effectively realized, and additional support in arch expansion or compression therapies can be successfully provided by crown tipping, which accounts for all teeth in both jaws, regardless of the Invisalign® system applied. Thus, our hypothesis that these aspects might negatively impact the efficiency and treatment success of orovestibular tooth movement can be neglected.

Aligners secure effective translational orovestibular movements. Nonetheless, treatment planning should take individual parameters into account.

These data provide the basis and represent a benchmark for future investigations in this field of research. Furthermore, the results of our study serve as reliable basis for treatment planning by practicing clinicians that can be implemented in patient therapy with aligners.

Author Contributions: L.K. interpreted the data and supervised the measurements. L.B. conducted the measurements. J.S. treated the patients and supervised the clinical processes. W.S. treated the patients and supervised the clinical processes. C.B. conceptualized the study and revised the manuscript. A.K. supervised the analyses and the data interpretation, and wrote the manuscript. All authors have read and agreed to the published version of the manuscript.

Funding: This research did not receive any specific grant from funding agencies in the public, commercial, or not-for-profit sectors.

Institutional Review Board Statement: The study was conducted in accordance with the Declaration of Helsinki. All authors adhered to the principles of good research practice.

Informed Consent Statement: The protocol did not need approval by the Ethics Committee since this was a non-interventional retrospective study. The patients had given their written consent to the treatment in advance.

Data Availability Statement: The raw data supporting the conclusions of this article will be made available by the authors on request.

Conflicts of Interest: The authors declare no conflicts of interest.

References

1. Phan, X.; Ling, P.H. Clinical limitations of Invisalign. *J. Can. Dent. Assoc.* **2007**, *73*, 263–266. [PubMed]
2. Boyd, R.L.; Waskalic, V. Three-dimensional diagnosis and orthodontic treatment of complex malocclusions with the invisalign appliance. *Semin. Orthod.* **2001**, *7*, 274–293. [CrossRef]
3. Abbate, G.M.; Caria, M.P.; Montanari, P.; Mannu, C.; Orrù, G.; Caprioglio, A.; Levrini, L. Periodontal health in teenagers treated with removable aligners and fixed orthodontic appliances. *J. Orofac. Orthop.* **2015**, *76*, 240–250. [CrossRef] [PubMed]
4. Azaripour, A.; Weusmann, J.; Mahmoodi, B.; Peppas, D.; Gerhold-Ay, A.; Van Noorden, C.J.; Willershausen, B. Braces versus Invisalign®: Gingival parameters and patients' satisfaction during treatment: A cross-sectional study. *BMC Oral Health* **2015** *15*, 69. [CrossRef] [PubMed]
5. Houle, J.P.; Piedade, L.; Todescan, R., Jr.; Pinheiro, F.H. The predictability of transverse changes with Invisalign. *Angle Orthod* **2017**, *87*, 19–24. [CrossRef]
6. Krieger, E.; Seiferth, J.; Marinello, I.; Jung, B.A.; Wriedt, S.; Jacobs, C.; Wehrbein, H. Invisalign® treatment in the anterior region Were the predicted tooth movements achieved? *J. Orofac. Orthop.* **2012**, *73*, 365–376. [CrossRef]
7. Nedwed, V.; Miethke, R.R. Motivation, acceptance and problems of invisalign patients. *J. Orofac. Orthop.* **2005**, *66*, 162–173 [CrossRef]
8. Schott, T.C.; Göz, G. Color fading of the blue compliance indicator encapsulated in removableclear Invisalign TeenHaligners *Angle Orthod.* **2011**, *81*, 185–191. [CrossRef]
9. Tuncay, O.C.; Bowman, S.J.; Nicozisis, J.L.; Amy, B.D. Effectiveness of a compliance indicator for clear aligners. *J. Clin. Orthod* **2009**, *43*, 263–268.
10. Djeu, G.; Shelton, C.; Maganzini, A. Outcome assessment of Invisalign and traditional orthodontic treatment compared with the American Board of Orthodontics objective grading system. *Am. J. Orthod. Dentofac. Orthop.* **2005**, *128*, 292–298; discussion 298 [CrossRef] [PubMed]
11. Kassam, S.K.; Stoops, F.R. Are clear aligners as effective as conventional fixed appliances? *Evid. Based Dent.* **2020**, *21*, 30–31 [CrossRef]
12. Ke, Y.; Zhu, Y.; Zhu, M. A comparison of treatment effectiveness between clear aligner and fixed appliance therapies. *BMC Oral Health* **2019**, *19*, 24. [CrossRef] [PubMed]
13. Sfondrini, M.F.; Gandini, P.; Castroflorio, T.; Garino, F.; Mergati, L.; D'Anca, K.; Trovati, F.; Scribante, A. Buccolingual Inclination Control of Upper Central Incisors of Aligners: A Comparison with Conventional and Self-Ligating Brackets. *Biomed. Res. Int* **2018**, *2018*, 9341821. [CrossRef] [PubMed]
14. Gu, J.; Tang, J.S.; Skulski, B.; Fields, H.W., Jr.; Beck, F.M.; Firestone, A.R.; Kim, D.G.; Deguchi, T. Evaluation of Invisalign treat-ment effectiveness and efficiency compared with conventional fixed appliances using the Peer Assessment Rating index. *Am. J. Orthod Dentofac. Orthop.* **2017**, *151*, 259–266. [CrossRef] [PubMed]
15. Hennessy, J.; Garvey, T.; Al-Awadhi, E.A. A randomized clinicaltrial comparing mandibular incisor proclination produced by fixedlabial appliances and clear aligners. *Angle Orthod.* **2016**, *86*, 706–712. [CrossRef] [PubMed]
16. Baldwin, D.K.; King, G.; Ramsay, D.S.; Huang, G.; Bollen, A.M. Activation time and material stiffness of sequential removable orthodontic appliances. Part 3: Premolar extraction patients. *Am. J. Orthod. Dentofac. Orthop.* **2008**, *133*, 837–845. [CrossRef] [PubMed]
17. Bollen, A.M.; Huang, G.; King, G.; Hujoel, P.; Ma, T. Activation time and material stiffness of sequential removable orthodontic appliances. Part 1: Ability to complete treatment. *Am. J. Orthod. Dentofac. Orthop.* **2003**, *124*, 496–501. [CrossRef] [PubMed]
18. Kravitz, N.D.; Kusnoto, B.; Agran, B.; Viana, G. Influence of attachments and interproximal reduction on the accuracy of canine rotation with Invisalign. A prospective clinical study. *Angle Orthod.* **2008**, *78*, 682–687. [CrossRef]
19. Simon, M.; Keilig, L.; Schwarze, J.; Jung, B.A.; Bourauel, C. Treatment outcome and efficacy of an aligner technique—Regarding incisor torque, premolar derotation and molar distalization. *BMC Oral Health* **2014**, *14*, 68. [CrossRef]
20. Weckmann, J.; Scharf, S.; Graf, I.; Schwarze, J.; Keilig, L.; Bourauel, C.; Braumann, B. Influence of attachment bonding protocol on precision of the attachment in aligner treatments. *J. Orofac. Orthop.* **2020**, *81*, 30–40. [CrossRef]
21. Boyd, R.L.; Miller, R.; Vlaskalic, V. The invisalign system in adult orthodontics: Mild crowding and space closure cases. *J. Clin Orthod.* **2000**, *34*, 203–213.

22. Charalampakis, O.; Iliadi, A.; Ueno, H.; Oliver, D.R.; Kim, K.B. Accuracy of clear aligners: A retrospective study of patients who needed refinement. *Am. J. Orthod. Dentofac. Orthop.* **2018**, *154*, 47–54. [CrossRef]
23. Morales-Burruezo, I.; Gandía-Franco, J.L.; Cobo, J.; Vela-Hernández, A.; Bellot-Arcís, C. Arch expansion with the Invisalign system: Efficacy and predictability. *PLoS ONE* **2020**, *15*, e0242979. [CrossRef] [PubMed]
24. Solano-Mendoza, B.; Sonnemberg, B.; Solano-Reina, E.; Iglesias-Linares, A. How effective is the Invisalign® system in expansion movement with Ex30′ aligners? *Clin. Oral Investig.* **2017**, *21*, 1475–1484. [CrossRef] [PubMed]
25. Zhou, N.; Guo, J. Efficiency of upper arch expansion with the Invisalign system. *Angle Orthod.* **2020**, *90*, 23–30. [CrossRef] [PubMed]
26. Kravitz, N.D.; Kusnoto, B.; BeGole, E.; Obrez, A.; Agran, B. How well does Invisalign work? A prospective clinical study evaluating the efficacy of tooth movement with Invisalign. *Am. J. Orthod. Dentofac. Orthop.* **2009**, *135*, 27–35. [CrossRef] [PubMed]
27. Keilig, L.; Piesche, K.; Jäger, A.; Bourauel, C. Applications of surface-surface matching algorithms for determination of orthodontic tooth movements. *Comput. Methods Biomech. Biomed. Eng.* **2003**, *6*, 353–359. [CrossRef]
28. Condo', R.; Pazzini, L.; Cerroni, L.; Pasquantonio, G.; Lagana', G.; Pecora, A.; Mussi, V.; Rinaldi, A.; Mecheri, B.; Licoccia, S.; et al. Mechanical properties of "two generations" of teeth aligners: Change analysis during oral permanence. *Dent. Mater. J.* **2018**, *37*, 835–842. [CrossRef] [PubMed]
29. Zhang, Y.; Hui, S.; Gui, L.; Jin, F. Effects of upper arch expansion using clear aligners on different stride and torque: A three-dimensional finite element analysis. *BMC Oral Health* **2023**, *23*, 891. [CrossRef]
30. Yao, S.; Jiang, W.; Wang, C.; He, Y.; Wang, C.; Huang, L. Improvements of tooth movement efficiency and torque control in expanding the arch with clear aligners: A finite element analysis. *Front. Bioeng. Biotechnol.* **2023**, *11*, 1120535. [CrossRef]
31. Rocha, A.S.; Gonçalves, M.; Oliveira, A.C.; Azevedo, R.M.S.; Pinho, T. Efficiency and Predictability of Coronal Maxillary Expansion Repercussion with the Aligners System: A Retrospective Study. *Dent. J.* **2023**, *11*, 258. [CrossRef] [PubMed]
32. Gonçalves, A.; Ayache, S.; Monteiro, F.; Silva, F.S.; Pinho, T. Efficiency of Invisalign First® to promote expansion movement in mixed dentition: A retrospective study and systematic review. *Eur. J. Paediatr. Dent.* **2023**, *24*, 112–123. [PubMed]

Disclaimer/Publisher's Note: The statements, opinions and data contained in all publications are solely those of the individual author(s) and contributor(s) and not of MDPI and/or the editor(s). MDPI and/or the editor(s) disclaim responsibility for any injury to people or property resulting from any ideas, methods, instructions or products referred to in the content.

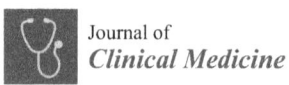 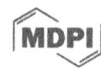

Article

Differential Recovery Patterns of the Maxilla and Mandible after Eliminating Nasal Obstruction in Growing Rats

Mirei Keitoku, Ikuo Yonemitsu *, Yuhei Ikeda, Huan Tang and Takashi Ono

Department of Orthodontic Science, Graduate School of Medical and Dental Sciences, Tokyo Medical and Dental University (TMDU), Tokyo 113-8510, Japan
* Correspondence: yoneman.orts@tmd.ac.jp; Tel.: +81-3-5803-5530

Abstract: Although nasal obstruction (NO) during growth causes maxillofacial growth suppression, it remains unclear whether eliminating the NO affects maxillary and mandibular growth differentially. We aimed to clarify whether eliminating NO can help regain normal maxillofacial growth and to determine the optimal intervention timing. Forty-two 4-week-old male Wistar rats were randomly divided into six groups. Their left nostril was sutured to simulate NO over different durations in the experimental groups; the sutures were later removed to resume nasal breathing. Maxillofacial morphology was assessed using microcomputed tomography. Immunohistochemical changes in hypoxia-inducible factor (HIF)-1α, osteoprotegerin (OPG), and receptor activator of nuclear factor kappa-B ligand (RANKL) of the condylar cartilage were evaluated to reveal the underlying mechanisms of these changes. Maxillary length was significantly lower in rats with NO for ≥5 weeks. In groups with NO for ≥7 weeks, the posterior mandibular length, ramus height, thickness of the hypertrophic cell layer in the condylar cartilage, HIF-1α levels, and RANKL levels were significantly lower and OPG levels and RANKL/OPG were significantly higher than those in the control group. Our findings suggest that eliminating NO is effective in regaining maxillofacial growth. Moreover, the optimal timing of intervention differed between the maxilla and mandible.

Keywords: nasal obstruction; recovery; optimal timing; maxillofacial growth; mouth breathing

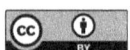

1. Introduction

Nasal obstruction (NO) induces mouth breathing and decreases percutaneous oxygen saturation (SpO_2). The hypoxic condition adversely affects the entire body. Clinical studies have shown that chronic NO induces a variety of symptoms, such as headache, fatigue, sleep disturbances, daytime drowsiness, and distraction, causing the quality of life (QoL) to be abrogated [1,2]. Furthermore, NO affects the hippocampus, leading to memory and learning deficits [3], and also affects taste cells, leading to impaired sweet taste perception [4]. In the orofacial region, mouth breathing is known to cause malocclusion. Several clinical studies have shown that mouth breathing due to NO propels downward migration of the palatal plane [5], narrowing of the maxilla, elevation of the palate [6], and vertical growth of the mandible [7]. A clinical study showed that nasal congestion leads to functional modulation of the neuromuscular system that alters craniofacial bone structure, tongue and mandible position, and soft tissues, causing "adenoid face" features [8]. These findings indicate that NO causes deterioration of growth, particularly in the maxillofacial region.

One of the factors that change the maxillofacial configuration due to NO is the physiological effect of the muscles. NO has been shown to inhibit masticatory muscle formation and contractile properties and suppress bone growth at muscle attachment sites [9]. Another factor is an increase in the hypoxia-inducible factor (HIF) in the mandibular cartilage [10]. HIF is a transcription factor that plays a pivotal role in the adaptive response of cells to hypoxic stress, which increases when systemic SpO_2 decreases due to hypoxia [11]. HIF-1α promotes osteoblast and osteoclast differentiation, regulates chondrocyte apoptosis [12], and exerts osteoclast activation mechanisms [13]. We previously found increased HIF-1α levels in the condyles of rats with NO, which promotes degeneration of the condylar cartilage and inhibits growth of the condyle [10]. In addition, the activation of osteoclasts occurs in conjunction with an increase in the ratio of osteoprotegerin (OPG), which is involved in osteoclast activation, and receptor activator of nuclear factor kappa-B ligand (RANKL), which suppresses osteoclast activity. Although NO has been reported to significantly affect the growth of the maxillofacial region through several proposed mechanisms, few studies have investigated the aftereffects of eliminating NO.

With regard to the effect of obstruction of the upper airway (UA), maxillofacial growth following treatment of hypertrophied adenoids has been investigated [14,15]. Adenoids are located in the posterior part of the nose, and their enlargement narrows the air passage and interferes with nasal breathing. Adenoids are often enlarged between the ages of 3–6 years, and adenoidectomy is performed in this age group in severe cases when complications, such as NO, sleep-disordered breathing, recurrent acute otitis media, and chronic rhinosinusitis, are present [16,17]. It has been reported that after adenoidectomy and recovery of normal nasal breathing, the reduced mandibular growth is eventually restored to the level in the control group [18], and labial tilting of the upper and lower incisors is improved [19]. Although adenoidectomy is effective between the ages of 4–7 years [16], it is necessary to clarify the maximum age at which intervention for NO can be expected to improve volumetric craniofacial growth.

In humans, maxillary growth peaks at around 10–11 years, while mandibular growth peaks at 12–14 years old [20,21]. Owing to the differential growth between the maxilla and mandible [22], the maxillary growth spurt occurs earlier than that of the mandible. Therefore, the critical periods of therapeutic intervention may differ between the maxilla and mandible. Although improvement in nasal breathing was reported to restore the maxillary growth after elimination of NO in 9-week-old rats [23], few comparative studies have clarified the morphological and histological effects on the maxillary and mandibular bones and investigated the optimal timing of eliminating NO. Therefore, the purpose of this study was to clarify whether the maxillofacial morphology could attain normal growth after elimination of NO and to determine the optimal timing of intervention for NO using an experimental model in growing rats.

2. Materials and Methods

2.1. Experimental Animal Model

The study protocol was approved by the Institutional Animal Care and Use Committee of Tokyo Medical and Dental University (TMDU) (Approval No. A2019-004C), and experimental procedures were performed in accordance with the TMDU Animal Care Standards and ARRIVE guidelines.

Forty-two 4-week-old male Wistar rats were randomly divided into 6 groups (n = 7 each), as shown in Figure 1. The experimental schedule was as follows: control group, 1-week recovery group (hereafter, W1 group), W3 group, W5 group, W7 group, and W9 group according to differences in the timing of NO elimination (Figure 1a). The left side of the nose of the rats in W1, W3, W5, W7, and W9 groups was sutured with a silk thread under isoflurane inhalation anesthesia (Figure 1b), and NO was eliminated by suture removal in each group every 2 weeks. All rats were euthanized after 13 weeks using CO_2 gas. The body weight of the rats and SpO_2 were measured every week at 10:00 a.m. throughout the experimental period. To avoid fluctuations in SpO_2 caused by body movement, a mouse pulse oximeter (Mouse OX; STARR Life Sciences, Oakmont, PA, USA) was used while administering 4% isoflurane (inhalation anesthetic) (SFMBX1; DS Pharma Biomedical, Osaka, Japan). The heads of the rats were fixed in 4% paraformaldehyde in 0.1 M phosphate buffer, pH 7.4, for 24 h at 4 °C.

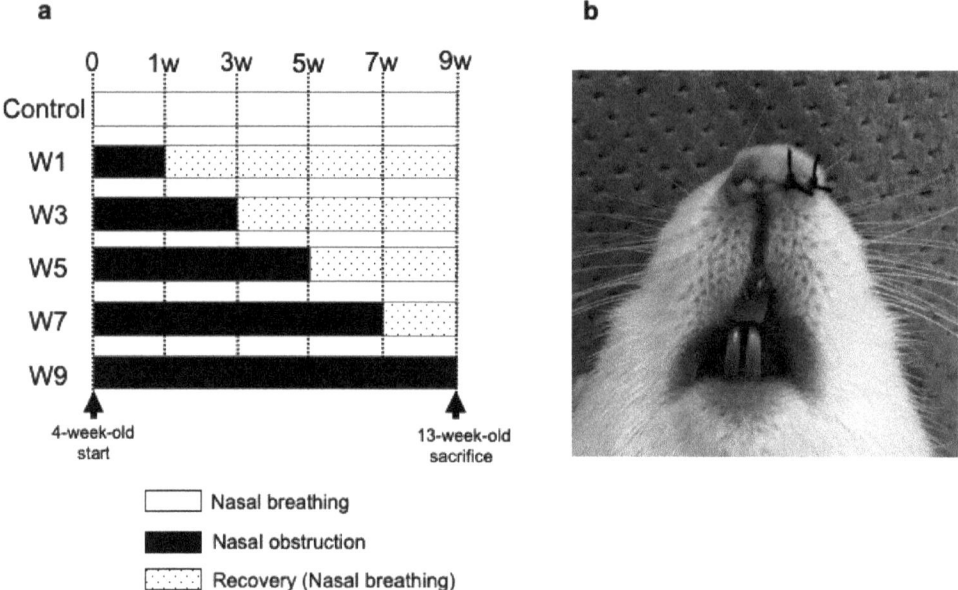

Figure 1. Time schedule of the experiment and implementation of NO. (**a**) Forty-two 4-week-old male Wistar rats were divided randomly into 6 groups (control group, 1-week recovery group (hereafter referred to as W1 group), W3 group, W5 group, W7 group, and W9 group ($n = 7$)). At the time of recovery in the schedule (W1, W3, W5, and W7 groups), the nasal sutures were removed, and the nasal obstruction was eliminated. In the W9 group, the nasal obstruction was maintained throughout the experimental period. All rats were sacrificed at 13 weeks of age; (**b**) the left side of the nostril of 35 rats in the W1, W3, W5, W7, and W9 groups were sutured with two stitches of silk thread.

2.2. Morphological Evaluation of Maxillofacial Bones

Maxillofacial morphological changes were measured using microcomputed tomography (micro-CT; SMX-100CT; Shimadzu, Kyoto, Japan). Scans were obtained with a source voltage of 75 kV and a source current of 30 mA. Various parts of the maxilla and mandibular bone were measured using a three-dimensional image analysis software program (TRI/3D-BON; Ratoc System Engineering, Tokyo, Japan). The three-dimensional coordinate positions of the biologically relevant cranial landmarks and the line connecting them are defined (Figure 2a,b; Tables 1 and 2). The air-occupied part was extracted from the CT image (Figure 2c) using 3D-BON, as shown in Figure 2d, and the UA volume was measured.

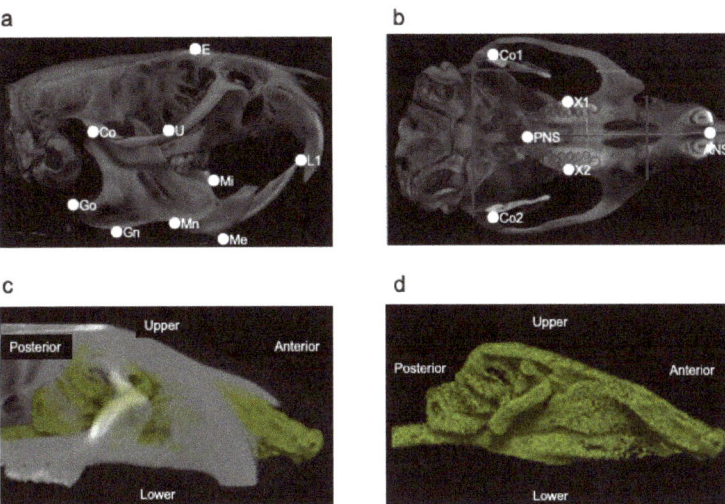

Figure 2. The landmarks used for measurements. (**a**) Landmarks are shown in lateral view. Abbreviations: E—the intersection between the frontal bone and the most superior and anterior point of the ethmoid; U—the intersection between the maxillary sinus and the distal surface of the third superior molar tooth; Co—the most posterior and superior point on the mandibular condyle; Go—the most posterior point on the mandibular ramus; Mn—the most concave portion of the concavity on the inferior border of the mandibular corpus; Gn—the most inferior point on the ramus that lies on a perpendicular bisector of the line Go–Mn; Me—the most inferior and anterior point of the lower border of the mandible; L1—the most anterior and superior point on the alveolar bone of the mandibular incisor; Mi—the junction of the alveolar bone and the mesial surface of the first mandibular molar. (**b**) Landmarks are shown in vertical view. Abbreviations: ANS—the most anterior part of the palate; PNS—the most posterior part of the palate; X1—the most anterior and superior point in the molar process of the right maxilla; X2—the most anterior and superior point in the molar process of the left maxilla. (**c**) The volume of the nasal cavity was measured by extracting the air part (yellow part) from the computed tomography image. (**d**) The air-occupied part extracted from (**c**).

Table 1. Definition of landmarks.

Landmarks	Definition
E	The intersection between the frontal bone and the most superior and anterior point of the ethmoid
U	The intersection between the maxillary sinus and the distal surface of the third superior molar tooth
Co	The most posterior and superior point on the mandibular condyle (Co, right; Co2, left)
Go	The most posterior point on the mandibular ramus
Mn	The most concave portion of the concavity on the inferior border of the mandibular corpus
Gn	The most inferior point on the ramus that lies on a perpendicular bisector of the line Go–Mn
Me	The most inferior and anterior point of the lower border of the mandible
L1	The most anterior and superior point on the alveolar bone of the mandibular incisor
Mi	The junction of the alveolar bone and the mesial surface of the first mandibular molar
ANS	The most anterior part of the palate
PNS	The most posterior part of the palate
X1	The most anterior and superior point in the molar process of the right maxilla
X2	The most anterior and superior point in the molar process of the left maxilla

Table 2. Measurements and interpretation.

Measurements	Interpretation
X1–X2	Maxillary width
ANS–PNS	Maxillary length
U–E	Maxillary height
Co–L1	Total mandibular length
Mi–L1	Anterior mandibular length
Go–Mn	Posterior mandibular length
Co–Gn	Ramus height
Co–Me	Mandibular body length
Co1–Co2	Mandibular width

2.3. Tissue Preparation

After morphological evaluation by micro-CT, the temporomandibular joints of both sides and their surrounding tissues were decalcified with Osteosoft (Merck Millipore, Burlington, MA, USA) for 3 weeks. They were then embedded in paraffin and cut sagittally into 6 µm thick sections with a microtome.

2.4. Histomorphometry with Toluidine Blue Staining

Sections from the center of the condyles were selected and stained with toluidine blue to measure the width of the mandibular condylar cartilage layers and observe the chondrocytes. From the articular surface down, the cartilage of the condyle was divided into four histological layers: fibrous, proliferating cell, mature cell, and hypertrophic cell layers, based on a previous study [24]. The thickness of the four layers in the superior region was measured using image analysis software (NIS-Elements Analysis D, National Institutes of Health, Bethesda, MD, USA) ($n = 7$ each group).

2.5. Immunohistochemistry for HIF-1α, OPG, and RANKL

Immunostaining for HIF-1α, OPG, and RANKL was performed using mandibular cartilage samples of the rats ($n = 7$ each group). The site and thickness of the cartilage were the same as those used for toluidine staining. Deparaffinized sections were pressurized with an antigen activator (Histro VT One; Nacalai Tesque, Kyoto, Japan) at a high temperature for 20 min. Endogenous peroxidase was removed by treatment with a hydrogen peroxide blocking reagent. After washing, the specimens were incubated overnight at 4 °C with the following primary antibodies: monoclonal mouse anti-HIF-1α (1:300, Gene Tex, GTX628480, clone GT10211, Irvine, TX, USA), monoclonal mouse anti-OPG (1:300, Santa Cruz Biotechnology, SC-390518, Dallas, TX, USA), and monoclonal mouse anti-RANKL (1:300, Santa Cruz Biotechnology, SC-377079, Dallas, TX, USA). The slides were then incubated with a secondary antibody (Vectastain ABC Mouse IgG Kit, Vector, PK-4002, Newark, NJ, USA). In each section, the number of HIF-1α-, OPG-, and RANKL-positive cells was counted at least three times within the region of interest (ROI; 150 µm × 200 µm) and averaged. The ROI was selected to cover the total thickness of the proliferative and hypertrophic layers in the superior region of the mandibular condyle. The RANKL/OPG ratio was also calculated to reveal the changes in osteoclastogenesis.

2.6. Statistical Analysis

Results are expressed as the mean ± standard deviation (SD). The data were analyzed using Tukey's test after testing for normality and equal variances. Moreover, correlations were determined between UA volume and its affected area and between mandibular height and thickness of the hypertrophic cell layer using Pearson's correlation. In all analyses, statistical significance was set at $p < 0.05$.

3. Results

3.1. Systemic Changes

There were no significant differences in body weight change between the control and any of the experimental groups of rats throughout the experiment (Figure S1). In the control group, the SpO$_2$ remained almost stable throughout the experimental period. SpO$_2$ levels were significantly lower in the W1, W3, and W5 groups during the NO period than those in the control group. In contrast, in groups W7 and W9, SpO$_2$ significantly decreased throughout the experimental period, regardless of the NO period (Figure 3).

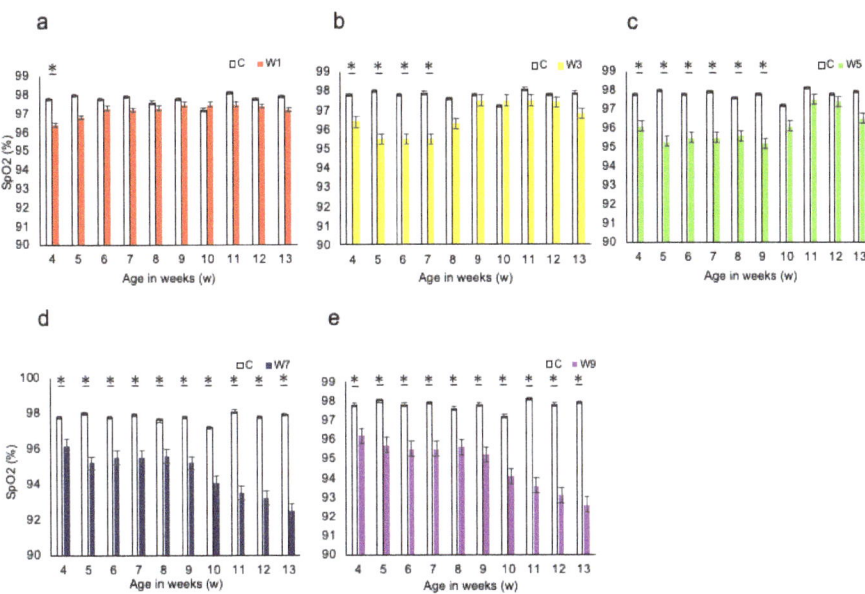

Figure 3. Changes in body weight and SpO$_2$. (**a**) Comparison of SpO$_2$ between the W1 and control groups throughout the experimental period, *: $p < 0.05$; (**b**) comparison of SpO$_2$ between the W3 and control groups throughout the experimental period, *: $p < 0.05$; (**c**) comparison of SpO$_2$ between the W5 and control groups throughout the experimental period, *: $p < 0.05$; (**d**) comparison of SpO$_2$ between the W7 and control groups throughout the experimental period, *: $p < 0.05$; (**e**) comparison of SpO$_2$ between the W9 and control groups throughout the experimental period, *: $p < 0.05$. Abbreviation: SpO$_2$—oxygen saturation.

3.2. Measurement of the Maxillofacial and UA Morphology

Figure 4 shows the changes in maxillofacial morphology with respect to reopening of the nasal airway during the experimental period. The anterior-posterior length of the maxilla was significantly lower in the W5, W7, and W9 groups than in the control group (Figure 4a). The UA volume was significantly lower in the W1, W3, W5, W7, and W9 groups than in the control group. The UA volume indicated difficulty in catching up with the normal growth pattern even after recovery of the nasal passage. The posterior mandibular length and ramus height were significantly lower in the W7 and W9 groups than in the control group (Figure 4b). The UA volume was significantly correlated with the maxillary length and posterior mandibular length (Figure 5), whereas there was no significant correlation between the total mandibular length and anterior mandibular length.

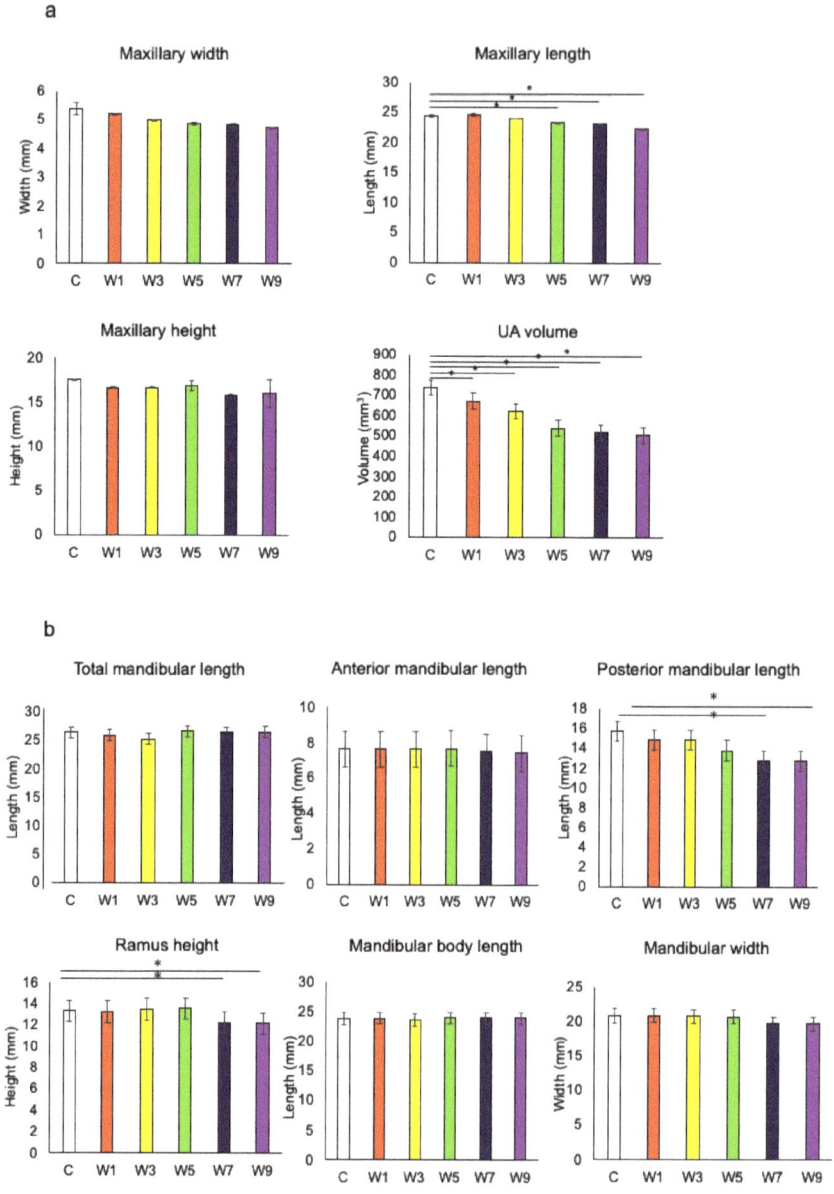

Figure 4. Measurement of the maxillofacial morphology. (**a**) Comparison of the maxillary size in three dimensions and upper airway volume, *: $p < 0.05$. Abbreviation: UA—upper airway; (**b**) comparison of the mandibular size in six dimensions, *: $p < 0.05$.

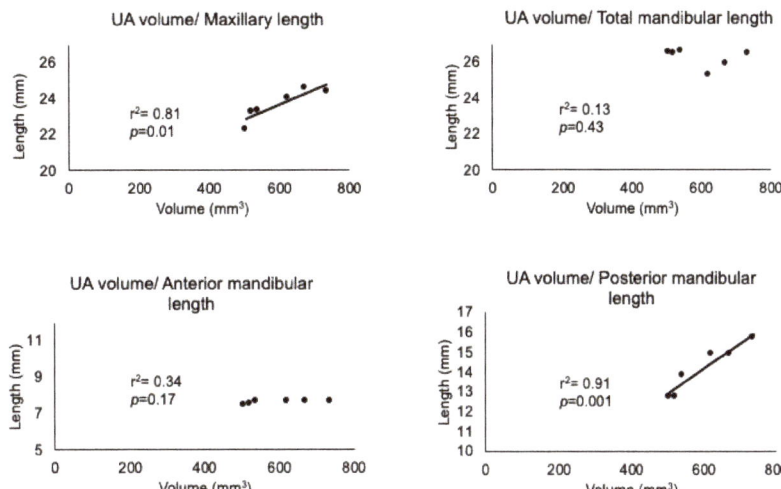

Figure 5. Correlations between upper airway volume and maxillomandibular measurements. Correlations between UA volume and variables in the maxillomandibular skeleton were determined. Abbreviations: UA—upper airway; r^2—squared correlation coefficient; p—probability.

3.3. Histomorphometry with Toluidine Blue Staining

In all groups, the fibrous layer, proliferating cell layer, mature cell layer, and hypertrophic cell layer of condylar cartilages were clearly observed by toluidine blue staining (Figure 6). However, there was a difference in the thickness of each layer, with the hypertrophic cell layer being the thickest. The thickness of the hypertrophic cell layer significantly decreased when the timing of recovery to nasal breathing was delayed (Figure 7). In particular, a significant decrease was observed in the W7 and W9 groups. However, there was no significant change in the thicknesses of the other layers. The thickness of the hypertrophic cell layer showed a significant positive correlation with ramus height (Figure 8).

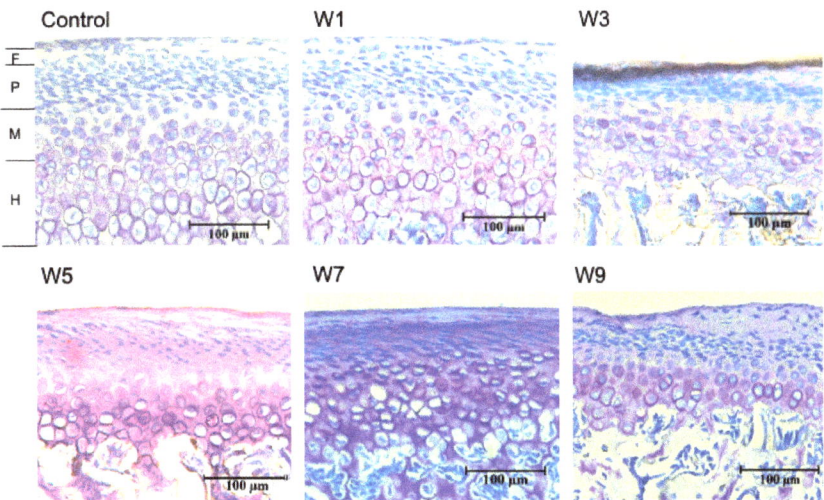

Figure 6. Histomorphometry with toluidine blue staining. Histological staining with toluidine blue in each of the 6 groups (C, W1, W3, W5, W7 and W9). The thickness of the four layers in the superior regions were measured using image analysis software. Abbreviations: F, fibrous layer; P, proliferating cell layer; M, mature cell layer; H, hypertrophic cell layer. Bar depicts 100 µm.

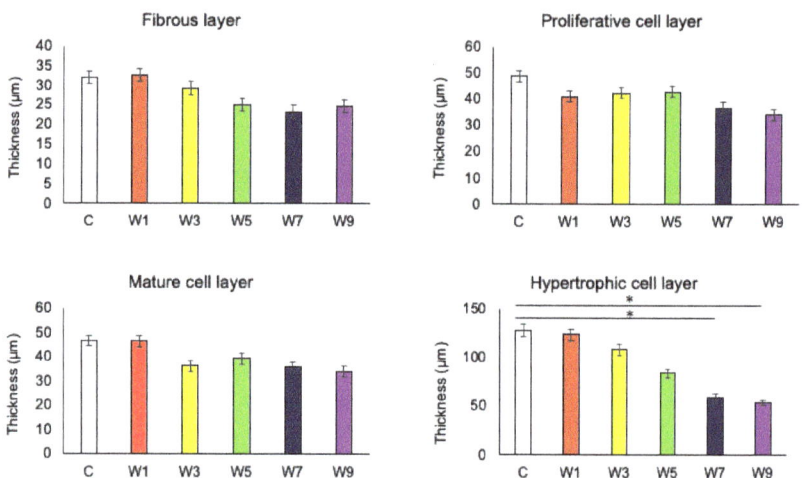

Figure 7. Comparison of the thickness of the four layers of mandibular cartilage in the six groups, *: $p < 0.05$.

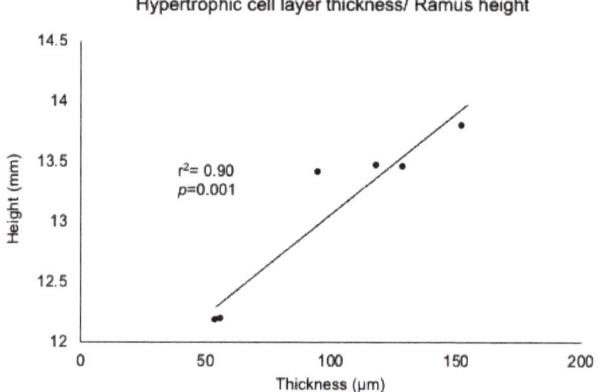

Figure 8. Correlation between ramus height and hypertrophic cell layer thickness. Correlations were determined between ramus height and hypertrophic cell layer thickness for each of the six groups. Abbreviations: r^2 = squared correlation coefficient; p = probability.

3.4. Expression of HIF-1α, OPG, and RANKL Protein in the Articular Cartilage

HIF-1α was specifically expressed in hypertrophic cell layers (Figure 9). This was observed in both experimental and control groups. In contrast, OPG and RANKL were specifically expressed at the border between the hypertrophic cell layer and subchondral bone (Figures 10 and 11), which was found in both control and experimental groups. The percentage of HIF-1α-positive cells increased as the NO exposure period increased. It was significantly higher in the W5, W7, and W9 groups than that in the control group (Figure 12). OPG was highly expressed in the control group; however, it showed a significant decrease when the NO persisted for 7 and 9 weeks. Conversely, RANKL was only slightly expressed in the control group and showed a significant increase as the NO period increased from 7 to 9 weeks. The RANKL/OPG ratio was significantly higher in the W7 and W9 groups than in the control group (Figure 12). The percentage of HIF-1α-positive cells showed a significant negative correlation with the thickness of the hypertrophic cell layer (Figure S2). Moreover, SpO$_2$ showed significant negative correlations with the percentage of HIF-1α and RANKL-positive cells, and with the RANKL/OPG ratio. In contrast, SpO$_2$ showed a significant positive correlation with the percentage of OPG-positive cells (Figure S3).

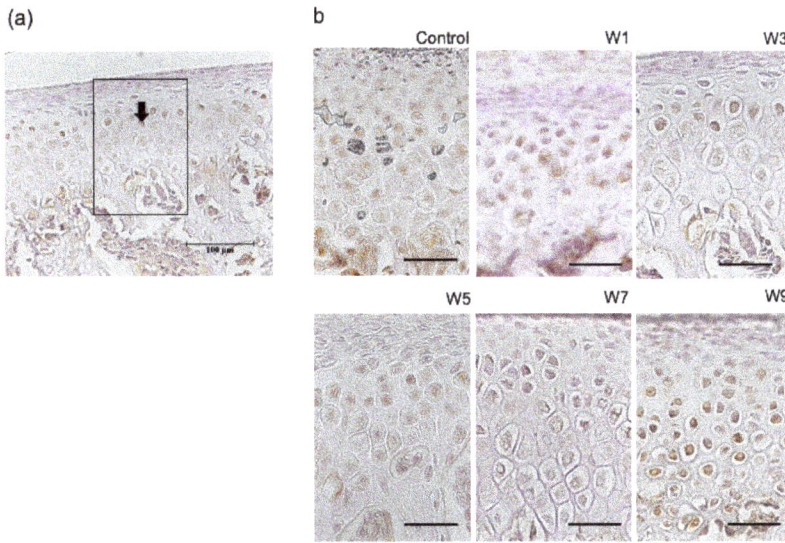

Figure 9. Immunohistochemical staining with anti-HIF-1α antibody. (**a**) HIF-1α-positive cells (arrows) were counted in the six groups using a fixed measuring frame (150 μm × 200 μm) indicated by the region of interest (black square). Bar depicts 100 μm; (**b**) immunohistochemically-stained images of the region of interest for the six groups. Images for HIF-1α in each of the 6 groups. Bar depicts 50 μm. Abbreviation: HIF-1α—hypoxia-inducible factor-1α.

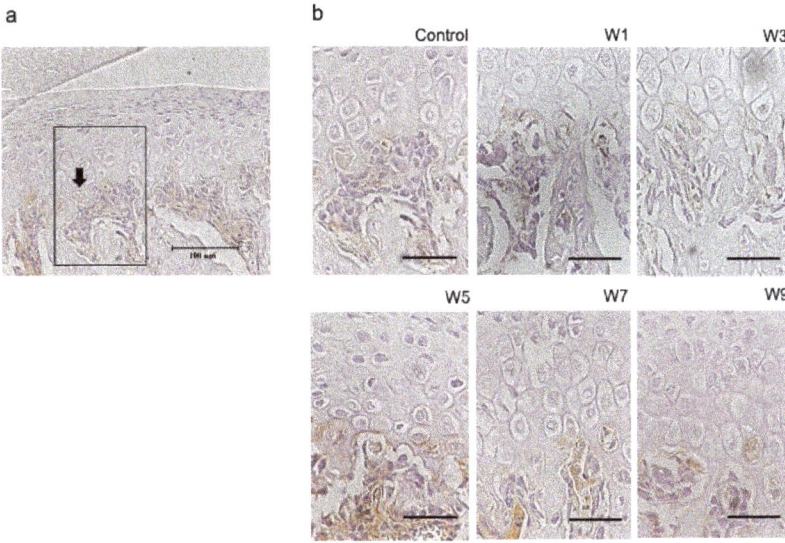

Figure 10. Immunohistochemical staining with RANKL. (**a**) RANKL-positive cells (arrows) were counted in the six groups using a fixed measuring frame (150 μm × 200 μm) indicated by the region of interest (black square); (**b**) immunohistochemically-stained images of the region of interest for the six groups. Images for RANKL in each of the 6 groups. Bar depicts 50 μm. Abbreviation: RANKL—receptor activator of nuclear factor kappa-B ligand.

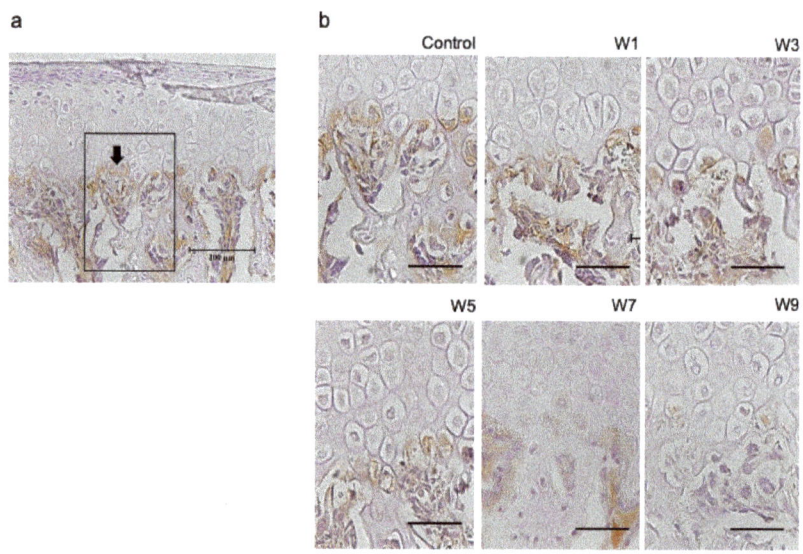

Figure 11. Immunohistochemical staining with OPG. (**a**) OPG-positive cells (arrows) were counted in the six groups using a fixed measuring frame (150 μm × 200 μm) indicated by the region of interest (black square); (**b**) immunohistochemically-stained images of the region of interest for the six groups. Images for OPG in each of the 6 groups. Bar depicts 50 μm. Abbreviation: OPG—osteoprotegerin.

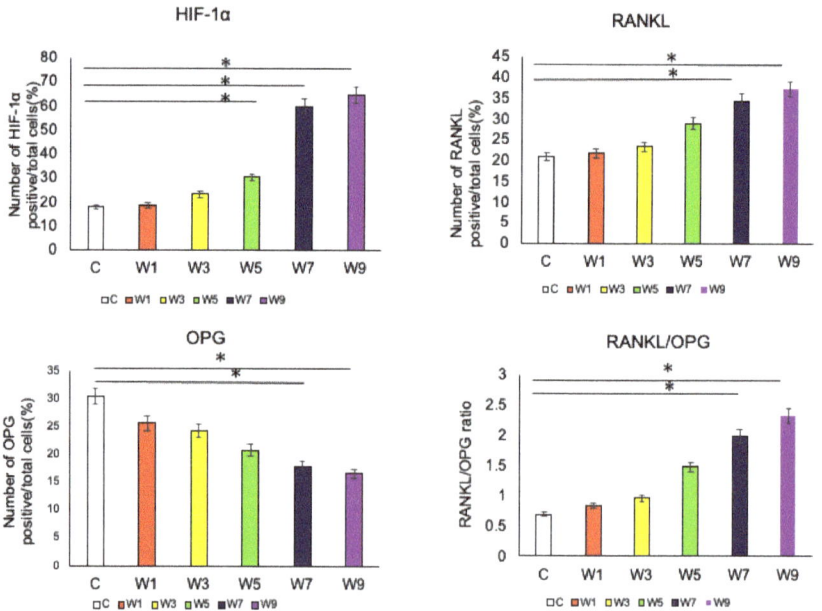

Figure 12. Changes in the percentages of immunohistochemically-positive cells. Comparison of the number of positive cells for antibodies against HIF-1α, RANKL, and OPG in the six groups. A comparison of the RANKLE/OPG ratios is also shown, *: $p < 0.05$. Abbreviations: HIF-1α—hypoxia-inducible factor-1α; RANKL—receptor activator of nuclear factor kappa-B ligand; OPG—osteoprotegerin.

4. Discussion

In this study, we focused on whether it was possible to regain maxillofacial growth by recovery of nasal breathing in growing rats and to determine the optimal timing of intervention for NO based on the growth patterns of the maxilla and mandible. The maxillary length and UA volume were significantly lower in rats with NO for ≥ 5 weeks and ≥ 1 week, respectively, as compared with those in the control rats. On the other hand, in the groups with NO for 7 weeks, the posterior mandibular length, ramus height, thickness of the hypertrophic cell layer in the condylar cartilage, HIF-1α levels, and RANKL levels were significantly lower and OPG levels were higher than those in the control group. These different time courses indicate that the maxilla requires earlier elimination of NO to catch up with the normal growth pattern than does the mandible.

Previous studies have investigated the effects of nasal breathing disorders by blocking only one nostril to decrease SpO_2 and induce hypoxia [3–8,10,25,26]. It has also been found that unilateral NO has little or no effect on the whole body of rats [8,10,27,28]. Similarly, there was no significant difference in body weight between the control and experimental groups in this study, indicating that there was no significant effect on whole-body growth. To observe the effect of eliminating NO, we developed a transient NO model by first suturing the nose with a thread and then inducing recovery by removing the thread, instead of the conventional method of burning one side of the nostril. In fact, during the period of NO, the SpO_2 of the experimental group was significantly lower than that of the control group. Thus, the transient NO model seems to be appropriate for investigating the effect of recovery from unilateral NO on craniofacial growth.

As for morphological changes in the NO model, the UA volume was significantly smaller in all experimental groups compared with that in the control group. This indicates that it is difficult for the UA to regain its physiological volume even after a short period of NO. Furthermore, the UA volume appeared to have decreased in proportion with the duration of NO. Previous studies have shown that the volume of space inside the nasomaxillary complex varies with the amount of airflow into the nasal cavity [29,30] and that increased external force on the central palatal suture cartilage promotes chondrogenic differentiation [31]. Thus, the findings may be attributable to an insufficient increase in the depth of the nasal cavity and contraction of the maxilla due to the reduced airflow caused by NO, regardless of the duration of SpO_2 reduction. With regard to maxillary morphological changes, the decrease in the anterior–posterior dimension was the most obvious finding in the three dimensions, with significant reduction in the W5, W7, and W9 groups. A previous study showed that the lateral growth of the maxilla is nearly complete by 4 weeks of age in rats, while the anteroposterior growth of the maxilla is not completed by 4 weeks of age and continues to increase slowly until 10 weeks [32]. In this study, a significant decrease in the anterior–posterior dimension was observed in the W5 group, which comprised 9-week-old rats. This suggests that presence of NO at the age of 9 weeks inhibits anterior–posterior maxillary growth, which is consistent with the age of maxillary growth in rats shown in a previous study [33].

On the other hand, morphometric measurements of the mandible showed that the posterior mandibular length and ramus height were significantly decreased in the W7 and W9 groups. There was also a correlation between the posterior mandibular length and UA volume. Thus, the reduction in UA volume is thought to be a factor for mandibular morphological changes. Other causes of mandibular morphological changes due to NO have been reported extensively [9,10,33] in relation to muscles and SpO_2. One study suggested that NO causes physiological and functional changes in the muscles attached to the mandible, resulting in mandibular muscular hypoplasia, which is particularly significant in the superficial layer of the masseter muscle [9]. Previous studies have revealed that mandibular muscle and bony growth of the mandible influence each other [34–36]. Muscle hypoplasia regulates bone growth during muscle attachment [37]. In our study, the posterior mandible, which was significantly reduced in length in groups W7 and W9, encompassed the vicinity of the gonion. Since the masseter muscle inserts at the site near the gonion, it is inferred that the amount of bone growth at the attachment site is reduced.

In groups W7 and W9, SpO_2 levels decreased significantly throughout the experimental period, regardless of the NO period. A significant reduction in posterior mandibular length was also observed in groups W7 and W9. This suggests that the SpO_2 level may be involved in mandibular morphological changes, as previously suggested [10]. The timing of the decrease in SpO_2 levels also coincided with a significant decrease in the condylar cartilage thickness, especially in the hypertrophic cell layer, as shown by toluidine blue staining. The hypertrophic cell layer plays a particularly important role in the progressive stages of osteogenesis [38]. In this study, a significant correlation was observed between the thickness of the hypertrophic cell layer and ramus height. If the physiological process of hypertrophy is jeopardized by any factor, the next critical step is osteogenesis [39]. Thus, maintenance of the SpO_2 level could contribute to the development of hypertrophy [40]. HIF-1α, which is induced by hypoxia [11], was found to be localized in the hypertrophic cell layer. This is consistent with the findings of a previous study [41]. This study also revealed a significant negative correlation between the percentage of HIF-1α-positive cells and the thickness of the hypertrophic cell layer, suggesting that HIF-1α has a significant influence on the growth of the condylar cartilage.

RANKL is expressed by osteoblasts and promotes osteoclast differentiation and bone resorption [42], and OPG is a de novo receptor for RANKL that binds to RANKL and inhibits bone resorption [43]. The RANKL/OPG ratio, calculated from RANKL and OPG expression, is a useful index for predicting the osteoclast environment [44]. In the present study, there was a significant increase in the HIF-1α and RANKL levels and significant decrease in OPG levels occurred significantly in the W7 and W9 groups. Previous studies have shown that increased HIF-1α levels promote an increase in RANKL production and a decrease in OPG production, osteoclast differentiation, and bone resorption [45,46]. In the present study, the timing of the changes in these three factors coincided with the timing of changes in mandibular growth, suggesting that they are associated with bone formation. The percentage of positive cells of HIF-1α, RANKL, OPG, and RANKL/OPG ratio were all found to be significantly correlated (HIF-1α, negative; RANKL, negative; OPG, positive; and RANKL/OPG ratio, negative) with systemic SpO_2. This suggests that systemic hypoxia affects the local area, the condylar cartilage, and it may be inferred that the osteogenic and osteoclastic systems of the mandible operate sensitively to systemic oxygen deprivation.

There are several limitations to this study. First, rats cannot breathe through their mouths. Because their bodily structures differ from those of humans, the findings of our study cannot be completely extrapolated to humans. Second, the effects of NO before 4 weeks of age were not evaluated. Therefore, it is necessary to develop methods to simulate NO in rats less than 4 weeks old. The rats used should be as young as possible if the effects of growth are to be examined. Finally, the sample size of this study was small. Because we wanted to elucidate the timing of recovery, the increased number of groups forced us to minimize the sample size for each group. Nevertheless, this study suggests that to enable the maxilla and mandible recover the normal growth pattern, the NO should be eliminated by 7 weeks of age for the maxilla and by 9 weeks of age for the mandible. A previous study showed that maxillary growth precedes mandibular growth in rats [47], and this difference in the growth peak may have caused the difference in the recovery time in this study. Likewise, maxillary growth also precedes mandibular growth in humans [48], suggesting that early recovery from NO is necessary for maxillary bone growth.

5. Conclusions

Recovery from NO in growing rats restored morphological growth in the anterior-posterior dimension of the maxilla and posterior mandibular length. Our findings also suggest that the optimal timing for intervention was before 7 weeks of age for the maxilla and before 9 weeks of age for the mandible in growing rats. In humans, the growth of the maxilla occurs before that of the mandible same as that in rats. This suggests that early intervention for the maxilla is necessary. The increase in HIF-1 and RANKL levels and decreased in OPG levels with increasing NO duration suggests that NO may affect the osteoclast environment of the mandibular cartilage. Similar changes in the osteoclast environment may occur in humans, and further research is necessary for confirmation.

Supplementary Materials: The following supporting information can be downloaded at: https://www.mdpi.com/article/10.3390/jcm11247359/s1, Figure S1: Changes in body weight of animals in the six groups during the experimental period; Figure S2: Correlation between the percentage of HIF-1α-positive cells and hypertrophic cell layer thickness; Figure S3: Correlation between SpO$_2$ and the percentage of positive cells of HIF-1α, RANKL, OPG and the RANKL/OPG ratio at 13 weeks of age.

Author Contributions: Conceptualization, M.K., I.Y., Y.I. and T.O.; Methodology, M.K. and H.T.; Validation, M.K.; Formal Analysis, M.K.; Investigation, M.K.; Data Curation, M.K.; Writing—Original Draft Preparation, M.K.; Writing—Review and Editing, I.Y., Y.I., H.T. and T.O.; Visualization, M.K.; Supervision, I.Y. and T.O.; Project Administration, M.K. and I.Y.; Funding Acquisition, I.Y. and Y.I. All authors have read and agreed to the published version of the manuscript.

Funding: This research was funded by a Grant-in-Aid for Scientific Research (16K11782, 18K17245, 20K10198) from the Ministry of Education, Culture, Sports, Science and Technology of Japan.

Institutional Review Board Statement: The animal study protocol was approved by the Ethics Committee of Tokyo Medical and Dental University (TMDU) (protocol code A2019-004C).

Informed Consent Statement: Not applicable.

Data Availability Statement: Not applicable.

Conflicts of Interest: The authors declare no conflict of interest.

References

1. Udaka, T.; Suzuki, H.; Kitamura, T.; Shiomori, T.; Hiraki, N.; Fujimura, T.; Ueda, N. Relationships among nasal obstruction, daytime sleepiness, and quality of life. *Laryngoscope* **2006**, *116*, 2129–2132. [CrossRef] [PubMed]
2. Rhee, J.S.; Book, D.T.; Burzynski, M.; Smith, T.L. Quality of life assessment in nasal airway obstruction. *Laryngoscope* **2003**, *113*, 1118–1122. [CrossRef] [PubMed]
3. Ogawa, T.; Okihara, H.; Kokai, S.; Abe, Y.; Karin Harumi, U.K.; Makiguchi, M.; Kato, C.; Yabushita, T.; Michikawa, M.; Ono, T. NO during adolescence induces memory/learning impairments associated with BDNF/TrkB signaling pathway hypofunction and high corticosterone levels. *J. Neurosci. Res.* **2018**, *96*, 1056–1065. [CrossRef] [PubMed]
4. Ren, E.; Watari, I.; Jui-Chin, H.; Mizumachi-Kubono, M.; Podyma-Inoue, K.A.; Narukawa, M.; Misaka, T.; Watabe, T.; Ono, T. Unilateral airway obstruction alters sweet taste preference and sweet taste receptors in rat circumvallate papillae. *Acta Histochem.* **2019**, *121*, 135–142. [CrossRef]
5. Posnick, J.C.; Agnihotri, N. Consequences and management of nasal airway obstruction in the dentofacial deformity patient. *Curr. Opin. Otolaryngol. Head Neck Surg.* **2010**, *18*, 323–331. [CrossRef]
6. Williams, R.; Patel, V.; Chen, Y.F.; Tangbumrungtham, N.; Thamboo, A.; Most, S.P.; Nayak, J.V.; Liu, S.Y.C. The upper airway nasal complex: Structural contribution to persistent nasal obstruction. *Otolaryngol. Head Neck Surg.* **2019**, *161*, 171–177. [CrossRef]
7. Zhao, Z.; Zheng, L.; Huang, X.; Li, C.; Liu, J.; Hu, Y. Effects of mouth breathing on facial skeletal development in children: A systematic review and meta-analysis. *BMC Oral Health* **2021**, *21*, 108. [CrossRef]
8. Harari, D.; Redlich, M.; Miri, S.; Hamud, T.; Gross, M. The effect of mouth breathing versus nasal breathing on dentofacial and craniofacial development in orthodontic patients. *Laryngoscope* **2010**, *120*, 2089–2093. [CrossRef]
9. Tang, H.; Yonemitsu, I.; Ikeda, Y.; Watakabe, K.; Shibata, S.; Hosomichi, J.; Ono, T. Effects of unilateral NO on the characteristics of jaw-closing muscles in growing rats. *Angle Orthod.* **2018**, *89*, 102–110. [CrossRef]
10. Watakabe, K.; Yonemitsu, I.; Ikeda, Y.; Tang, H.; Ono, T. Unilateral airway obstruction induces morphological changes of the mandibular condyle in growing. *Orthod. Waves* **2018**, *77*, 157–168. [CrossRef]
11. Palazon, A.; Goldrath, A.W.; Nizet, V.; Johnson, R.S. HIF transcription factors, inflammation, and immunity. *Immunity* **2014**, *41*, 518–528. [CrossRef] [PubMed]
12. Schipani, E.; Maes, C.; Carmeliet, G.; Semenza, G.L. Regulation of osteogenesis-angiogenesis coupling by HIFs and VEGF. *J. Bone Miner. Res.* **2009**, *24*, 1347–1353. [CrossRef] [PubMed]
13. Knowles, H. Hypoxic regulation of osteoclast differentiation and bone resorption activity. *Hypoxia* **2015**, *3*, 73–82. [CrossRef] [PubMed]
14. Wang, H.; Qiao, X.; Qi, S.; Zhang, X.; Li, S. Effect of adenoid hypertrophy on the upper airway and craniomaxillofacial region. *Transl. Pediatr.* **2021**, *10*, 2563–2572. [CrossRef] [PubMed]

15. Zhu, Y.; Li, J.; Tang, Y.; Wang, X.; Xue, X.; Sun, H.; Nie, P.; Qu, X.; Zhu, M. Dental arch dimensional changes after adenoidectomy or tonsillectomy in children with airway obstruction: A meta-analysis and systematic review under PRISMA guidelines. *Medicine* **2016**, *95*, e4976. [CrossRef] [PubMed]
16. Schupper, A.J.; Nation, J.; Pransky, S. Adenoidectomy in children: What is the evidence and what is its role? *Curr. Otorhinolaryngol Rep.* **2018**, *6*, 64–73. [CrossRef]
17. Greenfeld, M.; Tauman, R.; DeRowe, A.; Sivan, Y. Obstructive sleep apnea syndrome due to adenotonsillar hypertrophy in infants. *Int. J. Pediatr. Otorhinolaryngol.* **2003**, *67*, 1055–1060. [CrossRef]
18. Zettergren-Wijk, L.; Forsberg, C.M.; Linder-Aronson, S. Changes in dentofacial morphology after adeno-/tonsillectomy in young children with obstructive sleep apnoea—A 5-year follow-up study. *Eur. J. Orthod.* **2006**, *28*, 319–326. [CrossRef]
19. Becking, B.E.; Verweij, J.P.; Kalf-Scholte, S.M.; Valkenburg, C.; Bakker, E.W.P.; Merkesteyn, J.P.R. Impact of adenotonsillectomy on the dentofacial development of obstructed children: A systematic review and meta-analysis. *Eur. J. Orthod.* **2017**, *39*, 509–518. [CrossRef]
20. Proffit, W.R.; Fields, H.W.; Larson, B.S.; Sarver, D.M. *Contemporary Orthodontics*, 3rd ed.; Mosby: St. Louis, MI, USA, 2000.
21. Kusumoto, K.; Sato, K.; Mitani, H. The evaluation of the orthopedic appliances by using standard growth curves of maxilla and mandible. *J. Jpn. Orthod. Soc.* **1996**, *55*, 311–321.
22. Ranly, D.M. Craniofacial growth. *Dent. Clin. North Am.* **2000**, *44*, 457–470. [CrossRef] [PubMed]
23. Sato, T.; Yamaguchi, M.; Murakami, Y.; Horigome, Y.; Negishi, S.; Kasai, K. Changes in maxillofacial morphology due to improvement of nasal obstruction in rats. *Orthod. Craniofac. Res.* **2018**, *21*, 84–89. [CrossRef] [PubMed]
24. Ikeda, Y.; Yonemitsu, I.; Takei, M.; Shibata, S.; Ono, T. Mechanical loading leads to osteoarthritis-like changes in the hypofunctional temporomandibular joint in rats. *Arch. Oral Biol.* **2014**, *59*, 1368–1376. [CrossRef] [PubMed]
25. Ishidori, H.; Okihara, H.; Ogawa, T.; Abe, Y.; Kato, C.; Phyo, T.A.; Fujita, A.; Kokai, S.; Ono, T. Nasal obstruction during the growth period modulates the Wnt/beta-catenin pathway and brain-derived neurotrophic factor production in association with tyrosine kinase receptor B mRNA reduction in mouse hippocampus. *Eur. J. Neurosci.* **2022**, *55*, 5–17. [CrossRef]
26. Abe, Y.; Kato, C.; Uchima, K.; Okihara, H.; Ishida, T.; Fujita, K.; Yabushita, T.; Kokai, S.; Ono, T. Unilateral NO affects motor representation development within the face primary motor cortex in growing rats. *J. Appl. Physiol.* **2017**, *122*, 1494–1503. [CrossRef]
27. Padzys, G.S.; Martrette, J.M.; Tankosic, C.; Thornton, S.N.; Trabalon, M. Effects of short term forced oral breathing: Physiological changes and structural adaptation of diaphragm and orofacial muscles in rats. *Arch. Oral Biol.* **2011**, *56*, 1646–1654. [CrossRef]
28. Padzys, G.S.; Tankosic, C.; Trabalon, M.; Martrette, J.M. Craniofacial development and physiological state after early oral breathing in rats. *Eur. J. Oral. Sci.* **2012**, *120*, 21–28. [CrossRef]
29. Moss-Salentijn, L.; Melvin, L. Moss and the functional matrix. *J. Dent. Res.* **1997**, *76*, 1814–1817. [CrossRef]
30. Kilic, N.; Oktay, H. Effects of rapid maxillary expansion on nasal breathing and some naso-respiratory and breathing problems in growing children: A literature review. *Int. J. Pediatr. Otorhinolaryngol.* **2008**, *72*, 1595–1601. [CrossRef]
31. Saitoh, S.; Takahashi, I.; Mizoguchi, I.; Sasano, Y.; Kagayama, M.; Mitani, H. Compressive force promotes chondrogenic differentiation and hypertrophy in midpalatal suture cartilage in growing rats. *Anat. Rec.* **2000**, *260*, 392–401. [CrossRef]
32. Abed, G.S.; Buschang, P.H.; Taylor, R.; Hinton, R.J. Maturational and functional related differences in rat craniofacial growth. *Arch. Oral Biol.* **2007**, *52*, 1018–1025. [CrossRef] [PubMed]
33. Wang, X.; Sun, H.; Zhu, Y.; Tang, Y.; Xue, X.; Nie, P.; Zhu, M.; Wang, B. Bilateral intermittent NO in adolescent rats leads to the growth defects of mandibular condyle. *Arch. Oral Biol.* **2019**, *106*, 104473. [CrossRef] [PubMed]
34. Yonemitsu, I.; Muramoto, T.; Soma, K. The influence of masseter activity on rat mandibular growth. *Arch. Oral Biol.* **2007**, *52*, 487–493. [CrossRef] [PubMed]
35. Kitagawa, Y.; Hashimoto, K.; Enomoto, S.; Shioda, S.; Nojyo, Y.; Sano, K. Maxillofacial deformity and change in the histochemical characteristics of the masseter muscle after unilateral sectioning of the facial nerve in growing rabbits. *Acta Histochem. Cytochem.* **2002**, *35*, 305–313. [CrossRef]
36. Kiliaridis, S. Masticatory muscle influence on craniofacial growth. *Acta Odontol. Scand.* **1995**, *53*, 196–202. [CrossRef]
37. Hamrick, M.W.; McNeil, P.L.; Patterson, S.L. Role of muscle-derived growth factors in bone formation. *J. Musculoskelet. Neuronal Interact* **2010**, *10*, 64–70.
38. Yang, L.; Tsang, K.Y.; Tang, H.C.; Chan, D.; Cheah, K.S. Hypertrophic chondrocytes can become osteoblasts and osteocytes in endochondral bone formation. *Proc. Natl. Acad. Sci. USA* **2014**, *111*, 12097–12102. [CrossRef]
39. Chung, U.I. Essential role of hypertrophic chondrocytes in endochondral bone development. *Endocr. J.* **2004**, *51*, 19–24. [CrossRef]
40. Leijten, J.C.; Moreira Teixeira, L.S.; Landman, E.B.; van Blitterswijk, C.A.; Karperien, M. Hypoxia inhibits hypertrophic differentiation and endochondral ossification in explanted tibiae. *PLoS ONE* **2012**, *7*, e49896. [CrossRef]
41. Shirakura, M.; Tanimoto, K.; Eguchi, H.; Miyauchi, M.; Nakamura, H.; Hiyama, K.; Tanimoto, K.; Tanaka, E.; Takata, T.; Tanne K. Activation of the hypoxia-inducible factor-1 in overloaded temporomandibular joint, and induction of osteoclastogenesis. *Biochem. Biophys. Res. Commun.* **2010**, *393*, 800–805. [CrossRef]
42. Grimaud, E.; Soubigou, L.; Couillaud, S.; Coipeau, P.; Moreau, A.; Passuti, N.; Gouin, F.; Redini, F.; Heymann, D. Receptor activator of nuclear factor κB ligand (RANKL)/osteoprotegerin (OPG) ratio is increased in severe osteolysis. *Am. J. Pathol.* **2003**, *163*, 2021–2031. [CrossRef] [PubMed]

3. Lacey, D.L.; Timms, E.; Tan, H.L.; Kelley, M.J.; Dunstan, C.R.; Burgess, T.; Elliott, R.; Colombero, A.; Elliott, G.; Scully, S.; et al. Osteoprotegerin ligand is a cytokine that regulates osteoclast differentiation and activation. *Cell* **1998**, *93*, 165–176. [CrossRef] [PubMed]
4. Meng, X.; Wielockx, B.; Rauner, M.; Bozec, A. Hypoxia-inducible factors regulate osteoclasts in health and disease. *Front. Cell Dev. Biol.* **2021**, *9*, 658893. [CrossRef] [PubMed]
5. Corso, P.F.C.L.; Meger, M.N.; Petean, I.B.F.; Souza, J.F.; Brancher, J.A.; da Silva, L.A.B.; Rebelatto, N.L.B.; Kluppel, L.E.; Sousa-Neto, M.D.; Küchler, E.C.; et al. Examination of OPG, RANK, RANKL and HIF-1α polymorphisms in temporomandibular joint ankylosis patients. *J. Craniomaxillofac. Surg.* **2019**, *47*, 766–770. [CrossRef]
6. Zhu, J.; Tang, Y.; Wu, Q.; Ji, Y.C.; Feng, Z.F.; Kang, F.W. HIF-1α facilitates osteocyte-mediated osteoclastogenesis by activating JAK2/STAT3 pathway in vitro. *J. Cell. Physiol.* **2019**, *234*, 21182–21192. [CrossRef]
7. Vandeberg, J.R.; Buschang, P.H.; Hinton, R.J. Craniofacial growth in growth hormone-deficient rats. *Anat. Rec. A Discov. Mol. Cell. Evol. Biol.* **2004**, *278*, 561–570. [CrossRef]
8. Ochoa, B.K.; Nanda, R.S. Comparison of maxillary and mandibular growth. *Am. J. Orthod. Dentofacial. Orthop.* **2004**, *125*, 148–159. [CrossRef]

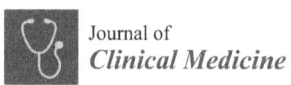 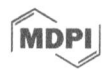

Article

Lip Bumper Therapy Does Not Influence the Sagittal Mandibular Incisor Position in a Retrospective CBCT Study

Olivia Griswold [1,†], Chenshuang Li [1,*,†], Justin C. Orr [1], Normand S. Boucher [1], Shalin R. Shah [2] and Chun-Hsi Chung [1]

1 Department of Orthodontics, School of Dental Medicine, University of Pennsylvania, Philadelphia, PA 19104, USA
2 Private Practice, Princeton Junction, West Windsor, NJ 08550, USA
* Correspondence: lichens@upenn.edu
† These authors contributed equally to this work.

Abstract: Lip bumper (LB) therapy is used as a treatment approach for mild to moderate crowding without extraction of teeth. Previous studies demonstrated that LB increases arch length through molar uprighting and lateral expansion. However, the effects of LB on mandibular incisors are inconclusive. The controversial results from different studies may be due to limitations including absence of a control group and/or use of 2D radiography. To address this issue, the current retrospective longitudinal CBCT study compared a rapid maxillary expansion (RME) group with no lower treatment [16 patients (9 females, 7 males); median age 8.86 years at T1 and 11.82 years at T2] and an RME + LB group [18 patients (13 females, 5 males); median age 9.46 years at T1 and 12.10 years at T2]. The CBCTs taken before and after phase 1 treatment were 3D superimposed based on the mandibular structure and were measured to determine the angular and linear changes of the mandibular incisors over the course of LB treatment. For comparisons between different timepoints within a group, a Wilcoxon matched-pairs signed rank test was used. For intergroup comparisons, a Mann–Whitney U test was used. Both groups showed eruption and protrusion of the mandibular incisors during the observation period, while there was no significant change in proclination of the lower incisors. When comparing the discrepancy of change between groups, there was no statistically significant difference detected. In summary, by utilizing a longitudinal 3D database, the current study demonstrated that the effect of LB on the position of the mandibular incisors is limited.

Keywords: interceptive orthodontics; lip bumper; CBCT; mandibular incisor

Citation: Griswold, O.; Li, C.; Orr, J.C.; Boucher, N.S.; Shah, S.R.; Chung, C.-H. Lip Bumper Therapy Does Not Influence the Sagittal Mandibular Incisor Position in a Retrospective CBCT Study. *J. Clin. Med.* **2022**, *11*, 6032. https://doi.org/10.3390/jcm11206032

Academic Editors: Vincenzo Grassia, Letizia Perillo and Fabrizia d'Apuzzo

Received: 18 September 2022
Accepted: 12 October 2022
Published: 13 October 2022

Publisher's Note: MDPI stays neutral with regard to jurisdictional claims in published maps and institutional affiliations.

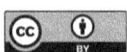

Copyright: © 2022 by the authors. Licensee MDPI, Basel, Switzerland. This article is an open access article distributed under the terms and conditions of the Creative Commons Attribution (CC BY) license (https://creativecommons.org/licenses/by/4.0/).

1. Introduction

Lip bumpers are functional, removable devices that utilize the force of the circumoral musculature to cause tooth movement [1]. Lip bumpers can also be used as a habit-breaking appliance in patients with a lip-sucking habit [1]. According to the literature, a lip bumper has the effects of increasing arch circumference through lateral and anterior-posterior expansion [2–4]. Thus, a lip bumper (LB) in conjunction with rapid maxillary expansion (RME) is a common tool in the orthodontic armamentarium to gain arch circumference in cases with mild to moderate crowding, which offers an opportunity to gain the necessary space as an alternative to extraction treatment [4].

Regarding the specific effects of lip bumpers on the mandibular dentition, it has been reported to increase transverse arch width, cause labial movement of the lower incisors and molar uprighting [5–11]. The lip bumper appliance can be customized by adjusting the arch wire to provide more posterior expansion or lower incisor flaring [1]. In as early as the 1970s, Bergersen et al. stated 95% of lip bumper cases exhibit forward migration of the lower incisors and distal movement of the first molar [12]. Later, Grossen et al. had similar findings of mandibular incisor protrusion and proclination along with mandibular molar distal tipping [6]. O'Donnell et al. also reported that following one year of lip bumper therapy, there was proclination and protrusion of the lower incisors as well as distal tipping of the first and second molars [5]. In agreement with these findings, Davidovitch et al. performed a prospective controlled study and found that lower incisors in the lip bumper group had a six times greater change in inclination and significant distal crown tip of the first molars compared to the control group [7]. While Subtelny et al. found that the majority of cases treated with a lip bumper had molar uprighting and distal movement, contrary to much of the literature, only 44% of cases had lower incisor protrusion [13]. Jacob et al. found the distal tip of the mandibular first molars, lower incisor tip protrusion and for the first time, reported 1.5 mm of first molar and lower incisor vertical development [8]. Thus, the effects of lip bumpers on mandibular molars are consistent across all these studies, but the effect on mandibular incisors varies in different studies.

It is worth noting that, all prior literatures have only utilized 2D lateral cephalograms or lateral tomographs to provide cephalometric measurements and to analyze changes over the course of lip bumper treatment. Multiple studies lacked a control group [5,6,8], and in some studies, the lip bumper was not the only orthodontic device applied to the mandibular arch [12]. Lip bumpers are routinely used in early mixed dentition and during this age, a significant amount of mandibular dentoalveolar growth and development is expected. A control group that is age-matched without mandibular treatment allows for assessment of natural changes due to growth and development over an experimental treatment period. In the prior studies that lack a control group, we cannot distinguish if the changes observed over the course of LB therapy are outcomes due to treatment effect, expected growth and development, or a combination of both. In 2009 and 2020, systematic reviews were performed to determine the strength of the evidence regarding lip bumper treatment effects. The 2009 systematic review by Hashish et al. found one study that met the inclusion criteria [14]. The 2020 systematic review by Santana et al. included 6 studies, no meta-analysis was performed due to heterogeneity and it was determined that the level of certainty regarding present data on lip bumper therapy was low [15].

As the orthodontic field continues to increase its use of CBCT technology, the availability of new data continues to grow. CBCT images allow for more precise measurement of the dentoskeletal complex and visual access to measurements not previously observable on 2D radiography [16,17]. CBCT technology offers us the opportunity to reinvestigate previous findings without the distortion, overlap and magnification of formerly studied 2D images [17,18]. Therefore, the aims of this study are to evaluate the changes of the mandibular incisors in response to lip bumper therapy, to help clinicians better understand the treatment effects of the lip bumper and in turn, optimize treatment plans and outcomes in orthodontics.

2. Materials and Methods

The study was conducted in accordance with the Declaration of Helsinki, and approved by the Institutional Review Board of the University of Pennsylvania (protocol # 850683 and date of approval: 31 January 2022). The study is a retrospective longitudinal CBCT study utilizing data from two private practice orthodontic clinics. Two separate groups were studied. The inclusive criteria are: patients (1) presented with mixed dentition; (2) had all four lower incisors erupted at T1; (3) skeletal class I or mild class II ($0° <$ ANB angle $< 6°$); (4) had RME or RME + LB as phase I orthodontic treatment; (5) had no orthodontic treatment prior to their T1 CBCT. The exclusive criteria are: patients (1) had craniofacial syndrome; (2) had history of trauma to craniofacial region; (3) had missing, impacted, large caries lesion, periapical lesion, ankylosis or trauma to mandibular incisors; (4) had orthodontic devices other than RME or LB delivered during the phase I treatment. The T2 CBCT was taken as the initial records for comprehensive phase II treatment (Table 1). The Voxel size of all the CBCT images was 0.400 mm $\times$ 0.400 mm $\times$ 0.400 mm.

Table 1. The demographic information of the two groups. RME: rapid maxillary expansion; LB: lip bumper; F: female; M: male; yrs: years. The Chi-square test was performed for the gender distribution comparison between groups. The Mann–Whitney U test was performed for the age and time interval comparisons between groups.

	RME Group	RME + LB Group	p-Value
Patient Number	16 (9 F, 7 M)	18 (13 F, 5 M)	0.3307
Age at T1 (yrs, median [Min, Max])	8.86 [7.62, 10.48]	9.46 [8.29, 10.29]	0.0581
Age at T2 (yrs, median [Min, Max])	11.82 [10.81, 13.82]	12.10 [10.98, 12.99]	0.0928
Time Interval (yrs, median [Min, Max])	2.98 [2.11, 3.84]	2.62 [1.75, 3.66]	0.2772

The RME group was treated with bonded RME (with occlusal platforms covering all posterior teeth) and no mandibular arch treatment. The group contained 16 subjects, 9 females and 7 males. The median age at T1 was 8.86 years (range: 7.62 to 10.48 years). The median age at T2 was 11.82 years (range: 10.81 to 13.82 years). The CBCT images for this experimental group were taken a median of 2.98 years apart (range: 2.11 to 3.84 years).

The RME + LB group was treated with bonded RME for the maxilla and LB for the mandible. The group contained 18 subjects, 13 females and 5 males. The median age at T1 was 9.46 years (8.29 to 10.29 years). The median age at T2 was 12.10 years (10.98 to 12.99 years). The CBCT images for this experimental group were taken a median of 2.62 years apart (range: 1.75 to 3.66 years). Prefabricated CG lip bumpers (Dentsply GAC international, NY, USA) were used. The lip bumpers were activated transversely by expanding the wire facially to 1 mm wider than the buccal tubes on the mandibular first molars at every visit until the mandibular molars were fully uprighted. Anteriorly, the lip bumpers were adjusted each visit in order to ensure they were positioned in the middle-third and 2 mm labial to the facial surface of the lower incisors. The median length of time in lip bumper treatment was 1.79 years (range: 1.16 to 2.66 years).

The CBCT DICOM files were imported into Dolphin 3D software (Dolphin Imaging version 11.95 Premium, Chatsworth, CA, USA) and oriented by using the Frankfort plane as the horizontal plane in the "Orientation" module. In addition, the orientation was adjusted axially so that the posterior borders of the orbits from a lateral view overlapped each other and coronally so that the inferior borders of both orbits sat on the same plane from a frontal view. In the "Superimposition of Volumes" module of the Dolphin 3D software, the T1 and T2 CBCT images were superimposed according to American Board of Orthodontics (ABO) standards of mandibular superimposition and in accordance with methods followed by previous research studies [16,18].

Utilizing the superimposed CBCTs within the "Superimposition of Volumes" module, data collection of both linear measurements and angular measurements was completed using a sagittal slice that was a best fit through the center of the mandibular central incisors using coronal and axial views (Figure 1). The thickness of the sagittal slice was set to a 1-voxel slice.

The mandibular incisor inclination was measured as a best fit line through the incisal tip and apex to the true vertical of the superimposition. Buccally angulated measurements were deemed to be positive while lingually angulated measurements were deemed negative. Over the time period, a positive value was indicative of proclination while a negative value was indicative of retroclination.

The protrusion of the mandibular incisor was measured at three levels: incisor tip cementoenamel junction (CEJ) and 5 mm apical to CEJ. The protrusion was measured by the distance between the buccal surface of the tooth to the true vertical line established at 10 mm ahead of the T1 symphysis. Both T1 and T2 incisor anterior–posterior positions were measured to the T1 true vertical line to eliminate mandibular bony structure changes due to the normal growth and development. Teeth anteriorly positioned to the true vertical line was recorded with a positive value while posteriorly positioned to the line was recorded with a negative value. Over the time period, a positive value was indicative of protrusion while a negative value was indicative of retrusion.

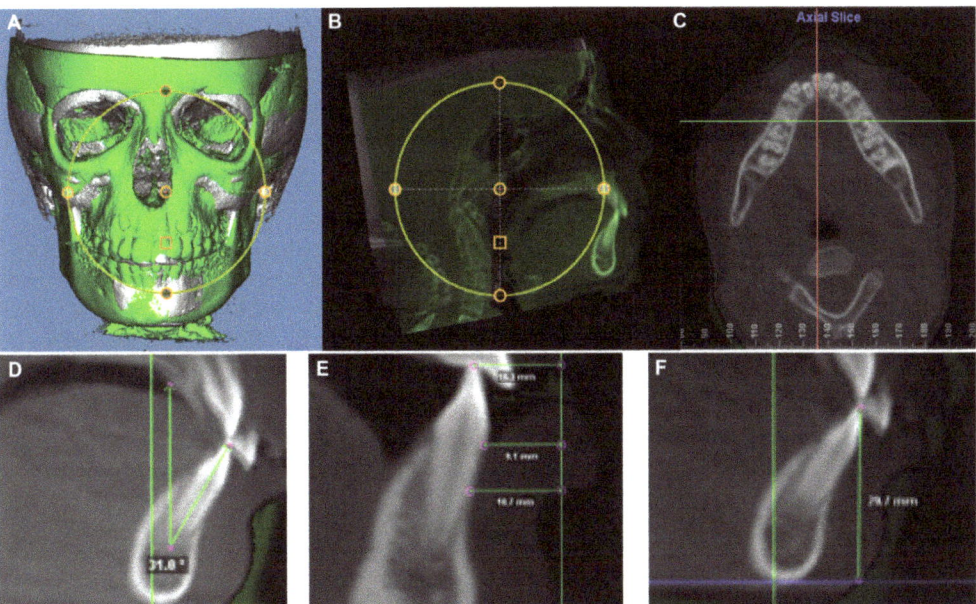

Figure 1. The demography of CBCT image analysis utilized in current study. (**A**) A screenshot of the superimposition of T1 and T2 CBCT images in a 3D reconstructed view. Th T1 CBCT image is represented in white and the T2 CBCT image is presented in green. (**B**) A screenshot of the superimposition of T1 and T2 CBCT images in midline sagittal slice view. The superimposition was performed based on the mandibular structure. The T1 CBCT image is represented in white and the T2 CBCT image is presented in green. (**C**) The axial slice was used to find the sagittal slice (red line) that was a best fit through the center of the mandibular central incisors. (**D**) Mandibular central incisor inclination measurement on the sagittal slice: Best fit line from tip of incisor through root apex measured to true vertical. (**E**) Mandibular central incisor protrusion measurement on the sagittal slice: The buccal surface of the tooth to true vertical line established at 10 mm ahead of the T1 symphysis (green vertical line). (**F**) Mandibular central incisor vertical position measurement on the sagittal slice: Tip of incisor to true horizontal line established at the T1 inferior border of symphysis (blue line).

The vertical position of the mandibular incisors was measured by the distance between the incisal edge and the true horizontal line established at the T1 inferior border of symphysis. Both T1 and T2 incisor vertical position were measured to the T1 true horizontal line to eliminate the difference of the inferior border of symphysis between T1 and T2 due to the normal growth and development of the mandible. Over the time period, a positive value was indicative of an eruption while a negative value was indicative of an intrusion.

All measurements were performed on both left and right sides of each sample. Thus, the sample size was 32 for the RME group and 36 for the RME + LB group. All the measurements were taken by the same examiner (O.G.), and 9 samples were randomly selected and remeasured at a 1-week interval to test the reliability and repeatability of the current measurement protocol. The interclass correlation coefficient (ICC) of each parameter was calculated utilizing the IBM SPSS software (Statistical Package for Social Sciences version 26.0, Chicago, IL, USA). Due to the large range of treatment times and the considerable difference in the time ranges between T1 and T2 of the samples included in the study, it was determined that statistics should be evaluated on both total changes as well as an average change per year. In doing so, the authors hoped to eliminate skewing of the results that may occur from a patient undergoing the expected changes from growth over a longer T1 to T2 time period. The Shapiro–Wilk normality test was performed using OriginPro 8 (Origin Lab Corp., Northampton, MA, USA). Some data did not follow normal distribution so all data are presented as raw data overlapped with a Median ± 95% confidence interval. For comparisons between different timepoints within a group, Wilcoxon matched-pairs signed rank test was used. For intergroup comparisons, Mann–Whitney U test was used. For all data presented in this manuscript, $p < 0.05$ (*) was considered as a statistically significant difference.

3. Results

3.1. Patient Demographic Information Comparison between Groups

For the sample population included in the current study, there was no significant difference in T1 age, T2 age and time intervals between T1 and T2 (Table 1). There was also no significant difference in gender distribution of the samples enrolled in each group (Table 1). This supports the comparability of the two groups.

For all the measurements, the lowest ICC was 0.922, which suggests high consistency and reliability of the current measurement protocol (Table 2).

Table 2. The Interclass Correlation test results of each parameter.

	Interclass Correlation	ICC (Absolute Agreement) 95% Confidence Interval [Lower Bound, Upper Bound]
L1 Inclination (o)	0.989	[0.978, 0.994]
L1 Protrusion-Incisal Edge (mm)	0.922	[0.983, 0.996]
L1 Protrusion-CEJ (mm)	0.991	[0.975, 0.996]
L1 Protrusion-CEJ5 (mm)	0.973	[0.948. 0.986]
L1 Vertical (mm)	0.994	[0.989, 0.997]

3.2. Mandibular Central Incisor Inclination Change

The majority of the previous studies concluded that significant amounts of proclination of the mandibular central incisors was observed after lip bumper therapy. In the current study, both RME and RME + LB groups did not show significant change in mandibular incisor inclination when comparing T2 image with T1 image (Table 3). In addition, when comparing between groups, there was no statistically significant differences in total changes or yearly changes of the mandibular central incisor inclination (Table 3, Figure 2). Thus, in the current study, the lip bumper did not cause proclination of mandibular central incisors.

Table 3. The amount of total changes of each measurement parameters for both groups. For T1 vs. T2 comparisons within group, Wilcoxon matched-pairs singed rank test was used. For RME vs. RME + LB comparisons, Mann–Whitney U test was used.

	Total Change					
	RME Group		RME + LB Group			RME vs. RME + LB p-Value
	T2-T1 Changes (Median [Min, Max])	T1 vs. T2 p-Value	T2-T1 Changes (Median [Min, Max])	T1 vs. T2 p-Value		
L1 Inclination (o)	0.10 [−7.30, 10.80]	0.5732	0.20 [−6.00, 6.50]	0.3644		0.8142
L1 Protrusion-Incisal Edge (mm)	0.40 [−0.40, 3.00]	0.0006	0.65 [−0.60, 3.70]	<0.0001		0.6312
L1 Protrusion-CEJ (mm)	0.60 [−0.70, 2.90]	<0.0001	0.60 [−0.50, 3.00]	<0.0001		0.7433
L1 Protrusion-CEJ5 (mm)	0.60 [−0.90, 3.40]	<0.0001	0.85 [−1.40, 2.80]	<0.0001		0.4138
L1 Vertical (mm)	1.60 [−0.60, 4.20]	<0.0001	1.45 [0.20, 3.40]	<0.0001		0.5349

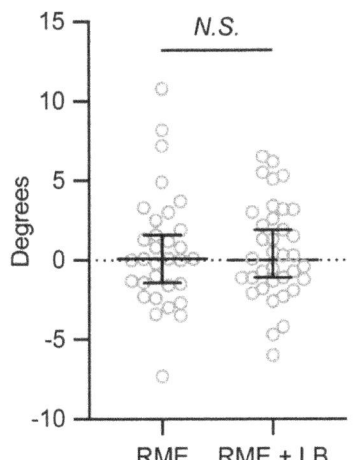 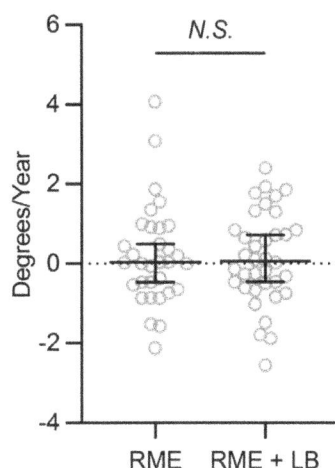

Figure 2. The (**A**) total change and (**B**) yearly change of the mandibular central incisors' inclination. The data are presented as raw data overlapped with Median ± 95% confidence interval. RME: rapid maxillary expansion; LB: lip bumper; N.S.: not significant.

3.3. Mandibular Central Incisor Anterior–Posterior Position Change

As some of the previous studies indicated, lip bumper treatment can cause protrusion of the mandibular central incisors. To further investigate, the anterior–posterior position of the mandibular central incisors was evaluated at three different vertical levels.

When comparing the T1 and T2 images, significant amounts of protrusion were detected in the RME + LB group at all three evaluation levels (Table 3). However, the amount of protrusion in the RME + LB group was not statistically significantly different than that in the RME group (Table 3, Figure 3). Thus, the amount of mandibular incisor protrusion observed in the RME + lip bumper groups may be from normal mandibular dentition growth and development instead of from treatment effect.

3.4. Mandibular Central Incisor Vertical Position Change

Lastly, we evaluated if the lip bumper caused a change in the vertical position of the mandibular central incisors.

As shown in Table 3, both RME and RME + LB groups showed statistically significant amounts of mandibular central incisor eruption during the phase I treatment. When comparing between these two groups, the amount of change was not statistically significantly different (Table 3, Figure 4). Thus, the amount of mandibular incisor eruption observed in the RME + lip bumper group may be from normal mandibular dentoalveolar growth and development instead of from treatment effect.

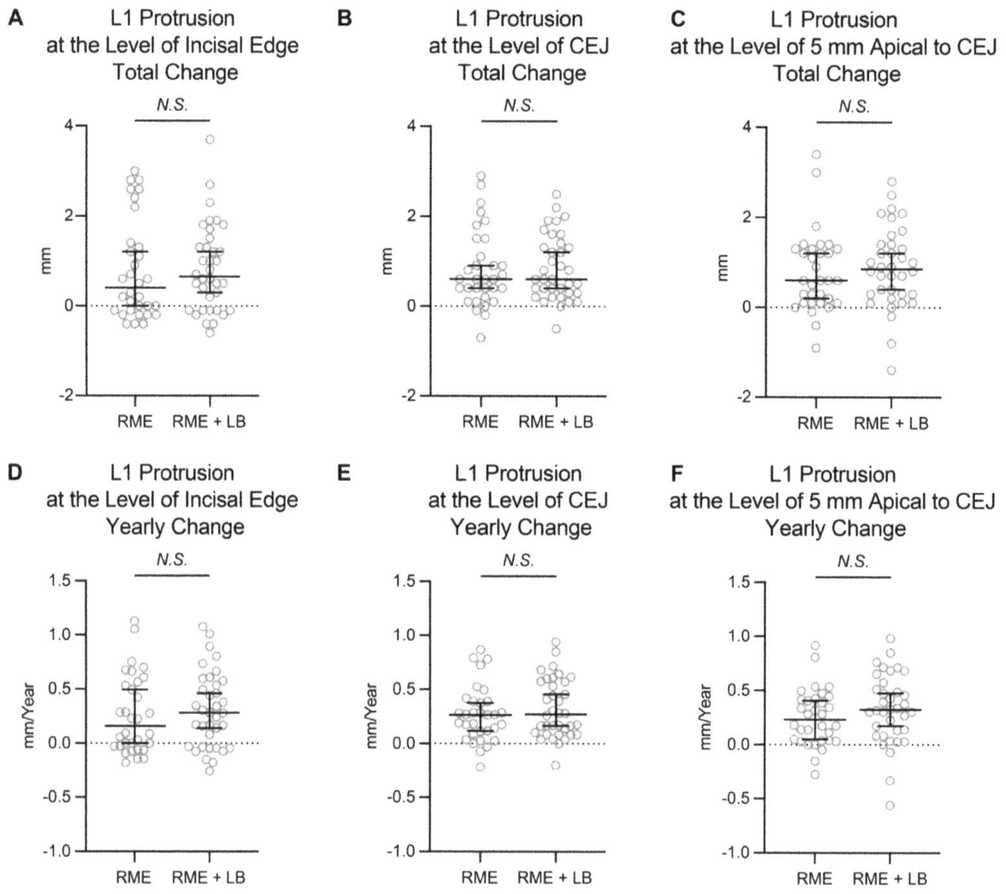

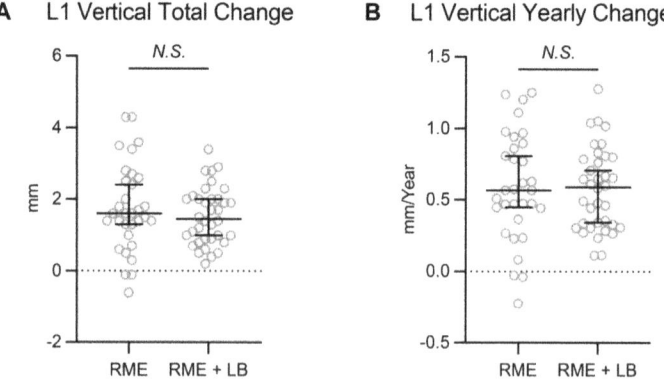

Figure 3. The total change and yearly change of the mandibular central incisors anterior–posterior position. The data are presented as raw data overlapped with Median ± 95% confidence interval CEJ: cementoenamel junction; RME: rapid maxillary expansion; LB: lip bumper; N.S.: not significant.

Figure 4. The (**A**) total change and (**B**) yearly change of the mandibular central incisors' vertical position. The data are presented as raw data overlapped with Median ± 95% confidence interval RME: rapid maxillary expansion; LB: lip bumper; N.S.: not significant.

4. Discussion

In the current study, a longitudinal CBCT database was utilized to evaluate the mandibular incisors' positional changes introduced by lip bumper therapy. This question has been previously evaluated and published in the literature utilizing lateral cephalograms. The novelty of the study comes from the use of CBCT images, which decreases magnification and distortion. Additionally, by utilizing 3D mandibular superimposition, discrepancies in measurements due to a tracing error between timepoints was reduced. Furthermore, by comparing with the control group, the study eliminated the effects of normal mandibular dentition growth and development.

Three positional changes were evaluated in this study: changes in inclination, changes in protrusion and vertical development of the mandibular incisors. Firstly, the central incisor inclination according to our study had no significant difference between the experimental group (RME + LB group) and the control group (RME group) in terms of total or annual change. This finding is contrary to numerous prior studies including O'Donnell et al., Grossen et al. and Davidovitch et al., who all found at least 2.5° of lower incisor proclination from lip bumper treatment [5–7]. On the other hand, the result of our study agreed with the study from Raucci et al. [9]. There are several possible explanations for this finding in our study. The first explanation is that the use of CBCT allowed for a more reliable measurement since there is no overlap of other anatomical structures over the lower incisor root [17]. Another explanation is that there were no control groups in either the O'Donnell et al. or Grossen et al. studies. Therefore, there is no way to determine if the proclination seen was just a normal part of growth and development in their subjects. Thirdly, the mandibular border has active modeling and remodeling during growth and development. Thus, using the changes of the incisal mandibular plane angle (IMPA) might not be a reliable parameter to evaluate the treatment effects. The most likely explanation for our finding of no change in lower incisor inclination compared to previously documented findings is that our study window was large, since the T2 image was not taken immediately after the lip bumper therapy. In the current study, the median time interval between lip bumper removal and T2 images was about 1.5 months. Thus, any treatment effect of incisor proclination introduced by the lip bumper had already relapsed and could not last until the timepoint when patients were ready for phase II comprehensive treatment.

Secondly, the anterior–posterior position change of the mandibular incisors was evaluated. About 0.6 mm of mandibular incisor protrusion was observed in the RME + LB group. This finding is different than the Jacob study, which found the lower incisor tip protruded 1.2 mm, and the O'Donnell study, which found a protrusion of 0.9 mm [5,8]. However, our findings were more closely similar to a different study which found the mandibular incisors protruded approximately 0.5 mm following lip bumper treatment [6]. When comparing the amount of mandibular incisor protrusion between RME and RME + LB groups, no statistically significant difference was detected. It is worth noting that the yearly change of mandibular incisor protrusion observed in the current study (0.16 mm/yr at the incisal edge of the RME group, 0.28 mm/year at the incisal edge of the RME + LB group) is close to the estimated yearly change (0.3 mm/year) of normal growth and development provided by Buschang et al. [19]. Overall, the current study indicated that the protrusion observed during the phase I treatment was entirely the result of normal mandibular dentition growth and development.

Another measurement evaluated in this study was the vertical eruption of the lower incisors. There was a statistically significant difference in the vertical position between T1 and T2 for both groups, but there was no statistically significant difference between groups. The total amount of vertical changes in our study (1.60 mm in the RME group, 1.45 mm in the RME + LB group) was similar to a previously reported study on lip bumper treatment that found eruption to be approximately 1.5 mm [8]. However, the previously reported study lacked a control group [8]. Thus, it is concluded that lip bumper therapy does not have a significant effect on vertical development of the lower incisors.

This study has multiple limitations that need to be discussed before accepting conclusions and interpreting the data's clinical relevance. The study was performed retrospectively on previously treated subjects. Due to the nature of the subjects, random allocation of treatment groups could not be performed. In addition, because of the retrospective nature of the data the exact delivery, the adjustment and design of the lip bumper was not controlled in the study. Furthermore, the length of lip bumper treatment varied within the experimental group. Most of the prior literature on the dentoalveolar effects of the lip bumper had treatment times not greater than one year. As previously cited in Murphy et al., the majority of treatment effects of lip bumper therapy are seen within the first 300 days [20]. In addition, as previously discussed there was a large variance in the total treatment time within groups and between the groups. Due to the age of the patient population, a significant amount of growth and development was expected to occur during the treatment period. Even though there were no statistically significant difference on T1 age, T2 age and the time interval between the two groups, the large variance in the length of total treatment of each individual could distort the results. Besides, atypical swallowing patterns have been proven to affect the upper and lower incisors' proclination in children and adolescents [21]. In the current study, we did not evaluate and compare the swallowing patterns of the involved subjects between the two groups. Future studies should try to have control and experimental groups with similar intervals between data timepoints, and consider the potential influence of atypical swallowing patterns. Finally, although the CBCT images provide the unique possibility to evaluate a 3D anatomic structure without the interference of overlapping structures, there are some detected differences within or between the groups that are near one voxel size and therefore, near the detection limit of the method used.

5. Conclusions

In the present study, the lip bumper did not cause significant proclination, protrusion or extrusion of the mandibular incisors. The dentoalveolar effects of lip bumper therapy need further evaluation with a well-controlled, prospective CBCT study in order to guide future treatment methodologies.

Author Contributions: Conceptualization, C.L. and C.-H.C.; methodology, O.G., C.L. and J.C.O.; software, O.G., C.L. and J.C.O.; validation, O.G.; formal analysis, O.G. and C.L.; investigation, O.G.; resources, S.R.S. and N.S.B.; data curation, O.G.; writing—original draft preparation, O.G. and C.L.; writing—review and editing, J.C.O., S.R.S., N.S.B. and C.-H.C.; visualization, O.G. and C.L.; supervision, C.L.; project administration, C.L.; funding acquisition, C.L. All authors have read and agreed to the published version of the manuscript.

Funding: This research was funded by the American Association of Orthodontists Foundation (AAOF) Orthodontic Faculty Development Fellowship Award (for C.L.), American Association of Orthodontists (AAO) Full-Time Faculty Fellowship Award (for C.L.), University of Pennsylvania School of Dental Medicine Joseph and Josephine Rabinowitz Award for Excellence in Research (for C.L.) and the J. Henry O'Hern Jr. Pilot Grant from the Department of Orthodontics, University of Pennsylvania School of Dental Medicine (for C.L.).

Institutional Review Board Statement: The study was conducted in accordance with the Declaration of Helsinki, and approved by the Institutional Review Board of the University of Pennsylvania (protocol # 850683 and date of approval: 31 January 2022).

Informed Consent Statement: Patient consent was waived as this is a retrospective study utilizing pre-exist database.

Data Availability Statement: The data presented in this study are contained within this article.

Conflicts of Interest: The authors declare no conflict of interest.

References

1. Ghafari, J. A lip-activated appliance in early orthodontic treatment. *J. Am. Dent. Assoc.* **1985**, *111*, 771–774. [CrossRef] [PubMed]
2. Buschang, P.H. Maxillomandibular expansion: Short-term relapse potential and long-term stability. *Am. J. Orthod. Dentofac. Orthop.* **2006**, *129*, S75–S79. [CrossRef] [PubMed]
3. Graber, L.W.; Vanarsdall, R.L.; Vig, K.W.L.; Huang, G.J. *Orthodontics: Current Principles and Techniques*; Elsevier: Amsterdam, The Netherlands, 2017.
4. Nevant, C.T.; Buschang, P.H.; Alexander, R.G.; Steffen, J.M. Lip bumper therapy for gaining arch length. *Am. J. Orthod. Dentofac. Orthop.* **1991**, *100*, 330–336. [CrossRef]
5. O'Donnell, S.; Nanda, R.S.; Ghosh, J. Perioral forces and dental changes resulting from mandibular lip bumper treatment. *Am. J. Orthod. Dentofac. Orthop.* **1998**, *113*, 247–255. [CrossRef]
6. Grossen, J.; Ingervall, B. The effect of a lip bumper on lower dental arch dimensions and tooth positions. *Eur. J. Orthod.* **1995**, *17*, 129–134. [CrossRef]
7. Davidovitch, M.; McInnis, D.; Lindauer, S.J. The effects of lip bumper therapy in the mixed dentition. *Am. J. Orthod. Dentofac. Orthop.* **1997**, *111*, 52–58. [CrossRef]
8. Jacob, H.B.; LeMert, S.; Alexander, R.G.; Buschang, P.H. Second molar impaction associated with lip bumper therapy. *Dent. Press J. Orthod.* **2014**, *19*, 99–104. [CrossRef] [PubMed]
9. Raucci, G.; Pacheco-Pereira, C.; Elyasi, M.; d'Apuzzo, F.; Flores-Mir, C.; Perillo, L. Short- and long-term evaluation of mandibular dental arch dimensional changes in patients treated with a lip bumper during mixed dentition followed by fixed appliances. *Angle Orthod.* **2016**, *86*, 753–760. [CrossRef]
10. Moin, K.; Bishara, S.E. An evaluation of buccal shield treatment. A clinical and cephalometric study. *Angle Orthod.* **2007**, *77*, 57–63. [CrossRef]
11. Werner, S.P.; Shivapuja, P.K.; Harris, E.F. Skeletodental changes in the adolescent accruing from use of the lip bumper. *Angle Orthod.* **1994**, *64*, 13–20, discussion 21–22. [CrossRef]
12. Bergersen, E.O. A cephalometric study of the clinical use of the mandibular labial bumper. *Am. J. Orthod.* **1972**, *61*, 578–602. [CrossRef]
13. Subtelny, J.D.; Sakuda, M. Muscle function, oral malformation, and growth changes. *Am. J. Orthod.* **1966**, *52*, 495–517. [CrossRef]
14. Hashish, D.I.; Mostafa, Y.A. Effect of lip bumpers on mandibular arch dimensions. *Am. J. Orthod. Dentofac. Orthop.* **2009**, *135*, 106–109. [CrossRef]
15. Santana, L.G.; de Campos Franca, E.; Flores-Mir, C.; Abreu, L.G.; Marques, L.S.; Martins-Junior, P.A. Effects of lip bumper therapy on the mandibular arch dimensions of children and adolescents: A systematic review. *Am. J. Orthod. Dentofac. Orthop.* **2020**, *157*, 454–465.e451. [CrossRef] [PubMed]
16. Li, C.; Lin, L.; Zheng, Z.; Chung, C.H. A User-Friendly Protocol for Mandibular Segmentation of CBCT Images for Superimposition and Internal Structure Analysis. *J. Clin. Med.* **2021**, *10*, 127. [CrossRef] [PubMed]
17. Kadioglu, O.; Currier, G.F. *Craniofacial 3D Imaging: Current Concepts in Orthodontics and Oral and Maxillofacial Surgery*; Springer International Publishing: Cham, Switzerland, 2019.
18. Ruellas, A.C.; Yatabe, M.S.; Souki, B.Q.; Benavides, E.; Nguyen, T.; Luiz, R.R.; Franchi, L.; Cevidanes, L.H. 3D Mandibular Superimposition: Comparison of Regions of Reference for Voxel-Based Registration. *PLoS ONE* **2016**, *11*, e0157625. [CrossRef] [PubMed]
19. Buschang, P.H.; Roldan, S.I.; Tadlock, L.P. Guidelines for assessing the growth and development of orthodontic patients. *Semin. Orthod.* **2017**, *23*, 321–335. [CrossRef]
20. Murphy, C.C.; Magness, W.B.; English, J.D.; Frazier-Bowers, S.A.; Salas, A.M. A longitudinal study of incremental expansion using a mandibular lip bumper. *Angle Orthod.* **2003**, *73*, 396–400. [CrossRef] [PubMed]
21. Begnoni, G.; Cadenas de Llano-Perula, M.; Dellavia, C.; Willems, G. Cephalometric traits in children and adolescents with and without atypical swallowing: A retrospective study. *Eur. J. Paediatr. Dent.* **2020**, *21*, 46–52. [CrossRef]

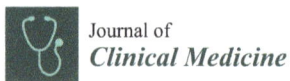

Article

Mini-Implant Rejection Rate in Teenage Patients Depending on Insertion Site: A Retrospective Study

Teodora Consuela Bungău [1], Luminița Ligia Vaida [1,*], Abel Emanuel Moca [1,*], Gabriela Ciavoi [1], Raluca Iurcov [1], Ioana Mihaela Romanul [1] and Camelia Liana Buhaș [2]

[1] Department of Dentistry, Faculty of Medicine and Pharmacy, University of Oradea, 10 Piața 1 Decembrie Street, 410073 Oradea, Romania
[2] Department of Morphological Disciplines, Faculty of Medicine and Pharmacy, University of Oradea, 410087 Oradea, Romania
* Correspondence: ligia_vaida@yahoo.com (L.L.V.); abelmoca@yahoo.com (A.E.M.)

Abstract: Mini-implants have undeniable advantages in Orthodontics. However, the use of mini-implants shows some limitations and disadvantages related to patient age, the quality of the bone tissue, the characteristics of the oral mucosa, implant site, the state of health of the organism and the quality of oral hygiene. The aim of this paper was to analyze the rejection rate of mini-implants in teenage patients, depending on their insertion site, and examine their stability up to three months after insertion. This retrospective study was conducted on dental charts belonging to patients aged between 12 and 17 years, from Oradea, Romania. The mini-implants were placed for various therapeutic reasons and were inserted in the following sites: buccal maxillary area, the infrazygomatic region, palatal area, buccal mandibular area and lingual area; they had a diameter of 1.6 mm (inter-radicular spaces) and of 2 mm (nonbearing tooth areas), and a length of 6–8 mm (mandible) or 8–10 mm (maxilla). The rejection rate was checked in the first month, second month, third month and after the third month from insertion. A total of 432 patients were included in the study, and they had a total of 573 mini-implants. Most implants were placed in the buccal region of the maxilla (27.7%) and most patients had one mini-implant placed (65.7%). The highest rejection rate was obtained in the first month (15.2%). The rejection rate between genders was similar. The mini-implants from the buccal mandibular region had a significantly higher rate of rejection in the first month (M1) in comparison to the mini-implants from the palatal region (24.4% vs. 8.3%). The mini-implants from the lingual region of the mandible had a significantly higher rate of rejection in the second month (M2) in comparison to the mini-implants from the infrazygomatic or the palatal region (10.5% vs 0%/0%). Mini-implants are very useful for carrying out various orthodontic treatments, but their stability should be enhanced.

Keywords: mini-implants; rejection rate; teenagers; insertion site

1. Introduction

In Orthodontics, anchorage is defined as the ability to resist undesired reactive tooth movements, and it can be obtained by using teeth, palate, head, neck and TADs (Temporary Anchorage Devices) [1]. TADs have become an increasingly used method for orthodontic treatments, and the skeletal anchorage they provide is fast replacing conventional anchorage [2]. In order to obtain an optimal anchorage, the ideal device should be easy to use, cheap, able to be loaded immediately, immobile, not require patient's compliance biocompatible and offer superior or comparable results to traditional anchorage systems [3]. Among the anchorage systems used in Orthodontics are osseointegrated implants, palatal implants, miniplates, miniscrew implants [4].

The miniscrew implants are also called mini-implants, this being the most used term in the orthodontic literature, and were developed as a mean to overcome the issue related to the large size of osseointegrated implants, which were used for orthodontic anchorage [5]. Mini-implants have undeniable advantages in Orthodontics [6]. They allowed for the reconsideration of anchorage principles and the biomechanics used in orthodontic treatment [7]. However, the use of mini-implants shows some limitations and disadvantages related to patient age [8], the quality of the bone tissue [9], the characteristics of the oral mucosa [10], implant site [11], the state of health of the organism [12] and the quality of patient oral hygiene [13].

Even though the failure rate shown in literature is approximately 10% [14], loose mini-implants during ongoing treatment, even for a minority of the cases, is a disadvantage. In addition to the factors listed above, mini-implant stability depends on the mechanical interlocking of threads and bony tissue and not on osseointegration. In order to obtain maximum efficiency, they should ideally remain immobile when orthodontic force is applied [15]. Literature shows that most miniscrew failure occurs in the first week after mini-implant insertion [16]. Moreover, loose mini-implants are often observed in teenagers [17]. This is likely to be related to active bone metabolism in growing children and to low maturation of the bone, including the maxillo-mandibular bone [18]. To the best of our knowledge, there are no recent studies that focus on investigating the mini-implant rejection rate in teenage patients, and research focusing on this age group was considered beneficial.

The aim of this paper was to analyze the distribution of the mini-implants according to the insertion site and gender in a sample of Romanian teenagers (12 to 17 years old). Another aim was to investigate the rejection rate of the mini-implants depending on the different insertion sites (buccal maxillary region, infrazygomatic region, palatal region, buccal mandibular region, lingual region) at one month, two months, three months and after three months from the insertion moment. Comparisons between boys and girls regarding the rejection rate of the mini-implants were also desired.

2. Materials and Methods

2.1. Ethical Considerations

The study was conducted in accordance with the 1964 Declaration of Helsinki and its later amendments and was approved by the Research Ethics Committee of the University of Oradea (IRB No. CEFMF/04 from 4 February 2022). All of the patients' parents or legal guardians that took part in this study have given their permission to be included in this research.

2.2. Sample Selection

This retrospective study was conducted on dental charts belonging to teenage patients from Oradea, North-Western Romania. The dental charts were analyzed between 4 February 2022 and 10 February 2022 and were collected from a private orthodontic office in Oradea, Romania. We analyzed all charts that belonged to adolescent patients treated in the last 5 years (1 October 2016 to 1 October 2021). The last mini-implant that was analyzed was placed in 10 June 2021, so that it could be evaluated after more than three months as well.

We included in this study generally healthy patients aged between 12 and 17 years who received orthodontic treatment with fixed appliance and mini-implants and have previously given their permission to take part in the study. Approval of study participation was also obtained from patients' parents or legal guardians.

Partially completed dental charts with missing information were excluded from the study. The excluded dental charts also belonged to patients from other countries or patients with local or general pathologies that could influence the maxillary bone structural integrity.

In order to avoid bias, all dental charts were initially examined by one author (T.C.B.) and were double checked by another author (A.E.M.). The inter-rater reliability was 93%. It showed a very good inter-rater agreement for the mini-implant failure, location of mini-implant, gender, age and purpose of mini-implants, respectively.

2.3. Mini-Implant Properties and Insertion Sites

Each patient that was included in this study had at least one mini-implant inserted and a maximum of 4 mini-implants, for various treatment reasons, such as:

- Correction of vertical dimension: molar intrusion in anterior open bite cases, lower molar intrusion in high angle patients, incisor intrusion in deep bite with excessive gingival display, and undesirable occlusal plane angulation;
- Correction of sagittal dimension: class II or class III biomechanics (intermaxillary elastic traction), anterior movement of the canine to substitute a missing lateral incisor (agenesis), distal or mesial movements of a single tooth or group of teeth for closing or opening up spaces, molar uprighting;
- Prosthetic cases which needed single tooth movement without a complete fixed appliance.

The following areas were used for mini-implant insertion:

- Buccal maxillary area: inter-radicular space between the maxillary second premolar and first molar; inter-radicular space between the upper lateral incisor and upper canine;
- The infrazygomatic region was analyzed separately considering the peculiarities of this area;
- Palatal area: midpalatal, paramedian area or inter-radicular space from the midline and up to and including the tuberosity space, depending on the purpose;
- Buccal mandibular area: interradicular space between lateral incisor and canine, up to mandibular first molar, mandibular second molar or the retromolar region;
- Lingual area: inter-radicular space from the lateral incisive to the retromolar area.

The diameter of the mini-implants was 1.6 mm for inter-radicular spaces and 2 mm for nonbearing tooth areas such as the midpalatal region or the zygomatic buttress. The length was 6–8 mm for the mandible and midpalatal area, and 8–10 mm for the maxilla or areas with thick mucosa (Table 1).

Table 1. Diameter and length used depending on the insertion site.

Location	Diameter (mm)	Length (mm)
Buccal maxilla	1.6	8–10
Infrazygomatic	2	8–10
Palatal	2	8–10
Buccal mandible	1.6	6–8
Lingual	1.6	6–8

As far as the insertion technique is concerned, the self-drilling method was used for all of the patients and it was performed by the same practitioner. After placement, the initial stability of the mini-implant was checked to ensure there were no signs of mobility.

All of the mini-implants (except for the infrazygomatic region) were placed in attached gingiva. The infrazygomatic mini-implants were placed in alveolar mucosa. All of the mini-implants were immediately loaded (maximum of 24–48 h post-insertion) with a force between 100 and 150 g (1–1.5 N). The force was measured using a Teclock Push Pull Gauge (PPN 750-5).

The removal or loss of a mini-implant due to the onset of mobility between the first 24 h and up to six months after insertion was considered a failure.

To serve the purpose of this study, a retrospective analysis was made to check the rejection rate of the mini-implants in the first-month post-insertion (M1), in the second month (M2), in the third month (M3) and after the third month. The distribution of the mini-implants according to the location and the rejection rate was also analyzed for each month.

2.4. Statistical Analysis

All the data from the study was analyzed using IBM SPSS Statistics 25 (IBM, Chicago, IL, USA) and illustrated using Microsoft Office Excel/Word 2013 (Microsoft, Redmond, WA, USA). Quantitative variables were tested for normal distribution using the Shapiro–Wilk Test and were written as averages with standard deviations or medians with interquartile ranges. Qualitative variables were written as counts or percentages and were tested using Fisher's Exact tests. Z-tests with Bonferroni correction were made to further detail the results obtained in the contingency tables. Odds ratio with 95% confidence intervals were used to illustrate the nature of association detected in contingency tables. Logistic regression models testing for goodness-of-fit and significance were used in prediction of the rejection rates in the first and second months. A p value of <0.05 was considered statistically significant.

3. Results

Initially, 485 patients were selected, but after applying the exclusion criteria, 432 patient dental charts were kept in this study. The 432 patients included in the study received a total of 573 mini-implants.

Regarding the distribution of the patients related to gender, most patients were girls. Out of the 432 selected patients, 243 were girls (56.2%) and 189 were boys (43.8%). The average age was 14.31 ± 1.625 years, with a median of 14 years, and the age range was between 12 and 17 years.

Data from Table 2 shows the distribution of the mini-implants according to their insertion site, with the most frequent insertion sites being the buccal part of the maxilla, the hard palate and the buccal part of the mandible.

Table 2. Distribution of the mini-implants according to the insertion site.

Location	No.	Percentage
Buccal maxilla	159	27.7%
Infrazygomatic	84	14.7%
Palatal	144	25.1%
Buccal mandible	123	21.5%
Lingual	63	11%

No., number.

Figure 1 shows the distribution of the mini-implants according to the insertion site, separately for girls and for boys. The distribution was relatively similar for the infrazygomatic, buccal mandibular and lingual mini-implants. Larger differences were identified for buccal maxillary and palatal mini-implants.

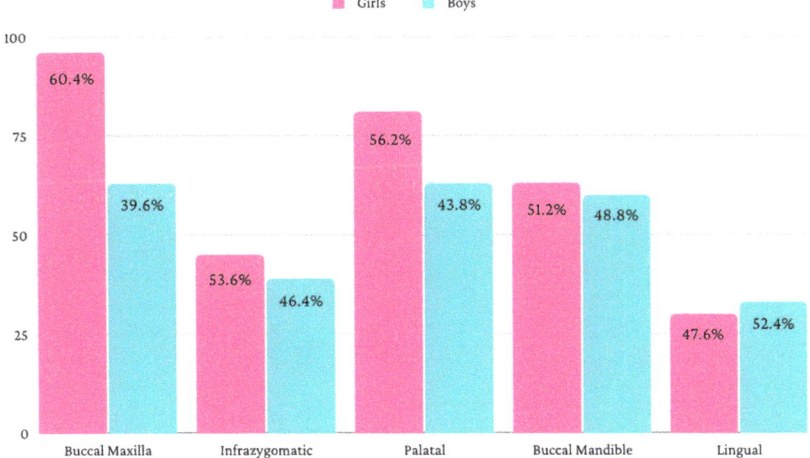

Figure 1. Distribution of the mini-implants for girls and for boys.

Most of the analyzed patients had only one mini-implant (65.7%, n = 284) or two mini-implants (32.9%, n = 142). Only a small percentage of 0.70% of patients received three (n = 3) or four (n = 3) mini-implants.

The first month showed the highest rejection rate of 15.2% (n = 87). After that, 3.7% (n = 18) of the mini-implants were rejected in the second month, 1.9% (n = 9) of the mini-implants were rejected in the third month, and 6.5% (n = 30) of the mini-implants were rejected after the third month. Figure 2 shows the number of mini-implants that remained in place, and the number of mini-implants that failed according to the insertion site.

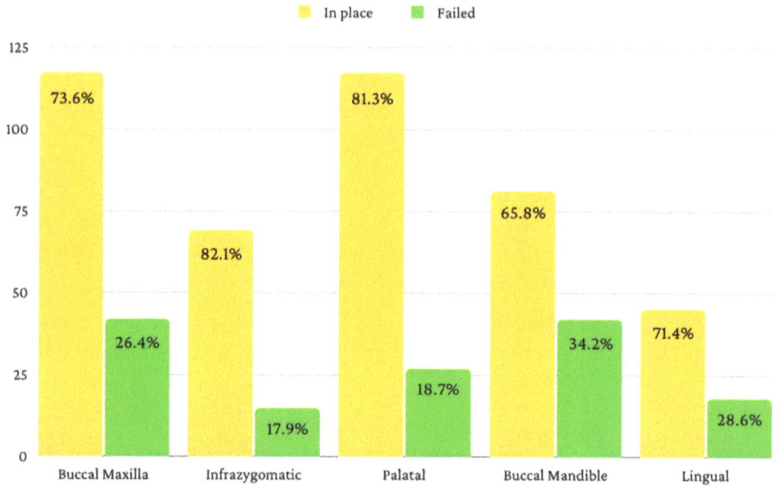

Figure 2. Mini-implants in place and rejected after more than three months.

Furthermore, the distribution of the mini-implants according to the location and the rejection rate was analyzed for each month (Table 3).

Table 3. Distribution of the mini-implants according to the location and the rejection rate in M1, M2 M3 and after M3.

Location (No. /%)	Buccal Maxilla	Infrazygomatic	Palatal	Buccal Mandible	Lingual	p *
M1						
In place	129 (81.1%)	75 (89.3%)	132 (91.7%)	93 (75.6%)	57 (90.5%)	0.002
Failed	30 (18.9%)	9 (10.7%)	12 (8.3%)	30 (24.4%)	6 (9.5%)	
M2						
In place	123 (95.3%)	75 (100%)	132 (100%)	87 (93.5%)	51 (89.5%)	<0.001
Failed	6 (4.7%)	0 (0%)	0 (0%)	6 (6.5%)	6 (10.5%)	
M3						
In place	120 (97.6%)	75 (100%)	129 (97.7%)	84 (96.6%)	51 (100%)	0.489
Failed	3 (2.4%)	0 (0%)	3 (2.3%)	3 (3.4%)	0 (0%)	
After M3						
In place	117 (97.5%)	69 (92%)	117 (90.7%)	81 (96.4%)	45 (88.2%)	0.056
Failed	3 (2.5%)	6 (8%)	12 (9.3%)	3 (3.6%)	6 (11.8%)	

No., number; %, percentage; * Fisher's Exact Test.

The global rejection rate of the mini-implants in the first month was 15.2%, the observed differences between groups were statistically significant according to Fisher's Exact Test (p = 0.002) and Z-tests with Bonferroni correction showed that the mini-implants from the buccal mandibular region had a significantly higher rate of rejection in the first month (M1) in comparison to the mini-implants from the palatal region (24.4% vs. 8.3%). Other differences between other regions were not statistically significant.

In the second month (M2), the global rejection rate of the mini-implants was 3.7%, and the observed differences between groups were statistically significant according to Fisher's Exact Test ($p < 0.001$) and Z-tests with Bonferroni correction showed that the mini-implants from the lingual region of the mandible had a significantly higher rate of rejection in the second month in comparison to the mini-implants from the infrazygomatic or the palatal region (10.5% vs. 0%/0%). Other differences between other regions were not statistically significant.

Because of the low rejection rates from the third month (M3) and after the third month, the observed differences between groups were not statistically significant according to Fisher's Exact Test.

A univariate logistic regression models used for the prediction of mini-implant rejection in the first month. Due to collinearity between implant length and implant region only univariate models were used. After testing for goodness-of-fit, the models had high significance ($p < 0.001$), showing the following results:

- In comparison to 10 mm implants, 6 mm implants had 2.283 higher odds of rejection in the first month (95% C.I.: 1.197–4.353) and 8 mm implants had 2.769 higher odds of rejection in the first month (95% C.I.: 1.601-4.788);
- In comparison to implants located in the vestibular maxilla, implants in the palatine region had 2.557 lower odds of rejection in the first month (95% C.I.: 1.254–5.208) and implants in the vestibular mandible had 1.779 higher odds of rejection in the first month (95% C.I.: 1.021–3.101).

Table 4 shows the distribution of mini-implants based on the patient's gender and rejection in M1, M2, M3, and after M3. The observed differences between groups were not statistically significant according to Fisher's Exact Test, the rejection rate being approximately similar between genders in M1, M3 and after M3. In the second month (M2) the rejection rate was significantly higher for girls than for boys (5.6% vs. 1.4%). As for the distribution of the mini-implants according to gender, insertion site and rejection rate (Table 5) the results obtained showed that most of the times the differences between gender were not statistically significant. However, the differences between genders were statistically significant for mini-implants inserted in the infrazygomatic region after M3, and for the mini-implants inserted in the lingual region at M1, M2, and after M3.

Table 4. Distribution of the mini-implants according to gender and the rejection rate in M1, M2, M3 and after M3.

Gender/Rejection	Girls		Boys		p *
	No.	%	No.	%	
		M1			
In place	270	85.7%	216	83.7%	0.559
Failed	45	14.3%	42	16.3%	
		M2			
In place	255	94.4%	213	98.6%	0.016
Failed	15	5.6%	3	1.4%	
		M3			
In place	249	97.6%	210	98.6%	0.520
Failed	6	2.4%	3	1.4%	
		After M3			
In place	249	97.6%	210	98.6%	0.520
Failed	6	2.4%	3	1.4%	

No., number; %, percentage; * Fisher's Exact Test.

Table 5. Distribution of the mini-implants according to gender, insertion site and rejection rate in M1, M2, M3 and after M3.

Location (No./%)	Buccal Maxilla		Infrazygomatic		Palatal		Buccal Mandible		Lingual	
	G	B	G	B	G	B	G	B	G	B
					M1					
In place	81 (84.4%)	48 (76.2%)	39 (86.7%)	36 (92.3%)	75 (92.6%)	57 (90.5%)	42 (66.7%)	45 (75%)	30 (100%)	27 (81.8%)
Failed	15 (15.6%)	15 (23.8%)	6 (13.3%)	3 (7.7%)	6 (7.4%)	6 (9.5%)	21 (33.3%)	15 (25%)	0 (0%)	6 (18.2%)
p *	0.218		0.494		0.764		0.329		0.025	
					M2					
In place	90 (93.8%)	63 (100%)	45 (100%)	39 (100%)	81 (100%)	63 (100%)	60 (95.2%)	57 (95%)	24 (80%)	33 (100%)
Failed	6 (6.2%)	0 (0%)	0 (0%)	0 (0%)	0 (0%)	0 (0%)	3 (4.8%)	3 (5%)	6 (20%)	0 (0%)
p *	0.082		-		-		1.000		0.009	
					M3					
In place	96 (100%)	60 (95.2%)	45 (100%)	39 (100%)	78 (96.3%)	63 (100%)	60 (95.2%)	60 (100%)	30 (100%)	33 (100%)
Failed	0 (0%)	3 (4.8%)	0 (0%)	0 (0%)	3 (3.7%)	0 (0%)	3 (4.8%)	0 (0%)	0 (0%)	0 (0%)
p *	0.060		-		0.257		0.244		-	
					After M3					
In place	96 (100%)	60 (95.2%)	45 (100%)	33 (84.6%)	75 (92.6%)	57 (90.5%)	63 (100%)	57 (95%)	24 (80%)	33 (100%)
Failed	0 (0%)	3 (4.8%)	0 (0%)	6 (15.4%)	6 (7.4%)	6 (9.5%)	0 (0%)	3 (5%)	6 (20%)	0 (0%)
p *	0.060		0.008		0.764		0.113		0.009	

No., number; %, percentage; * Fisher's Exact Test; G, girls; B, boys.

A univariate logistic regression models for the prediction of mini-implant rejection in the second month was performed. Due to collinearity between implant length and implant region only univariate models were used. After testing for goodness-of-fit and significance, only gender exhibited a significant prediction, showing that in comparison to male patients, implants in female patients had 4.25 higher odds of rejection in the second month (95% C.I.: 1.217–14.846).

The distribution of the mini-implants according to diameter and the rejection rate is shown in Table 6. The rejection rate was significantly more associated with 1.6 mm mini-implants in M1 and M2, and to 2 mm mini-implants after M3. The distribution of the mini-implants according to length and rejection rate is shown in Table 7. The rejection rate was significantly more associated with 6 or 8 mm mini-implants in M1 and M2.

Table 6. Distribution of the mini-implants according to implant diameter and the rejection rate in M1, M2, M3 and after M3.

Diameter (No./%)	1.6 mm	2 mm	p *
		M1	
In place	273 (79.1%)	207 (90.8%)	<0.001
Failed	72 (20.9%)	21 (9.2%)	
		M2	
In place	327 (94.8%)	228 (100%)	<0.001
Failed	18 (5.2%)	0 (0%)	
		M3	
In place	339 (98.3%)	225 (98.7%)	1.000
Failed	6 (1.7%)	3 (1.3%)	
		After M3	
In place	333 (96.5%)	210 (92.1%)	0.033
Failed	12 (3.5%)	18 (7.9%)	

No., number; %, percentage; * Fisher's Exact Test.

Table 7. Distribution of the mini-implants according to implant length and the rejection rate in M1, M2, M3 and after M3.

Length (No./%)	6 mm	8 mm	10 mm	p *
		M1		
In place	95 (81.2%)	178 (78.1%)	207 (90.8%)	0.001
Failed	22 (18.8%)	50 (21.9%)	21 (9.2%)	
		M2		
In place	108 (92.3%)	219 (96.1%)	228 (100%)	<0.001
Failed	9 (7.7%)	9 (3.9%)	0 (0%)	
		M3		
In place	116 (99.1%)	223 (97.8%)	225 (98.7%)	0.750
Failed	1 (0.9%)	5 (2.2%)	3 (1.3%)	
		After M3		
In place	112 (95.7%)	221 (96.9%)	210 (92.1%)	0.064
Failed	5 (4.3%)	7 (3.1%)	18 (7.9%)	

No., number; %, percentage; * Fisher's Exact Test.

4. Discussion

The indications for the use of mini-implants are numerous, and in many cases they can successfully replace other types of fixed orthodontic appliances, or sometimes they can be used as an alternative to orthognathic surgery [19]. They can also be used for the traction of transmigrated teeth [20]. Mini-implants do not require special surgical procedures, and are inserted easily. They can be inserted in various locations, do not require compliance from the patient and can be easily removed [21]. These advantages have led to an increase in the frequency of their use, but also to the extent of the indications of mini-implants [22].

The age of patients has proven to influence the success rate of mini-implants [23]. In this study, the group was composed of adolescent patients aged between 12 and 17 years. The age range was chosen because it is considered that growth spurts of the bone occur during infancy (1 to 4 years) and puberty (12 to 17 years) [24]. The lower limit of 12 years was also selected because some authors contraindicate the application of mini-implants in patients younger than 12 years old [25]. However, the chronological age of the patient is not always an indication of the skeletal development [26].

The mini-implants that were used in this study sample, had a diameter between 1.6 mm (inter-radicular spaces) and 2 mm (nonbearing tooth areas), and a length between 6–8 mm (mandible and midpalatal area) and 8–10 mm (maxilla and areas with thick mucosa). These dimensions fall within the limits recommended in the orthodontic literature. Suzuki et al. (2013) reached the conclusion that for a mini-implant with a diameter of 1.3 mm, the length of 5 mm (maxilla) and 6 mm (mandible) represent the minimum dimensions necessary for obtaining a good anchorage [27]. In general, mini-implants with a diameter smaller than 1.2 mm have higher chances of failure [28], and a short mini-implant placed in an insertion site with a thick mucosa has higher chances of being rejected, in these cases longer implants being recommended [29]. However, when it comes to skeletal anchorage, the length of the mini-implant is less important than the diameter of the mini-implant. The primary stability of a mini-implant is, also, better when the insertion angle is of 70 degrees [30]. The insertion technique used was the self-drilling technique because it reduces operative time, bone damage and patient discomfort, having a success rate similar to mini-implants inserted with the self-tapping technique [31]. The self-drilling technique, however, does not mean higher pressure. Applying excessive pressure while placing the mini-implant, can lead to mini-implant displacement, microfractures and alveolar bone enlargement [32].

In the investigated sample, most mini-implants were rejected in the first month of insertion (15.2%), and the fewest were rejected in the third month (1.9%). Alharbi et al. (2018) reported a rejection rate of 14.3% following the analysis of 11 studies with samples in which more than 100 implants were inserted [15], a result similar to that obtained in this study. Regarding adolescent patients, the same authors reported a failure rate of 8.6%, much lower than that obtained in this study [15]. Results closer to those obtained in this study sample were reported by Papageorgiou et al. (2012) who identified a failure rate of 12.6%, in patients under the age of 20 years [12]. Most mini-implants failed in the first month after insertion, a result consistent with those obtained by other authors who reported that most mini-implants fail in the first week after application [16].

In the first month after insertion, most mini-implants that failed were inserted in the buccal mandibular region (24.4% failure rate), and the fewest in the palatal region (8.3% failure rate). Failure rates of mini-implants placed in the buccal mandibular region of 7.2% were also reported, but those mini-implants were placed in the buccal mandibular shelf [33]. Higher failure rates, of 19.3%, have also been reported [33]. Some authors reported a failure rate of 39.1% of mini-implants placed in the buccal region of the mandible, and of 23.1% of mini-implants placed in the buccal region of the maxilla, at 12 months [34]. Regarding the failure rate of palatal mini-implants, this was similar to other studies that reported a failure rate of 6.1% [35] or 8.5% [34]. A single study reported a failure rate of 16.7%, much higher than that reported in this study [36].

Infrazygomatic placed mini-implants had a failure rate of 10.7% in the first month and 0% in the second and third month. Uribe et al. (2015) obtained a failure rate of 21.8% of mini-implants placed in the infrazygomatic region [37], while Liou et al. (2004) reported a 100% success rate of mini-implants placed in the infrazygomatic region [38].

The failure rates of the mini-implants depending on the gender of the patients were similar between boys and girls. In the first month, the failure rate was 14.3% for girls and 16.3% for boys and decreased in the second and third month. Some authors have reported bigger differences between genders, regarding the failure rate of mini-implants [39], but others have reported similar failure rates between the two genders [40].

Mini-implants were reported to have high success rates ($\geq$90%), which depended on device-related factors, patient-related factors, procedure-related factors, and orthodontic treatment-related factors [41,42]. Mini-implants are useful because they lead to a more efficient orthopedic development in patients with active growth [43]. The study of mini-implants must continue in order to discover the most effective application methods, the best insertion sites, but also the most suitable design, considering that their stability is affected by a variety of factors [44].

This study has some limitations. First of all, it is a retrospective study, so the accuracy regarding the age of the patients, the place of insertion and the dimensions of the mini-implants could have been erroneously recorded. Secondly, the group is limited to the patients of a single orthodontic office, so factors related to the insertion method, preference for certain mini-implants and other aspects related to therapeutic decisions may be specific to the operator.

5. Conclusions

In this study sample, the highest failure rate occurred in the first month, and the lowest in the third month. In the first month, mini-implants placed in the buccal mandibular region had a significantly higher rate of rejection in comparison to mini-implants placed in the palatal region, while in the second month mini-implants from the lingual region of the mandible had a significantly higher rate of rejection in comparison to the mini-implants from the infrazygomatic or the palatal region. Patients' gender did not influence the failure rate, with this being similar between girls and boys.

Author Contributions: Conceptualization, T.C.B. and A.E.M.; methodology, L.L.V.; software, G.C. validation, R.I., I.M.R. and C.L.B.; formal analysis, L.L.V.; investigation, T.C.B.; resources, L.L.V and I.M.R.; data curation, R.I. and G.C.; writing—original draft preparation, T.C.B. and A.E.M.. writing—review and editing, L.L.V. and C.L.B.; visualization, A.E.M.; supervision, C.L.B.; project administration, T.C.B.; funding acquisition, G.C. All authors contributed equally to this article. All authors have read and agreed to the published version of the manuscript.

Funding: This research received no external funding.

Institutional Review Board Statement: The study was conducted in accordance with the Declaration of Helsinki and approved by the Research Ethics Committee of the University of Oradea (IRB No. CEFMF/04 from 4 February 2022).

Informed Consent Statement: Informed consent was obtained from all subjects involved in the study.

Data Availability Statement: The data presented in this study are available on request from the corresponding authors. The data are not publicly available due to privacy reasons.

Conflicts of Interest: The authors declare no conflict of interest.

References

1. Feldmann, I.; Bondemark, L. Orthodontic anchorage: A systematic review. *Angle Orthod.* **2006**, *76*, 493–501. [CrossRef] [PubMed]
2. Leo, M.; Cerroni, L.; Pasquantonio, G.; Condò, S.G.; Condò, R. Temporary anchorage devices (TADs) in orthodontics: Review of the factors that influence the clinical success rate of the mini-implants. *Clin. Ter.* **2016**, *167*, e70–e77. [CrossRef]
3. Cope, J.B. Temporary anchorage devices in orthodontics: A paradigm shift. *Semin. Orthod.* **2005**, *11*, 3–9. [CrossRef]
4. McGuire, M.K.; Scheyer, E.T.; Gallerano, R.L. Temporary anchorage devices for tooth movement: A review and case reports. *J. Periodontol.* **2006**, *77*, 1613–1624. [CrossRef] [PubMed]
5. Reynders, R.; Ronchi, L.; Bipat, S. Mini-implants in orthodontics: A systematic review of the literature. *Am. J. Orthod. Dentofacial Orthop.* **2009**, *135*, e1–e19. [CrossRef] [PubMed]
6. Elias, C.N.; de Oliveira Ruellas, A.C.; Fernandes, D.J. Orthodontic implants: Concepts for the orthodontic practitioner. *Int. J. Dent.* **2012**, *2012*, 549761. [CrossRef]
7. Cousley, R.R.J. Mini-implants in contemporary orthodontics part 2: Clinical applications and optimal biomechanics. *Orthod. Update* **2015**, *8*, 56–61. [CrossRef]
8. Chen, Y.J.; Chang, H.H.; Huang, C.Y.; Hung, H.C.; Lai, E.H.; Yao, C.C. A retrospective analysis of the failure rate of three different orthodontic skeletal anchorage systems. *Clin. Oral Implant. Res.* **2007**, *18*, 768–775. [CrossRef]
9. Tseng, Y.C.; Hsieh, C.H.; Chen, C.H.; Shen, Y.S.; Huang, I.Y.; Chen, C.M. The application of mini-implants for orthodontic anchorage. *Int. J. Oral Maxillofac. Surg.* **2006**, *35*, 704–707. [CrossRef]
10. Kim, H.J.; Yun, H.S.; Park, H.D.; Kim, D.H.; Park, Y.C. Soft-tissue and cortical-bone thickness at orthodontic implant sites. *Am. J. Orthod. Dentofac. Orthop.* **2006**, *130*, 177–182. [CrossRef]
11. Wu, T.Y.; Kuang, S.H.; Wu, C.H. Factors associated with the stability of mini-implants for orthodontic anchorage: A study of 414 samples in Taiwan. *J. Oral Maxillofac. Surg.* **2009**, *67*, 1595–1599. [CrossRef]
12. Papageorgiou, S.N.; Zogakis, I.P.; Papadopoulos, M.A. Failure rates and associated risk factors of orthodontic miniscrew implants: A meta-analysis. *Am. J. Orthod. Dentofac. Orthop.* **2012**, *142*, 577–595. [CrossRef]
13. Kravitz, N.D.; Kusnoto, B. Risks and complications of orthodontic miniscrews. *Am. J. Orthod. Dentofac. Orthop.* **2007**, *131*, S43–S51. [CrossRef]
14. Park, H.S.; Jeong, S.H.; Kwon, O.W. Factors affecting the clinical success of screw implants used as orthodontic anchorage. *Am. J. Orthod. Dentofac. Orthop.* **2006**, *130*, 18–25. [CrossRef] [PubMed]
15. Alharbi, F.; Almuzian, M.; Bearn, D. Miniscrews failure rate in orthodontics: Systematic review and meta-analysis. *Eur. J. Orthod.* **2018**, *40*, 519–530. [CrossRef] [PubMed]
16. Kuroda, S.; Tanaka, E. Risks and complications of miniscrew anchorage in clinical orthodontics. *Jpn. Dent. Sci.* **2014**, *50*, 79–85. [CrossRef]
17. Park, H.S.; Lee, S.K.; Kwon, O.W. Group distal movement of teeth using microscrew implant anchorage. *Angle Orthod.* **2005**, *75*, 602–609. [CrossRef] [PubMed]
18. Motoyoshi, M.; Matsuoka, M.; Shimizu, N. Application of orthodontic mini-implants in adolescents. *Int. J. Oral Maxillofac. Surg.* **2007**, *36*, 695–699. [CrossRef]
19. Singh, K.; Kumar, D.; Jaiswal, R.K.; Bansal, A. Temporary anchorage devices—Mini-implants. *Natl. J. Maxillofac. Surg.* **2010**, *1*, 30–34. [CrossRef]
20. Vaida, L.; Todor, B.I.; Corega, C.; Băciuț, M.; Băciuț, G. A rare case of canine anomaly—A possible algorithm for treating it. *Rom. J. Morphol. Embryol.* **2014**, *55*, 1197–1202.
21. Papadopoulos, M.A.; Tarawneh, F. The use of miniscrew implants for temporary skeletal anchorage in orthodontics: A comprehensive review. *Oral Surg. Oral Med. Oral Pathol. Oral Radiol. Endod.* **2007**, *103*, e6–e15. [CrossRef] [PubMed]
22. Mizrahi, E. The Use of Miniscrews in Orthodontics: A Review of Selected Clinical Applications. *Prim. Dent. J.* **2016**, *5*, 20–27. [CrossRef] [PubMed]
23. Jing, Z.; Wu, Y.; Jiang, W.; Zhao, L.; Jing, D.; Zhang, N.; Cao, X.; Xu, Z.; Zhao, Z. Factors Affecting the Clinical Success Rate of Miniscrew Implants for Orthodontic Treatment. *Int. J. Oral Maxillofac. Implant.* **2016**, *31*, 835–841. [CrossRef] [PubMed]
24. Ohta, H. Growth spurts of the bone from infancy to puberty. *Clin. Calcium.* **2019**, *29*, 9–17. [PubMed]
25. Nausheer, A.; Rithika, J.; Abrar, Y.A.; Ranjan, R.B.K. Temporary anchorage devices in orthodontics: A review. *IJODR* **2020**, *6*, 222–228.

26. Moca, A.E.; Vaida, L.L.; Moca, R.T.; Țuțuianu, A.V.; Bochiș, C.F.; Bochiș, S.A.; Iovanovici, D.C.; Negruțiu, B.M. Chronological Age in Different Bone Development Stages: A Retrospective Comparative Study. *Children* **2021**, *8*, 142. [CrossRef]
27. Suzuki, M.; Deguchi, T.; Watanabe, H.; Seiryu, M.; Iikubo, M.; Sasano, T.; Fujiyama, K.; Takano-Yamamoto, T. Evaluation of optimal length and insertion torque for miniscrews. *Am. J. Orthod. Dentofacial Orthop.* **2013**, *144*, 251–259. [CrossRef]
28. Stanford, N. Mini-screws success rates sufficient for orthodontic treatment. *Evid. Based Dent.* **2011**, *12*, 19. [CrossRef]
29. Topouzelis, N.; Tsaousoglou, P. Clinical factors correlated with the success rate of miniscrews in orthodontic treatment. *Int. J. Oral Sci.* **2012**, *4*, 38–44. [CrossRef]
30. Tatli, U.; Alraawi, M.; Toroğlu, M.S. Effects of size and insertion angle of orthodontic mini-implants on skeletal anchorage. *Am. J. Orthod. Dentofac. Orthop.* **2019**, *156*, 220–228. [CrossRef]
31. Yi, J.; Ge, M.; Li, M.; Li, C.; Li, Y.; Li, X.; Zhao, Z. Comparison of the success rate between self-drilling and self-tapping miniscrews: A systematic review and meta-analysis. *Eur. J. Orthod.* **2017**, *39*, 287–293. [CrossRef] [PubMed]
32. Romano, F.L.; Consolaro, A. Why are mini-implants lost: The value of the implantation technique! *Dent. Press J. Orthod.* **2015**, *20*, 23–29. [CrossRef] [PubMed]
33. Chang, C.; Liu, S.S.; Roberts, W.E. Primary failure rate for 1680 extra-alveolar mandibular buccal shelf mini-screws placed in movable mucosa or attached gingiva. *Angle Orthod.* **2015**, *85*, 905–910. [CrossRef] [PubMed]
34. Arqub, S.A.; Gandhi, V.; Mehta, S.; Palo, L.; Upadhyay, M.; Yadav, S. Survival estimates and risk factors for failure of palatal and buccal mini-implants. *Angle Orthod.* **2021**, *91*, 756–763. [CrossRef]
35. Kakali, L.; Alharbi, M.; Pandis, N.; Gkantidis, N.; Kloukos, D. Success of palatal implants or mini-screws placed median or paramedian for the reinforcement of anchorage during orthodontic treatment: A systematic review. *Eur. J. Orthod.* **2019**, *41*, 9–20. [CrossRef]
36. Takaki, T.; Tamura, N.; Yamamoto, M.; Takano, N.; Shibahara, T.; Yasumura, T.; Nishii, Y.; Sueishi, K. Clinical study of temporary anchorage devices for orthodontic treatment–stability of micro/mini-screws and mini-plates: Experience with 455 cases. *Bull. Tokyo Dent. Coll.* **2010**, *51*, 151–163. [CrossRef]
37. Uribe, F.; Mehr, R.; Mathur, A.; Janakiraman, N.; Allareddy, V. Failure rates of mini-implants placed in the infrazygomatic region. *Prog. Orthod.* **2015**, *16*, 31. [CrossRef]
38. Liou, E.J.; Pai, B.C.; Lin, J.C. Do miniscrews remain stationary under orthodontic forces? *Am. J. Orthod. Dentofac. Orthop.* **2004**, *126*, 42–47. [CrossRef]
39. Manni, A.; Cozzani, M.; Tamborrino, F.; De Rinaldis, S.; Menini, A. Factors influencing the stability of miniscrews. A retrospective study on 300 miniscrews. *Eur. J. Orthod.* **2011**, *33*, 388–395. [CrossRef]
40. Lim, H.J.; Choi, Y.J.; Evans, C.A.; Hwang, H.S. Predictors of initial stability of orthodontic miniscrew implants. *Eur. J. Orthod.* **2011**, *33*, 528–532. [CrossRef]
41. Ramírez-Ossa, D.M.; Escobar-Correa, N.; Ramírez-Bustamante, M.A.; Agudelo-Suárez, A.A. An Umbrella Review of the Effectiveness of Temporary Anchorage Devices and the Factors That Contribute to Their Success or Failure. *J. Evid. Based Dent. Pract.* **2020**, *20*, 101402. [CrossRef] [PubMed]
42. Casaña-Ruiz, M.D.; Bellot-Arcís, C.; Paredes-Gallardo, V.; García-Sanz, V.; Almerich-Silla, J.M.; Montiel-Company, J.M. Risk factors for orthodontic mini-implants in skeletal anchorage biological stability: A systematic literature review and meta-analysis. *Sci. Rep.* **2020**, *10*, 5848. [CrossRef] [PubMed]
43. Bucur, S.-M.; Vaida, L.L.; Olteanu, C.D.; Checchi, V. A Brief Review on Micro-Implants and Their Use in Orthodontics and Dentofacial Orthopaedics. *Appl. Sci.* **2021**, *11*, 10719. [CrossRef]
44. Wilmes, B.; Rademacher, C.; Olthoff, G.; Drescher, D. Parameters affecting primary stability of orthodontic mini-implants. *J. Orofac. Orthop.* **2006**, *67*, 162–174. [CrossRef]

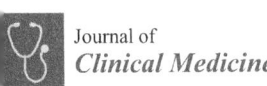

Skeletal, Dentoalveolar and Dental Changes after "Mini-Screw Assisted Rapid Palatal Expansion" Evaluated with Cone Beam Computed Tomography

Patricia Solano Mendoza *, Paula Aceytuno Poch, Enrique Solano Reina and Beatriz Solano Mendoza

Department of Orthodontics and Dentofacial Orthopedics, School of Dentistry, University of Seville, 41009 Sevilla, Spain
* Correspondence: patriciasolano83@hotmail.com

Abstract: The purpose of this study was to evaluate skeletal, dentoalveolar and dental changes after Mini-screw Assisted Rapid Palatal Expansion (MARPE) using tooth bone-borne expanders in adolescent patients after analyzing different craniofacial references by Cone beam computed tomography (CBCT) and digital model analysis. This prospective, non-controlled intervention study was conducted on fifteen subjects (mean age 17 ± 4 years) with transversal maxillary deficiency. Pre (T1) and post-expansion (T2) CBCTs and casts were taken to evaluate changes at the premolars and first molar areas. To compare means between two times, paired samples t- or Wilcoxon test were used following criteria. Significant *skeletal changes* were found after treatment for Nasal width and Maxillary width with means of 2.1 (1.1) mm and 2.5 (1.6) mm ($p < 0.00005$). Midpalatal suture showed a tendency of parallel suture opening in the axial and coronal view. For *dentoalveolar* changes, a significant but small buccal bone thickness (BBT) reduction was observed in all teeth with a mean reduction of 0.3 mm for the right and left sides, especially for the distobuccal root of the first molar on the left side (DBBTL1M) [IC95%: (−0.6; −0.2); $p = 0.001$] with 0.4 (0.4) mm. However, a significant augmentation was observed for the palatal bone thickness (PBT) on the left side. The buccal alveolar crest (BACL) and dental inclination (DI) showed no significant changes after treatment in all the evaluated teeth. MARPE using tooth bone-borne appliances can achieve successful skeletal transverse maxillary expansion in adolescent patients, observing small dentoalveolar changes as buccal bone thickness (BBT) reduction, which was not clinically detectable. Most maxillary expansions derived from skeletal expansion, keeping the alveolar bone almost intact with minor buccal dental tipping.

Keywords: micro implant-assisted rapid palatal expansion; maxillary transverse deficiency; Cone-beam computed tomography; alveolar bone; midpalatal suture; skeletal expansion; palatal expansion

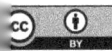

1. Introduction

Transversal maxillary deficiency (TMD) is a quite common condition that affects between 8–23% of deciduous and mixed dentitions. However, a lower prevalence has been reported in adult orthodontic patients [1–4]. This transverse deficiency [5], or maxillary hypoplasia [6], is one of the main problems related to facial growth that should be corrected as it is diagnosed, with the objective to reestablish a normal transverse skeletal relationship between maxillary and mandibular basal bones to obtain a stable occlusion [7].

Its etiology is multifactorial, frequently influenced by myofunctional disorders of the stomatognathic system and generally associated with oral breathing or deleterious habits such as thumb sucking [4,8,9]. Genetic and hereditary factors are also related, thus determining the development of maxillary transverse deficiencies. These factors promote structural changes in the maxilla which will generally lead to posterior crossbite (bilateral or unilateral), constriction of the nasal cavity and frequent dental crowding [8,10].

Traditionally, orthopedic rapid maxillary expansion (RME) has been performed to correct this matter during patient's growing period showing positive results with a better prognosis and treatment outcomes at early ages [5,11–14], producing a greater orthopedic effect in the deciduous and mixed dentition. As the patient grows, progressive calcification and craniofacial sutures interdigitation occur, including midpalatal suture closure. Consequently, skeletal expansion becomes a more difficult process due to increased mechanical resistance [15,16]. Limited skeletal orthopedic changes have been described after RME with the use of tooth-borne expanders observing undesirable side effects such as dental tipping, buccal bone thickness reduction, bone dehiscence and gingival recession in anchor teeth [17–22], limiting this treatment option to incomplete skeletal mature patients confirming the importance of early skeletal age treatment [23].

Skeletal support with the use of screws by means of mini-screw assisted rapid palatal expansion (MARPE) allows for a better distribution of applied forces when the palatal suture closure is incomplete, thus achieving a greater skeletal effect (orthopedic) by opening the mid-palatal suture and minimizing secondary effects derived from dentoalveolar (orthodontic) effects [24]. Cone-beam computed tomography (CBCT) images have revealed a significant increase in the skeletal dimension in adolescent and young adult patients treated with MARPE [25], reducing the aforementioned side effects when the intermaxillary suture is not completely closed [26–29], and, therefore, considering MARPE as a proper treatment option for correcting maxillary transversal discrepancies (MTD) [30–32] with potential skeletal effect [33,34]. Studies show conflicting results regarding the orthopedic effect MARPE and RME in young adult patients with different types of appliances [35].

Specifically, tooth bone-borne expanders with palatal minis crews and first molar anchorage have shown effective and positive results for maxillary expansion [33,36,37] with no risk of periodontal damage.

As studies using computed tomography (CT) report, buccal alveolar bone thinning after RME in anchored teeth [20,38], the use of CBCT seems to be fundamental, contributing to a more complete diagnosis of the transverse dimension [29,39] providing accurate tridimensional treatment outcomes evaluations of the maxillofacial complex and their dentoalveolar response.

This was the main reason that led us to hypothesize that MARPE using tooth bone-borne expanders could be a safe and effective treatment to correct maxillary transversal discrepancies in adolescent patients with incomplete ossification of the maxillary palatal suture achieving higher predictable skeletal effects with reduced dentoalveolar and dental effects

The purpose of this study is to evaluate skeletal, dentoalveolar and dental changes after MARPE using tooth bone-borne expanders in patients with incomplete maxillary palatal suture closure analyzing different craniofacial references by CBCT and digital model analysis in order to quantify maxillary transverse changes at the three levels after expansion treatment. Moreover, we tried to show the quantity of skeletal, alveolar and dental responses to treatment and compare these findings with those that are reported in the literature.

2. Material and Methods

This prospective, non-controlled intervention study was conducted on patients who needed maxillary expansion. Patients were recruited from three different centers in the same city, Seville (Spain): The Department of Orthodontics of the School Dentistry of the University of Seville, a private dental clinic (COINSOL) and a dental training institute IDEO All subjects met the following inclusion criteria: (1) presence of transverse skeletal maxillary deficiency with or without the presence of posterior crossbite as described by Tamburino et al. [40,41], (2) incomplete radiographic ossification of the midpalatal suture according to Angelieri's classification [42], (3) not having received previous orthodontic treatment, (4) presence of first and seconds upper premolars and first upper molars, (5) absence of any craniofacial irregularities, (6) and any bone defects, or systemic and periodontal disease, (7) not being pregnant (8) and having reached prepubertal development with less than 25 years of age. Palatal suture ossification was evaluated following this classification, categorizing the palatal maturation in five stages (A–E) through its CBCT analysis in an axial view. Patients who did not meet the inclusion criteria and those with a portion of the suture where the fusion had occurred (stage E in accordance with Angelieri's classification) and with no low-density spaces along the suture were excluded. Incomplete ossification of mid palatal suture was blindly evaluated in the initial CBCT (CbctT1) to confirm that the patient could be included in the study.

All subjects gave their informed consent before taking part in the study. This study was conducted in accordance with the Declaration of Helsinki, and the protocol was approved by the Ethics Committee of Vírgen Macarena-Virgen del Rocío University Hospitals in Seville (238e1b02c492fe6c37e2e9cf37c737297f4cf746).

An initial sample of 19 patients meeting the established inclusion criteria were selected. Four patients were not included in the analysis: two patients due to incomplete radiographic registers, one patient used other orthodontic appliance at the same time and one patient had a different screw positioning. The final sample consisted of 15 patients between 13 and 24 years of age (mean age: 17.0 ± 4.0), with transverse maxillary skeletal compression (mean:5.4 ± 2.1 mm) who completed maxillary expansion (Table 1).

Table 1. Sample age and maxillary compression distribution. Appliance's activation time. Age (years), Maxillar compression (mm), Appliance activation time (days).

	N	Min	Max	Mean Difference (SD)	IC 95% Mean	Median	Median (P_{25};P_{75})	IC95% Median
Age	15	13.0	24.0	17.0 (4.0)	15.0;19.0	16.0	(14.0;20.0)	16.0; 21.0
Maxillary compression	15	2.5	8.7	5.4 (2.1)	4.2; 6.5	5.1	(3.7;7.5)	3.8; 7.5
Appliance activation time	15	10.0	35.0	22.0 (8.0)	17.0; 26.0	20.0	(15.0;30.0)	15.0; 30.0

2.1. Methodology

Patients were treated by MARPE with a tooth-bone born expander using the MSE (maxillary skeletal expander designed by Dr. Moon from the University of UCLA) adapted to individual maxillary expansion requirements [43,44]. Four stainless steel arms of 1.5 mm in diameter emerged from a central main screw: two anterior arms extended symmetrically towards the palatal aspect of the first upper premolars near the most cervical part of the tooth (without support), and two posterior arms extended the palatal aspect of the first molars, which remained fixed to the bands placed on the first molars. A 0.7 mm thick steel lateral arm was connected to the expander's front arms (Figure 1).

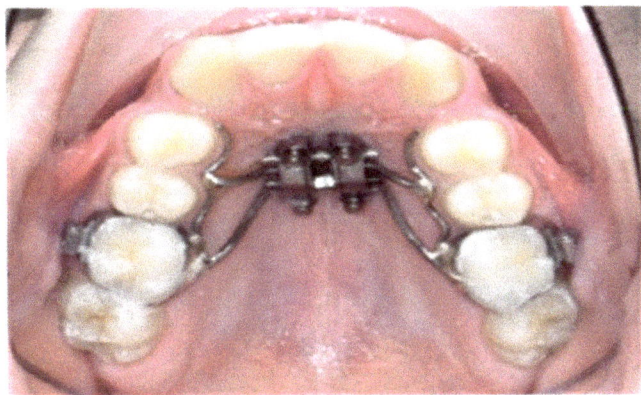

Figure 1. Tooth-bone-borne expander appliance.

Every device was adapted individually for each patient in the same laboratory through an initial impression with the bands positioned on the upper first molars.

The central screw expander had four holes of 1.8 mm in diameter for the retention and insertion of each mini screw of 1.74 mm in diameter and 9, 11 and 13 mm in length which were used for bone anchoring. Anterior and posterior mini-screws were positioned at the level the first premolar and the first molar, respectively (BMK micro-screws model ACR of Medical Resources). To ensure a bicortical anchorage, palatal gingiva thickness, bone height and distance between the expander and palatal gingiva were considered [45]. The central screw expander length was selected based on the patient's maxillary expansion needs to correct the transversal deficiency (8, 10 or 12 mm). The maxillary compression or maxillary transversal deficiency was calculated considering the difference between the mandibular and maxillary widths determined by the arch relationship according to Cantarella 2017 [44]. Expander placement and the first activation were performed in the same appointment, following the describe protocol suggested by Bruneto [8] according to patients age. The expander was activated by 1 turn per day (0.26 mm/turn) with subsequent biweekly visits until full expansion was achieved [8]. The total maxillary expansion was completed when the palatal cusp tips of the maxillary first molars were in contact with the corresponding buccal cusp tips of the mandibular first molars.

The same experienced examiner was present in the 3 centers (BSM) for the recruitment of patients enrolled in the study, confirming incomplete ossification of midpalatal suture and supervised successive visits until the expansion was completed, from February 2020 to December 2022 [46,47]. Radiographic CBCT (Cbct) and cast (Model) recordings were collected at two times: T1 (prior to expander placement) and T2 (immediately after maxillary expansion had been completed). The expander was removed before CbctT2 and ModelT2 to prevent image distortions, and immediately placed back without miniscrews, blocking it with ligature leaving the expansion device for a 6-month retention period. The patient's skeletal maturation was assessed via the cervical vertebral maturation index (CVM) in the initial teleradiograph (CbctT1) in accordance with Bacetti's classification and stratified in 6 stages from CVM I-VI [48,49] base of the presence or absence of concavity in the lower border of the body of C2, C3 and C4 and the body shape of C3 and C4.

Once the treatment was completed, all measurements were performed by two blinded, calibrated examiners. Radiographic measurements (PSM) and digital cast measurements (PAP) were performed, evaluating intraexaminer reproducibility. Skeletal and sutural maturation were assessed (PSM) from CbctT1 in accordance with the previously describe classifications [42,48,49]. Intraexaminer reproducibility was analyzed by using randomly selected patients. In order to assure a reliable reproducibility and blindness, each patient was assigned a unique code and measurements were recorded twice and spaced 1 week apart.

Stone casts were digitally scanned with Itero® Element 2 Scanner (Tel Aviv-Yafo, Israel) and analyzed for measurements with OrthoCAD® software (OrthoCAD iCast Orthodontic 3D Digital Modeling Study of Align Technology, Inc., IL, USA) to evaluate changes at the following levels: first and second premolar and first molar (1PM, 2PM, 1M): (1) *Palatal Gingival Width* (PGW): distance from the palatal gingival margin of the tooth of interest to its contralateral, (2) *Palatal Cusp Width* (PCW): distance from the palatal cusp of the tooth of interest to its contralateral, (3) right and left *Clinical Coronal Height* (CCH) to evaluate gingival margin position changes: distance from the center of the gingival margin to the buccal cusp for the premolars and to the center of the crown in the buccal aspect for the first molar.

CBCT scan images were obtained with i-CAT® Kavo 1723 flat panel model for IDEO and COINSOL patients, and with Planmeca Promax® 3D Sirona (Finlandia, Helsinki) for Dental School patients. For i-CAT® Kavo: 37 mA, 120 kV and 26 s scan time were set for T1 and T2. Voxel size of 0.2 mm. for both exposure times and a field of view of 16 × 13 cm FOV (cervical included). PlanMeca Promax 3D from Sirona system used same parameters for two evaluation periods T1 and T2, being: 14 mA, 90 KV, with a 12 s exposure time, 0.2 Vox and 8 × 8 FOV. Anatomage in Vivo 5,3. i-CAT® Kavo software was used to perform all radiographic measurements with a 1:1 scale, slice thickness 0.5 mm. All CBCT volume images were reoriented prior to radiographic measurements considering three-dimensional reference planes for craniofacial structures orientation and to standardize linear measurements in the sagittal section (y-plan), axial section (x-plane) and coronal section (z-plan):

a. Radiographs orientation: In the axial section (x-plane), the mid-palatine suture was used. In the midsagittal section (y-plane), the horizontal palatal plane was the selected reference, considering the anterior and posterior nasal spine. In the coronal section (z-plane), the image was oriented perpendicular to the patient's midsagittal plane tangent to the most inferior level of nasal floor [50].

b. Cuts standardization: Points were established in the coronal, axial and sagittal plane at selected teeth: first and second premolars and first molar (1 PM, 2 PM, 1 M) in line with previous validated cut Standardization and radiographic measurement method described by Podesser [50] on CT, and by Christie [51] and Toklu [29] on CBCT.

- In the coronal plane: For the first premolar and the first molar: cuts were made at the most anterior section where the crown and palatal root can be seen at their greatest length. For the second premolar: in the most anterior section showing maximum length of its root (Figure 2).

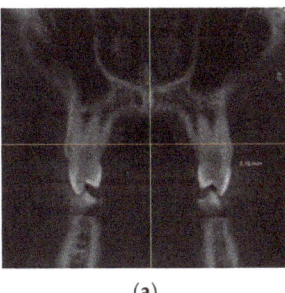
(a)

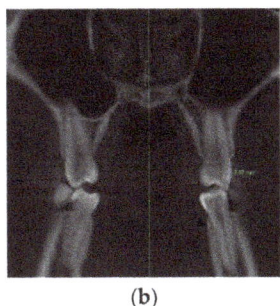
(b)

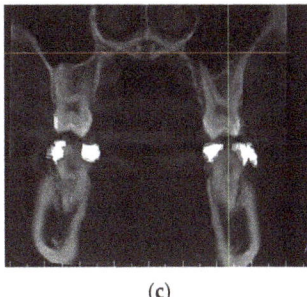
(c)

Figure 2. Selected cut-off points in the coronal plane at: (**a**) first premolar, (**b**) second premolar and (**c**) first molar.

- In the axial plane: at the level of the right and left first molar trifurcation for each side (Figure 3). (Maxillary right first molar furcation for the right posterior teeth and the maxillary left first molar furcation for the left posterior teeth) According to Toklu [29].

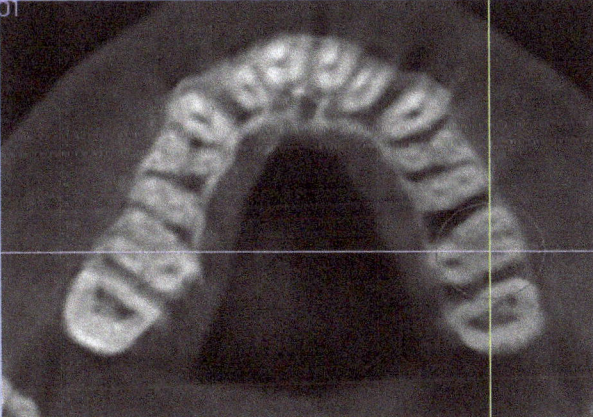

Figure 3. Cut in the axial plane for buccal and palatal bone thickness (BBT and PBT) measurements.

Radiographic changes were evaluated at selected teeth for the following variables: (1) **Skeletal changes**: *Nasal width, maxillary width, palatal suture opening, sutural expansion,* *nasal floor, palatal floor*, (2) **Dentoalveolar changes**: *buccal maxillary width and palatal maxillary width*, on left (L) and right (R) side of the upper arch: *buccal bone thickness, palatal bone thickness* and *buccal alveolar bone crest Level*, (3) **Dental changes**: *dental inclination* (Table 2).

Table 2. Description of radiographic CBCT measurements performed with In vivo software program. Standardized coronal and axial sections for radiographic measurements of first and second premolars and first molars.

Nasal width (NW)	Distance between right and left most lateral point of the nasal cavity in the coronal section at the level of first molar where total length of palatal root and crown are visualized.	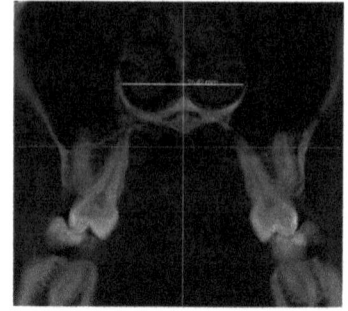
Maxillary width (MW)	Distance between the lowest point of lateral right and left contour concavities of the maxillary bone, on a coronal section, at the level of first molar where total length of palatal root and crown are visualized.	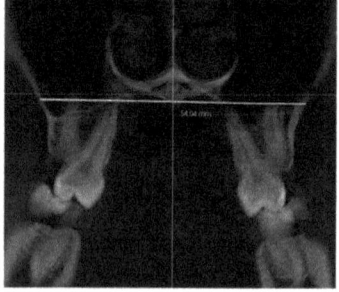
Palatal suture opening (SO)	Distance between the external right and left maxilla edges in the axial view generating a slice in the horizontal plane, allowing a good visualization of the midpalatal suture at first and second premolar, and first molar. The edges were identified with a small point on an axial cross-sectional slice at the level of the first molar trifurcation.	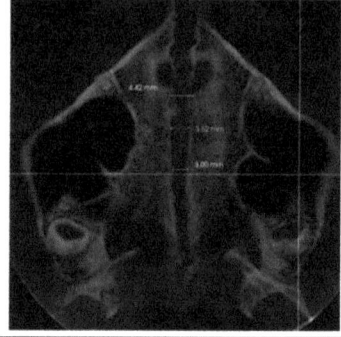

Table 2. Cont.

Buccal maxillary width (BMW)	Distance between right and left most prominent point of the buccal bone crest in first and second premolar, and first molar, in the first anterior coronal cut described for each tooth.	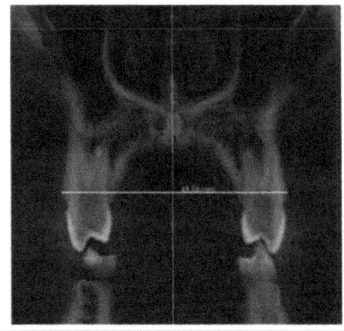
Palatal maxillary width (PMW)	Distance between right and left most prominent point of palatal bone crest in first and second premolar, and first molar, in the first anterior coronal slice as describe for each tooth. At the level of the buccal maxillary width.	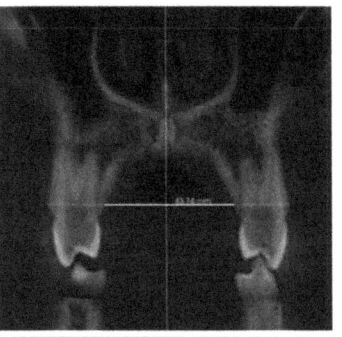
Buccal bone thickness (BBT)	Distance from the external border of the buccal cortical plate to the center of buccal aspect of first and second premolar root, and from the external border of buccal cortical plate to the center of the messiobuccal and distobuccal root of first molar, in an axial section parallel to the palatal plane, at the level of the first molar right (R) and left (L) trifurcation for each side.	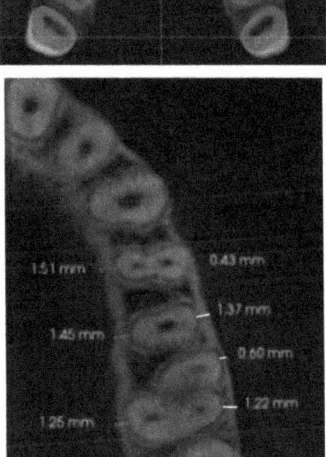

Table 2. *Cont.*

Palatal bone thickness (PBT)	Distance from the external border of palatal cortical plate to the center of palatal aspect of first and second premolar root, and first molar palatal root, in an axial section parallel to palatal plane, at the level of the first molar right (R) and left (L) trifurcation for each side.	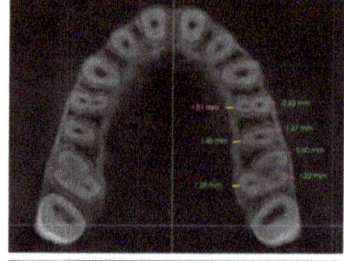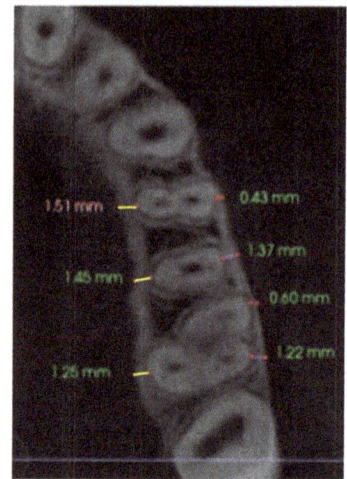
Buccal alveolar bone crest level (BACL)	Distance from the tip of buccal cusp to the buccal bone crest of first and second premolar, and from the mesiobuccal cusp of first molar crown, to the buccal bone crest in the first anterior coronal cut describe for each tooth, on the right (R) and left (L) side.	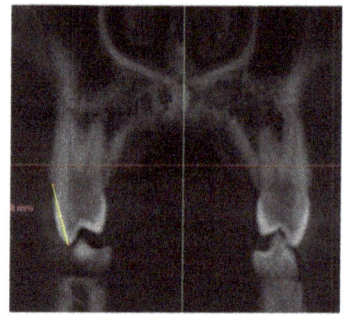
Dental inclination (INCL)	Angle formed by the intersection of two tangents that passed through the buccal and palatal cusps of the first and second premolars of both contralateral teeth, and through the messiobuccal and palatal cusp of the first molar, in the coronal section.	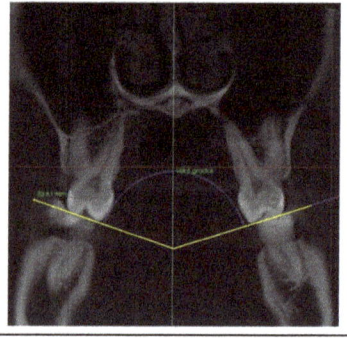

Midpalatal suture expansion was also assessed in the coronal view, measured in the middle of the palate as sutural expansion (SEM), and at the level of *nasal and palatal floor* on a coronal cross-sectional slice through the center of the first molar, by connecting the right and left external edges of the suture according to the previous method used by Ngan [34]. (Table 3). The suture external edges were verified in the axial cross-sectional slice for each tested position.

Table 3. Evaluation of the suture opening pattern in the coronal section and midpalatal suture expansion at the nasal and palatal floor levels.

Nasal Floor (NF)	Distance from right and left external edges of the palatine suture at the level of the nasal floor in the coronal view. On a coronal cross-sectional slice through the center of the first molar. The suture external edges were verified in the axial cross-sectional slice.	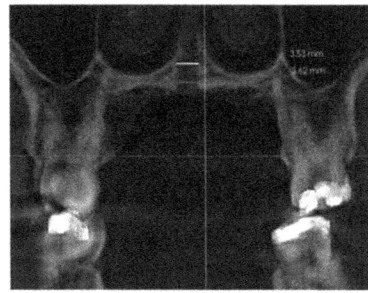
Palatal Floor (PF)	Distance from right and left external edges of the palatine suture at the level of the palatal floor. On a coronal cross-sectional slice through the center of the first molar. The suture external edges were verified in the axial cross-sectional slice.	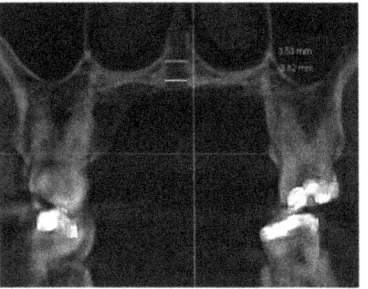

The skeletal expansion was calculated by the radiographic analysis of: *Sutural expansion* (SEM), *intermolar width* (IMW), and *palatal maxillary width* (PMW) in compliance with the method proposed by Ngan et al. 2018 [34] (Table 4).

Total expansion (TE) included the skeletal (separation of two maxillary halves at the midpalatal suture) and dentoalveolar expansion (alveolar bone bending and dental tipping). A mathematical equation was used to calculate the skeletal and dentoalveolar components of the Total expansion: TE = Skeletal (orthopedic) expansion: Midpalatal sutural separation + dentoalveolar (orthodontic) expansion (alveolar bone bending + dental tipping). Total expansion was defined as the change between the two time periods (T2–T1) in (1) *Intermolar width*, distance between the palatal cusp tip of the right and left first molars measured in a coronal cross-sectional slice through the midportion of the first molar. (2) *Sutural expansion* in the middle of the palate on the same coronal cross-sectional slice and (3) *palatal maxillary width*, measured at the first molar's furcation on the same coronal cross-sectional slice (Table 4). From the dentoalveolar expansion: Alveolar bone bending, and dental inclination were also determined for each patient. Alveolar bone bending was defined as any additional palatal alveolar expansion achieved apart from the sutural separation and was calculated by subtracting *Sutural Expansion* (SEM) from the change (T2–T1) in *palatal maxillary width* (PMW). Dental inclination was computed by subtracting *sutural expansion* and the calculated alveolar bone bending from total expansion [34].

Table 4. Radiographic CBCT measurements to quantify skeletal, dentoalveolar and dental expansion Sutural expansion, intermolar width and palatal maxillary width (SEM, IMW and PMW) were measured at first molar and quantified on the same coronal cross-sectional slice.

Sutural expansion (SEM)	The sutural expansion in the middle of the palate. Distance between the left and right external border of the palatal aspect of the maxilla, in the middle of the palate between the palatine bone and the nasal floor, on a coronal cross-sectional slice at first molar. Through the midportion of the first molar.	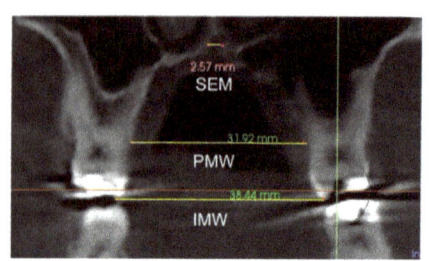
Intermolar width (IMW)	Distance between right and left tip of palatal cusp of first molars in a coronal cross-sectional slice through the midportion of first molar.	
Palatal maxillary width (PMW)	Distance between the right and left external border of the palatal maxillary bone, on a coronal cross-sectional slice at first molar. Through the midportion of the first molar.	

2.2. Statistical Analysis

The statistical analyses were performed with the Statistical Package, using SPSS 26.0 software for Windows (SPSS Inc. Chicago, IL, USA). For quantitative variables, those that presented a symmetric distribution, were presented as means and standard deviation (SD) and those that presented a very asymmetric distribution, as median and interquartile range (P_{25}, P_{75}) and frequency and percentages for the categorical variables. The 95% CIs have been calculated for all the statistics obtained. To assess changes after MARPE maxillary expansion at two evaluation moments, the *Student's t-test* was performed for paired data once the randomness and normality requirements had been confirmed. In cases of not meeting the normality requirement (*Shapiro–Wilks test*), the non-parametric test (*Wilcoxon test*) was applied. To compare the means between two independent groups, the *Student's t-test* was performed for independent data once the requirements of randomness normality (*Shapiro Wilks test*) and equality of variance (*Levene's t*) had been confirmed. If said requirements were not met, the *Student's t-test* was performed for independent data with *Welch's* correction. If the normality requirements were not met, a non-parametric test (*Mann–Whitney U*) was applied. Significance of the results was evaluated at the level of alpha < 0.05.

Based on the observed effect sizes, experimental statistical power analyses were conducted to determine the power of the study. The sample size was calculated to detect any clinically relevant differences in the reduction in buccal wall thickness of 0.5 mm after expansion [20,29]. Being the standard deviation of the differences 0.62, considering an alpha error of 0.05 and a power of 85%, the minimum number of subjects to be included in the study was 14 patients. ICCs assessment for intraexaminer reproducibility ranged between 0.85 and 0.98 for radiographic and cast measurement showing an important level of repeatability for all measurements.

3. Results

ICC were greater than 0.90 for most of the variables and greater than 0.83 for the second left premolar's clinical crown height, the first premolar's palatal maxillary width, the first premolar's suture opening, the second right premolar's buccal bone thickness, the first left molar's buccal bone thickness and the second left premolar's buccal bone thickness.

The initial maxillary transversal deficiency ranged from 2.5 to 8.7 mm with a mean of 5.4 (2.1) mm. The mean amount of screw expansion was 6.8 mm (1.8), ranging from 3.4 mm to 9.4 mm, with a mean of 22 (8.0) days, 95% CI: (17.0, 26.0). Sutural stage maturation evaluation according to Angelieri's classification [42] confirming all sutures were not completely ossified before maxillary expansion: 86.7% [95% CI: (86.7; 93.3) of the sample (n = 13) presented midpalatal suture stages type C and 6.7% (n = 1) stage type B and D

Regarding skeletal maturation (CVM) according to Baccetti [48,49], most patients presented stages IV and V with a distribution of 46.7% (n = 7) and 40% (n = 6), respectively, and 13.3% stage III (Table 5).

Table 5. Sample sex, cross bite, skeletal maturation and palatal sutural stage distribution.

		N Number (%)	95% CI
Sex	Male	3 (20)	6.0; 44.4
	Female	12 (80)	55.6; 94.0
Cross Bite	Absence	3 (20)	6.0; 44.4
	Bilateral	12 (80)	56.6; 94.0
Skeletal maturation	Stage I	0 (0)	0.0; 21.8
	Stage II	0 (0)	0.0; 21.8
	Stage III	2 (13.3)	2.9; 36.3
	Stage IV	7 (46.7)	23.9; 70.6
	Stage V	6 (40.0)	18.8; 64.7
	Stage VI	0 (0)	0.0; 21.8
Palatal Sutural Stage	Stage A	0 (0)	0.0; 21.8
	Stage B	1 (6.7)	0.7; 27.2
	Stage C	13 (86.7)	63.7; 97.1
	Stage D	1 (6.7)	0.7; 27.2
	Stage E	0 (0)	0.0; 21.8

3.1. Radiographic Measurements

CBCTs performed at the two evaluation times were needed to analyzed all evaluated parameters and existing changes after treatment at the skeletal, dentoalveolar and dental level.

Skeletal changes: The midpalatal suture was successfully opened showing a significant change in all patients. Suture opening (SO) in the axial view expressed a similar quantity at the premolar and molar areas, with a mean of 3.3 (1.3) mm for the first premolars, 2.9 (1.4) mm for the second premolars and 2.6 (1.3) mm for the first molars, showing a gradual opening tendency from the anterior to the posterior part with no statistically significant differences between teeth along the length of the midpalatal suture (Table 6).

Midpalatal suture expansion assessed on the coronal view showed a statistically significant change ($p < 0.000$) at the Nasal and Palatal Floor levels after maxillary expansion, not showing statistically significant differences between them.

Dentoalveolar changes: Statistically significant differences were found after maxillary expansion for buccal and palatal maxillary width in all analyzed teeth. Regarding buccal bone thickness (BBT), once the maxillary expansion was completed, all locations showed similar significant changes with a mean reduction of −0.3 mm for both sides (Table 7). Although these values show statistically significant differences, they are not clinically relevant. In the palatal aspect, bone thickness (PBT) only showed significant changes on the left side, on the first premolar and the molar, respectively. The buccal alveolar crest remained with hardly any changes, not being significant at any locations.

Table 6. Comparison of Pre and Posttreatment Skeletal measurements. Skeletal changes comparing CbcT1-CbcT2 measurements. BMW: Buccal maxillary width. PMW: Palatal maxillary width. NW: Nasal width. MW: Maxillary width. SO: suture opening. 1PM: first premolar; 2PM: second premolar and M1: first molar.

T1–T2	N	Min	Max	Mean Difference (SD) mm	IC95% Mean	Median (mm)	Median (P_{25}; P_{75})	IC95% Median	p-Value
NW	15	0.4	4.6	2.1 (1.1)	1.5; 2.7	2.3	1.1; 2.7	1.3; 2.7	0.00005
MW	15	0.4	6.2	2.5 (1.6)	1.6; 3.4	2.1	1.3; 3.8	1.9; 3.8	0.00005
SO1PM	15	1.7	6.0	3.3 (1.3)	2.5; 4.0	2.7	2.4; 4.4	2.4; 4.4	0.00005
SO2PM	15	1.2	6.0	2.9 (1.4)	2.1; 3.6	2.4	1.6; 3.8	1.7; 3.8	0.00005
SO1M	15	1.0	6.0	2.6 (1.3)	1.9; 3.3	2.2	1.8; 3.4	1.8; 3.4	0.00005
NF	15	1.1	4.7	2.4 (1.0)	1.9; 3.0	2.4	1.7; 3.1	1.7; 3.1	0.000
PF	15	1.0	4.5	2.4 (1.0)	1.8; 3.0	2.6	1.6; 3.2	1.8; 3.6	0.000
SEM	15	0.7	4.7	2.7 (1.0)	2.1; 3.1	2.6	1.9; 3.3	2.2; 3.3	0.000

Table 7. Comparison of Pre and Post treatment Dentoalveolar measurements. Dentoalveolar changes comparing CbctT1-CbctT2 measurements. BBT: buccal bone thickness. MB: messiobuccal root of first molar. DB: distobuccal root of first molar. R: right side. L: left side. PBT: Ppalatal bone thickness. BACL: bone alveolar crest level. 1PM: first premolar; 2PM: second premolar and M1: first molar.

T1–T2	N	Min	Max	Mean difference (SD) mm	IC95% Mean	Median (mm)	Median (P_{25};P_{75})	IC95% Median	p-Value
BMW1PM	15	0.6	7.8	3.7 (2.0)	2.6; 4.8	3.5	2.1; 5.0	2.2; 5.0	0.00005
BMW2PM	15	0.8	14.8	4.1 (3.6)	2.1; 6.1	2.6	2.2; 4.3	2.4; 4.3	0.001
BMW1M	15	1.1	9.7	3.7 (2.1)	2.6; 4.9	3.3	2.6; 4.0	3.1; 4.0	0.001
PMW1PM	15	1.0	8.4	3.7 (1.8)	2.7; 4.7	3.4	2.6; 4.8	2.9; 4.8	0.00005
PMW2PM	15	1.6	7.8	3.2 (1.6)	2.3; 4.1	3.0	2.2; 3.6	2.8; 4.4	0.001
PMW1M	15	−5.6	7.2	2.2 (2.6)	0.7; 3.6	2.3	1.7; 3.0	1.8; 3.0	0.009
BBTR1PM	15	−1.0	0.0	−0.3 (0.3)	−0.4; −0.1	−0.2	−0.4; 0.0	−0.2; −0.0	0.003
BBTR2PM	15	−0.4	0.3	−0.1 (0.2)	−0.2; −0.0	−0.2	−0.2; −0.0	−0.2; −0.0	0.013
MBBTR1M	15	−0.9	0.0	−0.3 (0.3)	−0.5; −0.2	−0.2	−0.6; −0.1	−0.3; −0.1	0.001
DBBTR1M	15	−0.9	0.0	−0.3 (0.3)	−0.5; −0.2	−0.3	−0.5; −0.2	−0.4; −0.2	0.00005
BBTL1PM	15	−1.3	−0.2	−0.3 (0.4)	−0.6; −0.1	−0.2	−0.5; −0.1	−0.5; −0.1	0.004
BBTL2PM	15	−0.6	0.0	−0.3 (0.2)	−0.3; −0.1	−0.3	−0.4; −0.1	−0.3; −0.1	0.00005
MBBTL1M	15	−1.1	0.0	−0.4 (0.4)	−0.6; −0.2	−0.3	−0.7; 0.0	−0.6; 0.0	0.003
DBBTL1M	15	−1.5	0.0	−0.4 (0.4)	−0.6; −0.2	−0.3	−0.7; −0.1	−0.5; −0.1	0.001
PBTR1PM	15	−1.8	1.1	0.1 (0.7)	−0.3; 0.5	0.2	−0.3; −0.4	−0.0; 0.4	0.552
PBTR2PM	15	−0.7	0.8	0.2 (0.4)	−0.4; 0.5	0.3	0.0; 0.4	0.0; 0.4	0.09
PBTR1M	15	−0.2	0.9	0.1 (0.3)	−0.0; 0.3	0.0	0.0; 0.3	0.0; 0.3	0.073
PBTL1PM	15	−0.4	0.6	0.2 (0.2)	0.0; 0.3	0.2	0.1; 0.3	0.1; 0.3	0.013
PBTL2PM	15	−0.3	0.5	0.1 (0.2)	0.0; 0.3	0.2	0.1; 0.3	0.1; 0.3	0.012
PBTL1M	15	−0.1	0.5	0.2 (0.2)	0.1; 0.3	0.1	0.0; 0.4	0.1; 0.4	0.003
BACLR1PM	15	−2.3	0.7	−0.1 (0.7)	−0.5; 0.3	0.0	−0.2; 0.2	0.0; 0.3	0.448
BACLR2PM	15	−1.1	0.5	−0.1 (0.5)	−0.4; 0.2	0.0	−0.4; 0.2	−0.1; 0.2	0.420
BACLR1M	15	−2.2	1.0	−0.0 (0.8)	−0.5; 0.5	0.2	−0.6; 0.6	−0.2; 0.6	0.493
BACLL1PM	15	−1.2	0.3	−0.2 (0.4)	−0.4; 0.0	0.0	−0.2; 0.1	−0.0; 0.1	0.012
BACLL2PM	15	−1.6	0.7	−0.2 (0.5)	−0.5; 0.1	−0.1	−0.6; 0.1	−0.5; 0.1	0.145
BACLL1M	15	−0.4	1.5	0.2 (0.6)	−0.1; 0.5	0.1	−0.1; 0.4	−0.1; 0.4	0.144

Dental changes: Dental inclination did not show significant variation after treatment being minimal on all the evaluated teeth. The reduction in the measured angle shows a tendency to positive tipping, slightly increasing from the first molar to the first premolar (Table 8).

Table 8. Comparison of Pre and Post treatment Dental inclination measurements. Dental inclination changes after maxillary expansion comparing CbctT1-CbctT2 measurements. INCL: inclination. 1PM: first premolar; 2PM: second premolar and M1: first molar.

T1–T2	N	Min	Max	Mean Difference (SD) mm	IC 95% Mean	Median mm	Median (P$_{25}$;P$_{75}$)	IC95% Median	p-Value
INCL1PM	15	−33.6	22.4	−1.6 (15.9)	−10.4; 7.3	−0.2	−13.2; 8.6	−2.0; 8.6	0.71
INCL2PM	15	−22.5	32.3	−2.0 (15.6)	−10.6; 6.7	−5.7	−14.0; 6.0	−12.9; 6.0	0.62
INCL1M	15	−15.3	21.7	−3.3 (9.4)	−8.5; 1.9	−3.7	−10.0; −1.3	−8.0; −1.3	0.200

3.2. Cast Measurements

Palatal gingival widths and palatal cusp widths showed significant changes in all the teeth after MARPE. Regarding the height of the clinical crown (CCH), significant minor changes were observed only on the left side, with a mean change of 0.2 (0.2) mm, 0.1 (0.2) mm and 0.1 (0.1) mm for premolars and the first molar, respectively. However, none of these small increases were clinically noticeable.

A total expansion of 4.5 (1.8) mm was obtained after MARPE, defined as the change in the IMW for the first molar. Greater expansion amount (2.7 (1.0) mm) corresponds to skeletal component and a lower proportion (1.8 (1.7) mm) to dentoalveolar expansion, both changes being statistically significant. Significant changes were observed for IMW, PMW and SEM. From the dentoalveolar expansion, the alveolar bone bending effect and the dental inclination showed reduced mean values of 0.7 (1.6) mm and 1.1 (1.3) mm, respectively. The amount of skeletal expansion achieved within the total expansion was 60 %, determined by mid-palatal suture expansion [2.7 (1.0) mm] in the center of the palate at the first's molar level, meaning 40% remaining corresponds to the dentoalveolar component (1.8 mm). Flexion of the alveolar bone accounted for 15,5% of TE. The remaining fraction of TE in the first molar resulted from dental inclination was 24.4%.

4. Discussion

It is generally accepted that chronological age is not a precise parameter to base the skeletal maturation diagnosis [32] due to the high variability of midpalatal suture development stages during a patients' life [52]. Skeletal effects derived from maxillary expansion have been observed to be greater in young patients, at the prepubertal stages, while pubertal or post pubertal stages can have greater dentoalveolar effects [49]. However, approximately 11% of adult population still present a pubertal stage 4 CVM. This percentage is not high, but it should be considered relevant from a clinical standpoint [53].

Garrett found similar values to our study for alveolar bending after RME with the use of tooth-borne expanders observing a 13% (0.84 mm) of alveolar bone bending, but higher dental tipping effect of 39% at the premolar (2.34 mm) and 49% (3.27 mm) at the first molar from the total expansion achieved in patients with a mean age of 13.8 years [54]. These data show a trend of decreasing orthopedic skeletal effect, increasing alveolar bending and orthodontic tipping from anterior to posterior in line with previous reports [55,56]. Compared to bone-borne maxillary expanders, tooth-born expanders showed as twice as large alveolar bone bending effect [57].

4.1. Skeletal Changes

In our study, a total expansion of 4.5 (1.8) mm was achieved after MARPE, defined as the change between the intermolar width at the level of the first molar (IMW). This change was slightly lower compared to other report values [34], but in line with other study [33]. This may be due to the fact that no overcorrection was performed, but enough to correct transversal discrepancy. Buccal and palatal maxillary width showed a significant increase in all the teeth, confirming earlier studies' results. Significant nasal and maxillary width changes were seen, thus explaining a disjunction effect in the nasal cavity as some studies show [13–15].

The highest proportion of the enhanced total expansion, corresponds to skeletal expansion (60%), determined by mean midpalatal suture expansion (SEM) measured in the middle of the palate at first molar level (2.7 (1.0) mm), coincident with other studies using the same measurements method and type of expander (2.55 ± 0.71 mm) [34] over skeletally mature patients (CVM 4) [49] similar to our sample. Ngan et al. [34] reports a 41% of skeletal expansion (SE), with a 2.55 ± 0.71 mm of midpalatal suture expansion (SEM), and a total expansion (TE) of 6.26 ± 1.31 mm, which means that proportionally we have enhanced a higher percentage of skeletal expansion considering that most of our patients where categorized as skeletally mature (stage IV, and V) [49] with a mean age of 17.1 ± 3.5 years. MARPE clinical efficacy and stability performed in young subjects (between 19 and 26 years) report success rates of 86.96%, maintaining achieved skeletal and dentoalveolar changes after disjunction, as well as periodontal structures solidity during retention period [31].

Regarding suture opening, the available literature reports a marked suture opening pattern [44] describing a tendency to result in a pyramidal pattern in the vertical aspect According to some studies, the triangular suture opening pattern presents the apex in the nasal area and the base in the dental cusps, regardless of the mechanism used [26,37,58] Lim et al. support MARPE is not only limited to the maxilla, involving also circummaxillary structures [25]. Studies using tooth-borne expanders tend to describe a triangular pattern on the sagittal view for suture opening, wider at the base of anterior maxillar portion [54,57,59] whereas a more parallel pattern was found for bone-borne expanders [57]. These findings could also could be influenced by the location of the appliance [34]. Expanders are tended to be placed in the intermediate palatal position, described as "palatal T zone" [36] in order to assure a higher bicortical anchoring and a more parallel suture opening pattern [60] From our results, we could describe a uniform almost parallel opening along the mid palatal suture in the axial view, not observing differences superior to 0.4 mm as we move to the molar area, consistent with previous studies using bone-borne or tooth bone-borne expanders [30,34,57,61].

The midpalatal suture expansion, on the coronal cross-sectional slice through the midportion of first molar, evaluated at the Nasal and Palatal Floor levels, showed no statistically significant differences between them, with a mean of 2.4 (1.0) mm, confirming a parallel opening suture pattern also on the coronal view. These values are in congruence with the dimension of suture expansion (SEM) at the first molar level on the axial view with a mean of 2.7 (1.0) mm.

4.2. Dentoalveolar Changes

A smaller proportion (40%) corresponds to the dentoalveolar component (1.8 mm) Alveolar bone bending (ABB) and dental inclination (DI) showed reduced mean values of 0.7 (1.6) mm and 1.1 (1.3) mm, respectively. Flexion of the alveolar bone accounted for 15.5% of the total expansion and 24.4% of the dental inclination corresponding to the first molar. Ngan [34] reported a higher dentoalveolar effect of 59%, observing 12% of alveolar bone bending and 47% of first molar dental tipping (2.98 ± 0.56 mm). These results are in agreement with Choi [31] who reported an 87% success for orthopedic expansion in an adolescent sample, where 43% of TE was derived from skeletal expansion [31].

Recent studies evaluating RME effect on periodontal structures found significant reductions in buccal bone thickness (BBT) [29,54], while others reports did not find any or only found minimal changes [62,63]. Garib [20] observed a buccal bone thickness (BBT) reduction from 0.6 to 0.9 mm after RME with no statistical differences between tooth tissue and tooth-borne expanders, regarding the buccal movement of the posterior teeth [20]. A retrospective study treated with MARPE with tooth bone-borne expanders [61] described a maxillary transverse deficiency correction reporting, 37.0% of skeletal expansion, 22.2% of alveolar expansion and 40.7% of dental expansion, observing buccal bone thickness (BBT) (0.6–1.1 mm) and buccal alveolar crest Level (BACL) (1.7–2.2 mm) reductions. Despite the decrease in thickness and height of the buccal bone accompanied with buccal tipping of the maxillary first molar, a high percentage of skeletal expansion was achieved (37%). Some of these changes are comparable to those observed after conventional RME [20,38,64].

Significant changes were found in our study regarding buccal bone thickness (BBT) reductions which ranged from 0.1 (0.2) to 0.4 (0.4) mm for the premolar and molars, but no significant changes were observed after treatment at any site with regards to buccal alveolar crest Height BACL. Ngan [34] reported similar slight changes with a mean buccal bone thickness reduction from 0.27 mm to 0.60 mm at the first molar where bands were placed. As for palatal bone thickness (PBT), there were significant increases from 0.1 to 0.2 mm on the left side for the three teeth, and a small buccal bone thickness (BBT) reduction <0.5 mm was observed in same location after maxillary expansion. Therefore we can deduce that these changes tended to show a more skeletal maxillar expansion pattern, coincident with other studies reporting bilateral palatal bone thickness augmentation after MARPE [29,65] or after RME [20,38]. Toklu et al. [29] found an equivalent reduction in buccal bone thickness, but a palatal bone thickness increase in the anchored teeth with the use of tooth borne and tooth bone-borne expanders after RME, observing a buccal bone thickness reduction in the banded first molars (approximately 0.7–1.2 mm) with both types of expanders in patients with a mean age of 13.8 years.

Dentoalveolar changes such as reduction in buccal bone thickness (BBT) and augmentation of alveolar bone height or vertical buccal alveolar crest Level (BACL) have been confirmed to be greater with the use of tooth-born expanders by one recent prospective comparative study on 60 adolescent patients treated with MARPE tooth bone-borne maxillary expanders or tooth-born expanders [66].

4.3. Dental Changes

Buccal teeth inclination and dentoalveolar structures flexion are common findings after RME. However, studies report small statistical relevance. When comparing dental effects related to the use of tooth and tooth bone-borne expanders, one study observed differences which are not statistically significant in terms of absolute dental tipping between groups for the first premolar when this was banded, finding a dental inclination increase of 2.33° (3.03)° with a tooth-borne expander, whereas it remained unchanged in the tooth bone borne expander group (not banded) [29]. However, this finding should be cautiously interpreted due to the great individual variability that has been observed for tipping as shown by previous studies [38,67].

In our study, dental inclination measured in degrees did not show any significant variation after treatment, being minimal on all the evaluated teeth, showing a tendency to positive tipping, slightly increasing from the first molar to the first premolar. Therefore, it could be said that MARPE with tooth bone-borne expanders is an effective and safe treatment to correct maxillary transversal discrepancy in adolescent patients when the midpalatal suture is still not fully ossified and partially open.

Some authors state that a 1–24° molar inclination increase is inevitable, probably due to alveolar bending and posterior teeth tipping effect [61,68]. A previous study evaluating this effect after RME observed a significant bilateral first molar buccal tipping with mean values of 5.6°–6.2° [51]. Park et al. [61] reported similar values after MARPE, observing a higher degree of buccal tipping in the first molar compared to the first premolar, related to the buccal bone thickness (BBT) and the crest height (BACL) reduction observed in their study. Perhaps these results can be influenced by a greater mean age of this sample (20.1 ± 2.4 years, range: 16–26 years) compared to our sample. In line with these results, other research reported similar inclination changes, but with lower tipping values of 2.5° [20], and 3.9°, respectively [69]. On the other hand, one recent study found greater first molar inclinations between 4.95°–6.99° after MARPE, but such differences were not significant when compared to first premolar inclinations [61]. Lim et al. [25]. observed a reduction of 0.23° per year for buccal tooth inclination after MARPE completion, which is associated to the previously explained remodeling of buccal bone apposition. In this same line of research, Lagraverè et al. [12] in a comparative study between tooth-borne and tooth bone-borne expander with control group, showed similar changes in the transverse dimension and a significant crown inclination in the posterior segments with both type of appliances.

The high potential of CBCT for evaluating maxillary structures has been confirmed. Good resolution, accuracy (only about 2% magnification), precision, non-invasiveness, lower effective radiation dose compared to other diagnostic methods, with shorter acquisition times have been described as its main advantages (60 s) [70–73].

Despite all efforts to minimize patient radiation exposure as much as possible, an optimal quality image is needed to perform accurate measurements. Voxel size influences the final image, thus affecting the accuracy of the performed measurements [74,75]. Several studies assessing linear measurements in skull and jaw bones in CBCT have been carried out [76–78]. Unfavorable effects such as poor image sharpness and artifacts derived from CBCT imaging are inevitable and can influence alveolar accuracy measurements [74,79]. Specifically related to alveolar bone dimensions, the study of Sun et al. concluded that alveolar bone-height and thickness measurements can be achieved with CBCT images with good to excellent repeatability, pointing out that decreasing voxel size from 0.4 to 0.25 mm can improve alveolar bone linear measurement accuracy, observing that measures with a voxel size of 0.25 mm were closer to the direct measurements than when using 0.4 mm [74].

However, another study evaluating bone height and width, showed that 0.4 mm voxel images provided results as accurate as 0.125 mm voxel images [80]. Moreover, Torres and coauthors did not find differences between voxel sizes of 0.2, 0.3 and 0.4 mm, when evaluating linear bone measurements, in agreement with previous results [81]. Although a higher radiation dose when using lower voxel size values is inevitable, this can be justified by its higher resolution needed for this type of measures. A 0.2 voxel size was used in our study in accordance with other similar research considered as reference [29,57].

Some limitations such as small sample size and the short-term follow up have been considered and discussed, though the desired goals have been fulfilled. Moreover, a control group could be used to compare different expander designs or treatments. However, no sufficient homogeneous sample could be collected. On the other hand, the high precision of quantitative analyses on CBCT images contributes to the reliability of the outcomes, making the small sample size acceptable [20]. Therefore, it would be interesting to confirm our results in future studies with longer retention periods and larger samples.

5. Conclusions

From the analysis of our results, we can conclude that:

1. MARPE with tooth bone-borne expanders is an effective method for treating maxillary deficiency in adolescent patients with incomplete ossification of the midpalatal suture, observing a significant maxillary expansion.
2. Although, some periodontal or dentoalveolar changes such as buccal bone thickness reduction were observed radiographically after treatment, none of these effects were clinically detectable.
3. Maxillary deficiency correction with MARPE resulted in a larger skeletal expansion, with reduced dentoalveolar and dental effects and the buccal alveolar crest remained practically unchanged.
4. Tendency of parallel midpalatal suture opening pattern was observed after treatment in the coronal and axial view.
5. Aside from the use of tooth bone support for maxillary expansion, no significant dental inclination effect was observed after treatment.

Author Contributions: Conceptualization, P.S.M. and B.S.M.; methodology, P.S.M.; software, P.S.M.; validation, P.S.M., E.S.R. and B.S.M.; investigation, P.S.M. and P.A.P.; resources, P.S.M.; data curation, P.A.P.; writing—original draft preparation, P.S.M.; writing—review and editing, P.S.M.; supervision, E.S.R. All authors have read and agreed to the published version of the manuscript.

Funding: This research received no external funding.

Institutional Review Board Statement: The study was conducted in accordance with the Declaration of Helsinki, and approved by the Ethics Committee of hospital universitario Vírgen Macarena-Virgen del Rocío (238e1b02c492fe6c37e2e9cf37c737297f4cf746) 14 December 2020.

Informed Consent Statement: Informed consent was obtained from all subjects involved in the study.

Conflicts of Interest: The authors declare no conflict of interest.

References

1. Hawes, R.; Kutin, G. Posterior Cross-Bites in the Deciduous and Mixed Dentitions. *Am. J. Orthod.* **1969**, *56*, 491–504.
2. Egermark-Eriksson, I.; Carlsson, G.E.; Magnusson, T.; Thilander, B. A Longitudinal Study on Malocclusion in Relation to Signs and Symptoms of Cranio-Mandibular Disorders in Children and Adolescents. *Eur. J. Orthod.* **1990**, *12*, 399–407. [CrossRef] [PubMed]
3. Brunelle, J.A.; Bhat, M.; Lipton, J.A. Prevalence and Distribution of Selected Occlusal Characteristics in the US Population, 1988–1991. *J. Dent. Res.* **1996**, *75*, 706–713. [CrossRef] [PubMed]
4. Da Silva Filho, O.G.; Santamaria, M.; Capelozza Filho, L. Epidemiology of Posterior Crossbite in the Primary Dentition. *J. Clin. Pediatr. Dent.* **2007**, *32*, 73–78. [CrossRef] [PubMed]
5. McNamara, J.A. Maxillary Transverse Deficiency. *Am. J. Orthod. Dentofac. Orthop.* **2000**, *117*, 567–570. [CrossRef]
6. Consolaro, A.; Consolaro, R.B. Jaws Can Be Referred to as Narrow or Hypoplastic, but the Term "Atresia" is Inaccurate! *Dental Press J. Orthod.* **2018**, *23*, 19–23. [CrossRef]
7. Andrucioli, M.C.D.; Matsumoto, M.A.N. Transverse Maxillary Deficiency: Treatment Alternatives in Face of Early Skeletal Maturation. *Dental Press J. Orthod.* **2020**, *25*, 70–79. [CrossRef]
8. Brunetto, D.P.; Sant'Anna, E.F.; Machado, A.W.; Moon, W. Non-Surgical Treatment of Transverse Deficiency in Adults Using Microimplant-Assisted Rapid Palatal Expansion (MARPE). *Dental Press J. Orthod.* **2017**, *22*, 110–125. [CrossRef]
9. Modéer, T.; Odenrtck, L.; Lindner, A. Sucking Habits and Their Relation to Posterior Cross-bite in 4-year-old Children. *Eur. J. Oral Sci.* **1982**, *90*, 323–328. [CrossRef]
10. Yllmaz, A.; Arman-Özçlrplcl, A.; Erken, S.; Polat-Özsoy, Ö. Comparison of Short-Term Effects of Mini-Implant-Supported Maxillary Expansion Appliance with Two Conventional Expansion Protocols. *Eur. J. Orthod.* **2015**, *37*, 556–564. [CrossRef]
11. Haas, A.J. The Treatment of Maxillary Deficiency by Opening the Midpalatal Suture. *Angle Orthod.* **1965**, *35*, 200–217. [PubMed]
12. Lagravère, M.O.; Carey, J.; Heo, G.; Toogood, R.W.; Major, P.W. Transverse, Vertical, and Anteroposterior Changes from Bone-Anchored Maxillary Expansion vs. Traditional Rapid Maxillary Expansion: A Randomized Clinical Trial. *Am. J. Orthod. Dentofac. Orthop.* **2010**, *137*, 304.e1–304.e12. [CrossRef]
13. Franchi, L.; Pavoni, C.; Faltin, K.; McNamara, J.A.; Cozza, P. Long-Term Skeletal and Dental Effects and Treatment Timing for Functional Appliances in Class II Malocclusion. *Angle Orthod.* **2013**, *83*, 334–340. [CrossRef] [PubMed]
14. Lin, Y.; Chen, G.; Fu, Z.; Ma, L.; Li, W. Cone-Beam Computed Tomography Assessment of Lower Facial Asymmetry in Unilateral Cleft Lip and Palate and Non-Cleft Patients with Class III Skeletal Relationship. *PLoS ONE* **2015**, *10*, e0130235. [CrossRef]
15. Melsen, B.; Melsen, F. The Postnatal Development of the Palatomaxillary Region Studied on Human Autopsy Material. *Am. J. Orthod.* **1982**, *82*, 329–342. [CrossRef]
16. Thilander, B. Palatal Suture Closure in Man from 15 to 35 Years of Age. *Am. J. Orthod.* **1977**, *72*, 42–52.
17. Erverdi, N.; Okar, I.; Kücükkeles, N.; Arbak, S. A Comparison of Two Different Rapid Palatalexpansion Techniques from the Point of Root Resorption. *Am. J. Orthod. Dentofac. Orthop.* **1994**, *106*, 47–51. [CrossRef]
18. Schuster, G.; Borel-Scherf, I.; Schop, P.M. Frequency of and Complications in the Use of RPE Appliances—Results of a Survey in the Federal State of Hesse, Germany. *J. Orofac. Orthop.* **2005**, *66*, 148–161. [CrossRef]
19. Harzer, W.; Schneider, M.; Gedrange, T.; Tausche, E. Direct Bone Placement of the Hyrax Fixation Screw for Surgically Assisted Rapid Palatal Expansion (SARPE). *J. Oral Maxillofac. Surg.* **2006**, *64*, 1313–1317. [CrossRef]
20. Garib, D.G.; Henriques, J.F.C.; Janson, G.; de Freitas, M.R.; Fernandes, A.Y. Periodontal Effects of Rapid Maxillary Expansion with Tooth-Tissue-Borne and Tooth-Borne Expanders: A Computed Tomography Evaluation. *Am. J. Orthod. Dentofac. Orthop.* **2006**, *129*, 749–758. [CrossRef]
21. Tausche, E.; Hansen, L.; Hietschold, V.; Lagravère, M.O.; Harzer, W. Three-Dimensional Evaluation of Surgically Assisted Implant Bone-Borne Rapid Maxillary Expansion: A Pilot Study. *Am. J. Orthod. Dentofac. Orthop.* **2007**, *131*, 92–99. [CrossRef] [PubMed]
22. Baysal, A.; Karadede, I.; Hekimoglu, S.; Ucar, F.; Ozer, T.; Veli, I.; Uysal, T. Evaluation of Root Resorption Following Rapid Maxillary Expansion Using Cone-Beam Computed Tomography. *Angle Orthod.* **2012**, *82*, 488–494. [CrossRef] [PubMed]
23. Fishman, L.S. Radiographic Evaluation of Skeletal Maturation. A Clinically Oriented Method Based on Hand-Wrist Films. *Angle Orthod.* **1982**, *52*, 88–112.
24. Lee, K.J.; Park, Y.C.; Park, J.Y.; Hwang, W.S. Miniscrew-Assisted Nonsurgical Palatal Expansion before Orthognathic Surgery for a Patient with Severe Mandibular Prognathism. *Am. J. Orthod. Dentofac. Orthop.* **2010**, *137*, 830–839. [CrossRef] [PubMed]
25. Lim, H.M.; Park, Y.C.; Lee, K.J.; Kim, K.H.; Choi, Y.J. Stability of Dental, Alveolar, and Skeletal Changes after Miniscrew-Assisted Rapid Palatal Expansion. *Korean J. Orthod.* **2017**, *47*, 313–322. [CrossRef] [PubMed]

26. Garib, D.G.; Henriques, J.F.C.; Janson, G.; Freitas, M.R.; Coelho, R.A. Rapid Maxillary Expansion—Tooth Tissue-Borne versus Tooth-Borne Expanders: A Computed Tomography Evaluation of Dentoskeletal Effects. *Angle Orthod.* **2005**, *75*, 548–557 [CrossRef]
27. Gurel, H.G.; Memili, B.; Erkan, M.; Sukurica, Y. Long-Term Effects of Rapid Maxillary Expansion Followed by Fixed Appliances *Angle Orthod.* **2010**, *80*, 5–9. [CrossRef]
28. Zhou, Z.; Chen, W.; Shen, M.; Sun, C.; Li, J.; Chen, N. Cone Beam Computed Tomographic Analyses of Alveolar Bone Anatomy at the Maxillary Anterior Region in Chinese Adults. *J. Biomed. Res.* **2014**, *28*, 498–505. [CrossRef]
29. Gunyuz Toklu, M.; Germec-Cakan, D.; Tozlu, M. Periodontal, Dentoalveolar, and Skeletal Effects of Tooth-Borne and Tooth-Bone-Borne Expansion Appliances. *Am. J. Orthod. Dentofac. Orthop.* **2015**, *148*, 97–109. [CrossRef]
30. Carlson, C.; Sung, J.; McComb, R.W.; MacHado, A.W.; Moon, W. Microimplant-Assisted Rapid Palatal Expansion Appliance to Orthopedically Correct Transverse Maxillary Deficiency in an Adult. *Am. J. Orthod. Dentofac. Orthop.* **2016**, *149*, 716–728 [CrossRef]
31. Choi, S.H.; Shi, K.K.; Cha, J.Y.; Park, Y.C.; Lee, K.J. Nonsurgical Miniscrew-Assisted Rapid Maxillary Expansion Results in Acceptable Stability in Young Adults. *Angle Orthod.* **2016**, *86*, 713–720. [CrossRef] [PubMed]
32. Jang, H.I.; Kim, S.C.; Chae, J.M.; Kang, K.H.; Cho, J.W.; Chang, N.Y.; Lee, K.Y.; Cho, J.H. Relationship between Maturation Indices and Morphology of the Midpalatal Suture Obtained Using Cone-Beam Computed Tomography Images. *Korean J. Orthod.* **2016**, *46*, 345–355. [CrossRef] [PubMed]
33. Wilmes, B.; Ludwig, B.; Vasudavan, S.; Nienkemper, M.; Drescher, D. Application and Effectiveness of a Mini-Implant- and Tooth-Borne Rapid Palatal Expansion Device: The Hybrid Hyrax. *World J. Orthod.* **2010**, *11*, 323–330.
34. Ngan, P.; Nguyen, U.K.; Nguyen, T.; Tremont, T.; Martin, C. Skeletal, Dentoalveolar, and Periodontal Changes of Skeletally Matured Patients with Maxillary Deficiency Treated with Microimplant-Assisted Rapid Palatal Expansion Appliances: A Pilot Study. *APOS Trends Orthod.* **2018**, *8*, 71–85. [CrossRef]
35. Silva-Ruz, I.; Tort-Barahona, F.; Acuña-Aracena, P.; Villalon-Pooley, P. Disyunción Maxilar Rápida Asistida Con Microtornillos En Pacientes En Crecimiento Con Deficiencia Maxilar Transversal. *Int. J. Interdiscip. Dent.* **2021**, *14*, 61–66. [CrossRef]
36. Wilmes, B.; Ludwig, B.; Vasudavan, S.; Nienkemper, M.; Drescher, D. The T-Zone: Median vs. Paramedian Insertion of Palatal Mini-Implants. *J. Clin. Orthod.* **2016**, *50*, 543–551.
37. Ludwig, B.; Baumgaertel, S.; Zorkun, B.; Bonitz, L.; Glasl, B.; Wilmes, B.; Lisson, J. Application of a New Viscoelastic Finite Element Method Model and Analysis of Miniscrew-Supported Hybrid Hyrax Treatment. *Am. J. Orthod. Dentofac. Orthop.* **2013**, *143*, 426–435. [CrossRef]
38. Rungcharassaeng, K.; Caruso, J.M.; Kan, J.Y.K.; Kim, J.; Taylor, G. Factors Affecting Buccal Bone Changes of Maxillary Posterior Teeth after Rapid Maxillary Expansion. *Am. J. Orthod. Dentofac. Orthop.* **2007**, *132*, 428.e1–428.e8. [CrossRef]
39. Vanarsdall, I.B.R.L.; Kocian, P. *Rapid Maxillary Expansion with Skeletal Anchorage vs. Bonded Tooth/Tissue Born Expanders: A Case Report Comparison Utilizing CBCT*; Rocky Mountain Orthodontics: Denver, CO, USA, 2012.
40. Simontacchi-Gbologah, M.S.; Tamburrino, R.K.; Boucher, N.S.; Vanarsdall, R.L.; Secchi, A.G. Comparison of Three Methods to Analyze the Skeletal Transverse Dimension in Orthodontic Diagnosis. Unpublished Thesis, University of Pennsylvania, Philadelphia, PA, USA, 2010.
41. Tamburrino, R.K.; Boucher, N.S.; Vanarsdall, R.L.; Secchi, A.G. The Transverse Dimension: Diagnosis and Relevance to Functional Occlusion. *RWISO J.* **2010**, *2*, 13–22.
42. Angelieri, F.; Cevidanes, L.H.S.; Franchi, L.; Gonçalves, J.R.; Benavides, E.; McNamara, J.A. Midpalatal Suture Maturation. Classification Method for Individual Assessment before Rapid Maxillary Expansion. *Am. J. Orthod. Dentofac. Orthop.* **2013**, *144*, 759–769. [CrossRef]
43. Suzuki, H.; Moon, W.; Previdente, L.H.; Suzuki, S.S.; Garcez, A.S.; Consolaro, A. Miniscrew-Assisted Rapid Palatal Expander (MARPE): The Quest for Pure Orthopedic Movement. *Dental Press J. Orthod.* **2016**, *21*, 17–23. [CrossRef] [PubMed]
44. Cantarella, D.; Dominguez-Mompell, R.; Mallya, S.M.; Moschik, C.; Pan, H.C.; Miller, J.; Moon, W. Changes in the Midpalatal and Pterygopalatine Sutures Induced by Micro-Implant-Supported Skeletal Expander, Analyzed with a Novel 3D Method Based on CBCT Imaging. *Prog. Orthod.* **2017**, *18*, 34. [CrossRef] [PubMed]
45. Nojima, L.I.; da Nojima, M.C.G.; da Cunha, A.C.; Guss, N.O.; Sant'anna, E.F. Mini-Implant Selection Protocol Applied to MARPE *Dental Press J. Orthod.* **2018**, *23*, 93–101. [CrossRef] [PubMed]
46. Shirazi, S.; Stanford, C.; Cooper, L. Testing for COVID-19 in Dental Offices Mechanism of Action, Application, and Interpretation of Laboratory and Point-of-Care Screening Tests. *J. Am. Dent. Assoc.* **2021**, *4*, 514–525.e8. [CrossRef]
47. Shirazi, S.; Stanford, C.; Cooper, L. Characteristics and Detection Rate of SARS-CoV-2 in Alternative Sites and Specimens Pertaining to Dental Practice: An Evidence Summary. *J. Am. Dent. Assoc.* **2021**, *10*, 1158. [CrossRef]
48. Baccetti, T.; Franchi, L.; McNamara, J.A. An Improved Version of the Cervical Vertebral Maturation (CVM) Method for the Assessment of Mandibular Growth. *Angle Orthod.* **2002**, *72*, 316–323. [CrossRef]
49. Baccetti, T.; Franchi, L.; McNamara, J.A. The Cervical Vertebral Maturation (CVM) Method for the Assessment of Optimal Treatment Timing in Dentofacial Orthopedics. *Semin. Orthod.* **2005**, *11*, 119–129. [CrossRef]
50. Podesser, B.; Williams, S.; Crismani, A.G.; Bantleon, H.P. Evaluation of the Effects of Rapid Maxillary Expansion in Growing Children Using Computer Tomography Scanning: A Pilot Study. *Eur. J. Orthod.* **2007**, *29*, 37–44. [CrossRef]

51. Christie, K.F.; Boucher, N.; Chung, C.H. Effects of Bonded Rapid Palatal Expansion on the Transverse Dimensions of the Maxilla: A Cone-Beam Computed Tomography Study. *Am. J. Orthod. Dentofac. Orthop.* **2010**, *137*, S79–S85. [CrossRef]
52. Angelieri, F.; Franchi, L.; Cevidanes, L.H.S.; McNamara, J.A. Diagnostic Performance of Skeletal Maturity for the Assessment of Midpalatal Suture Maturation. *Am. J. Orthod. Dentofac. Orthop.* **2015**, *148*, 1010–1016. [CrossRef]
53. Perinetti, G.; Braga, C.; Contardo, L.; Primozic, J. Cervical Vertebral Maturation: Are Postpubertal Stages Attained in All Subjects? *Am. J. Orthod. Dentofac. Orthop.* **2020**, *157*, 305–312. [CrossRef] [PubMed]
54. Garrett, B.J.; Caruso, J.M.; Rungcharassaeng, K.; Farrage, J.R.; Kim, J.S.; Taylor, G.D. Editor's Summary, Q & A, Reviewer's Critique. *Am. J. Orthod. Dentofac. Orthop.* **2008**, *134*, 8–9. [CrossRef]
55. Lamparski, D.G.; Rinchuse, D.J.; Close, J.M.; Sciote, J.J. Comparison of Skeletal and Dental Changes between 2-Point and 4-Point Rapid Palatal Expanders. *Am. J. Orthod. Dentofac. Orthop.* **2003**, *123*, 321–328. [CrossRef] [PubMed]
56. Davidovitch, M.; Efstathiou, S.; Sarne, O.; Vardimon, A.D. Skeletal and Dental Response to Rapid Maxillary Expansion with 2- versus 4-Band Appliances. *Am. J. Orthod. Dentofac. Orthop.* **2005**, *127*, 483–492. [CrossRef] [PubMed]
57. Lin, L.; Ahn, H.W.; Kim, S.J.; Moon, S.C.; Kim, S.H.; Nelson, G. Tooth-Borne vs. Bone-Borne Rapid Maxillary Expanders in Late Adolescence. *Angle Orthod.* **2015**, *85*, 253–262. [CrossRef]
58. Haas, A. Rapid Expansion of The Maxillary Dental Arch nd Nasal Cavity By Opening The Midpalatal Suture. *Angle Orthod.* **1961**, *31*, 73–90.
59. Lione, R.; Ballanti, F.; Franchi, L.; Baccetti, T.; Cozza, P. Treatment and Posttreatment Skeletal Effects of Rapid Maxillary Expansion Studied with Low-Dose Computed Tomography in Growing Subjects. *Am. J. Orthod. Dentofac. Orthop.* **2008**, *134*, 389–392. [CrossRef]
60. Ludwig, B.; Glasl, B.; Kinzinger, G.S.M.; Lietz, T.; Lisson, J.A. Anatomical Guidelines for Miniscrew Insertion: Vestibular Interradicular Sites. *J. Clin. Orthod.* **2011**, *45*, 165–173.
61. Park, J.J.; Park, Y.C.; Lee, K.J.; Cha, J.Y.; Tahk, J.H.; Choi, Y.J. Skeletal and Dentoalveolar Changes after Miniscrew-Assisted Rapid Palatal Expansion in Young Adults: A Cone-Beam Computed Tomography Study. *Korean J. Orthod.* **2017**, *47*, 77–86. [CrossRef]
62. Akyalcin, S.; Schaefer, J.S.; English, J.D.; Stephens, C.R.; Winkelmann, S. A Cone-Beam Computed Tomography Evaluation of Buccal Bone Thickness Following Maxillary Expansion. *Imaging Sci. Dent.* **2013**, *43*, 85–90. [CrossRef]
63. Starnbach, H.; Bayne, D.; Cleall, J.; Subtelny, J.D. Facioskeletal and Dental Changes Resulting from Rapid Maxillary Expansion. *Angle Orthod.* **1966**, *36*, 152–164. [PubMed]
64. Corbridge, J.K.; Campbell, P.M.; Taylor, R.; Ceen, R.F.; Buschang, P.H. Transverse Dentoalveolar Changes after Slow Maxillary Expansion. *Am. J. Orthod. Dentofac. Orthop.* **2011**, *140*, 317–325. [CrossRef] [PubMed]
65. Garib, D.G.; Navarro, R.; Francischone, C.E.; Oltramari, P.V. Rapid Maxillary Expansion Using Palatal Implants. *J. Clin. Orthod.* **2008**, *42*, 665–671.
66. Jia, H.; Zhuang, L.; Zhang, N.; Bian, Y.; Li, S. Comparison of Skeletal Maxillary Transverse Deficiency Treated by Microimplant-Assisted Rapid Palatal Expansion and Tooth-Borne Expansion during the Post-Pubertal Growth Spurt Stage: A Prospective Cone Beam Computed Tomography Study. *Angle Orthod.* **2021**, *91*, 36–45. [CrossRef] [PubMed]
67. Adkins, M.D.; Nanda, R.S.; Currier, G.F. Arch Perimeter Changes on Rapid Palatal Expansion. *Am. J. Orthod. Dentofac. Orthop.* **1990**, *97*, 194–199. [CrossRef]
68. Lione, R.; Franchi, L.; Fanucci, E.; Laganá, G.; Cozza, P. Three-Dimensional Densitometric Analysis of Maxillary Sutural Changes Induced by Rapid Maxillary Expansion. *Dentomaxillofacial Radiol.* **2013**, *42*, 71798010. [CrossRef]
69. Lagravère, M.O.; Heo, G.; Major, P.W.; Flores-Mir, C. Meta-analysis of immediate changes with rapid maxillary expansion treatment. *J. Am. Dent. Assoc.* **2006**, *137*, 44–53. [CrossRef] [PubMed]
70. Nada, R.M.; Van Loon, B.; Schols, J.G.J.H.; Maal, T.J.J.; de Koning, M.J.; Mostafa, Y.A.; Kuijpers-Jagtman, A.M. Volumetric Changes of the Nose and Nasal Airway 2 Years after Tooth-Borne and Bone-Borne Surgically Assisted Rapid Maxillary Expansion. *Eur. J. Oral Sci.* **2013**, *121*, 450–456. [CrossRef]
71. Nada, R.M.; van Loon, B.; Maal, T.J.J.; Bergé, S.J.; Mostafa, Y.A.; Kuijpers-Jagtman, A.M.; Schols, J.G.J.H. Three-Dimensional Evaluation of Soft Tissue Changes in the Orofacial Region after Tooth-Borne and Bone-Borne Surgically Assisted Rapid Maxillary Expansion. *Clin. Oral Investig.* **2013**, *17*, 2017–2024. [CrossRef]
72. Gauthier, C.; Voyer, R.; Paquette, M.; Kompré, P.; Papadakis, A. Periodontal Effects of Surgically Assisted Rapid Palatal Expansion Evaluated Clinically and with Cone-Beam Computerized Tomography: 6-Month Preliminary Results. *Am. J. Orthod. Dentofac. Orthop.* **2011**, *139*, 16–19. [CrossRef]
73. Camps-Perepérez, I.; Guijarro-Martínez, R.; Peiró-Guijarro, M.A.; Hernández-Alfaro, F. The Value of Cone Beam Computed Tomography Imaging in Surgically Assisted Rapid Palatal Expansion: A Systematic Review of the Literature. *Int. J. Oral Maxillofac. Surg.* **2017**, *46*, 827–838. [CrossRef] [PubMed]
74. Sun, Z.; Smith, T.; Kortam, S.; Kim, D.G.; Tee, B.C.; Fields, H. Effect of Bone Thickness on Alveolar Bone-Height Measurements from Cone-Beam Computed Tomography Images. *Am. J. Orthod. Dentofac. Orthop.* **2011**, *139*, e117–e127. [CrossRef] [PubMed]
75. Leung, C.C.; Palomo, L.; Griffith, R.; Hans, M.G. Accuracy and Reliability of Cone-Beam Computed Tomography for Measuring Alveolar Bone Height and Detecting Bony Dehiscences and Fenestrations. *Am. J. Orthod. Dentofac. Orthop.* **2010**, *137*, S109–S119. [CrossRef] [PubMed]
76. Lascala, C.A.; Panella, J.; Marques, M.M. Analysis of the Accuracy of Linear Measurements Obtained by Cone Beam Computed Tomography (CBCT-NewTom). *Dentomaxillofacial Radiol.* **2004**, *33*, 291–294. [CrossRef] [PubMed]

77. Berco, M.; Rigali, P.H.; Miner, R.M.; DeLuca, S.; Anderson, N.K.; Will, L.A. Accuracy and Reliability of Linear Cephalometric Measurements from Cone-Beam Computed Tomography Scans of a Dry Human Skull. *Am. J. Orthod. Dentofac. Orthop.* **2009**, *136*, 17.e1–17.e9. [CrossRef]
78. Hilgers, M.L.; Scarfe, W.C.; Scheetz, J.P.; Farman, A.G. Accuracy of Linear Temporomandibular Joint Measurements with Cone Beam Computed Tomography and Digital Cephalometric Radiography. *Am. J. Orthod. Dentofac. Orthop.* **2005**, *128*, 803–811. [CrossRef]
79. Scarfe, W.C.; Farman, A.G. What Is Cone-Beam CT and How Does It Work? *Dent. Clin. N. Am.* **2008**, *52*, 707–730. [CrossRef]
80. Patcas, R.; Müller, L.; Ullrich, O.; Peltomäki, T. Accuracy of Cone-Beam Computed Tomography at Different Resolutions Assessed on the Bony Covering of the Mandibular Anterior Teeth. *Am. J. Orthod. Dentofac. Orthop.* **2012**, *141*, 41–50. [CrossRef]
81. Torres, M.G.G.; Campos, P.S.F.; Segundo, N.P.N.; Navarro, M.; Crusoé-Rebello, I. Accuracy of Linear Measurements in Cone Beam Computed Tomography with Different Voxel Sizes. *Implant Dent.* **2012**, *21*, 150–155. [CrossRef]

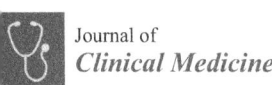

Journal of Clinical Medicine

Article

Validity and Reproducibility of the Peer Assessment Rating Index Scored on Digital Models Using a Software Compared with Traditional Manual Scoring

Arwa Gera [1], Shadi Gera [1], Michel Dalstra [1], Paolo M. Cattaneo [2] and Marie A. Cornelis [2,*]

[1] Section of Orthodontics, Department of Dentistry and Oral Health, Aarhus University, DC 8000 Aarhus, Denmark; arwa@dent.au.dk (A.G.); shadigera@dent.au.dk (S.G.); michel.dalstra@dent.au.dk (M.D.)
[2] Faculty of Medicine, Dentistry and Health Sciences, Melbourne Dental School, University of Melbourne, Carlton, VIC 3053, Australia; paolo.cattaneo@unimelb.edu.au
* Correspondence: marie.cornelis@unimelb.edu.au

Abstract: The aim of this study was to assess the validity and reproducibility of digital scoring of the Peer Assessment Rating (PAR) index and its components using a software, compared with conventional manual scoring on printed model equivalents. The PAR index was scored on 15 cases at pre- and post-treatment stages by two operators using two methods: first, digitally, on direct digital models using Ortho Analyzer software; and second, manually, on printed model equivalents using a digital caliper. All measurements were repeated at a one-week interval. Paired sample *t*-tests were used to compare PAR scores and its components between both methods and raters. Intra-class correlation coefficients (ICC) were used to compute intra- and inter-rater reproducibility. The error of the method was calculated. The agreement between both methods was analyzed using Bland-Altman plots. There were no significant differences in the mean PAR scores between both methods and both raters. ICC for intra- and inter-rater reproducibility was excellent (≥ 0.95). All error-of-the-method values were smaller than the associated minimum standard deviation. Bland-Altman plots confirmed the validity of the measurements. PAR scoring on digital models showed excellent validity and reproducibility compared with manual scoring on printed model equivalents by means of a digital caliper.

Keywords: orthodontics; CAD/CAM; PAR index; dental models; digital models; clinical

Citation: Gera, A.; Gera, S.; Dalstra, M.; Cattaneo, P.M.; Cornelis, M.A. Validity and Reproducibility of the Peer Assessment Rating Index Scored on Digital Models Using a Software Compared with Traditional Manual Scoring. *J. Clin. Med.* **2021**, *10*, 1646. https://doi.org/10.3390/jcm10081646

Academic Editor: Letizia Perillo

Received: 23 February 2021
Accepted: 10 April 2021
Published: 13 April 2021

Publisher's Note: MDPI stays neutral with regard to jurisdictional claims in published maps and institutional affiliations.

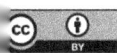

Copyright: © 2021 by the authors. Licensee MDPI, Basel, Switzerland. This article is an open access article distributed under the terms and conditions of the Creative Commons Attribution (CC BY) license (https://creativecommons.org/licenses/by/4.0/).

1. Introduction

For high standards of orthodontic treatment quality to be maintained, frequent monitoring of treatment outcomes is a prerequisite for orthodontists. The orthodontic indices widely used in clinical and epidemiological studies to evaluate malocclusion and treatment outcome [1–3] include the Index of Orthodontic Treatment Need (IOTN) [4], the Index of Complexity Outcome and Need (ICON) [5], the American Board of Orthodontics objective grading system (ABO-OGS) index [6], the Peer Assessment Rating (PAR) index [7], and the Dental Aesthetic Index (DAI) [8].

The PAR [7] is an occlusal index developed to provide an objective and standardized measure of static occlusion at any stage of treatment using dental models. Therefore, this index is widely used among clinicians whether it is in the private or the public sector, including educational institutions. In fact, in the UK, the use of this index is obligatory in all orthodontic clinics offering public service to audit orthodontic treatment outcome, and it is used as a measure for quality assurance. The assessment of malocclusion can be recorded at any stage of orthodontic treatment, such as pre- and/or post-treatment, whereas the difference in PAR scores between two stages evaluates treatment outcome. Its validity and reliability on plaster models have been reported in England [9], as well as in the United States [10]. It is also a valid tool for measuring treatment need [11].

The use of plaster models and digital calipers has been acknowledged as the gold standard for study model analyses and measurements [12,13]. Traditionally, PAR scoring is performed on plaster models by means of a PAR ruler or a combination of a digital caliper and a conventional ruler. Several studies have used this method to assess malocclusion, treatment need, treatment outcomes, and stability of occlusion [11,14–19]. However, the human-machine interface has evolved, influencing orthodontics significantly, shifting from a traditional clinical workflow towards a complete digital flow, where digital models have become more prevalent. Digital models enable patients' records to be stored digitally and for essential orthodontic assessments, such as diagnosis, treatment planning, and assessment of treatment outcome, to be carried out virtually through several built-in features, such as linear measurements [13,20], Bolton analysis, space analyses [21], treatment planning [22], and PAR scoring [12,23]. However, this modern paradigm demands adaptation and assessment of applicability in orthodontic clinical work. Nevertheless, assessments of the validity and reproducibility of 3-dimensional (3-D) digital measurement tools remain scarce.

Digital models can be obtained either directly or indirectly and can be printed or viewed on a computer display. Scanned-in plaster models are the indirect source of digital models and are as valid and reliable as conventional plaster models [12,13,24,25]. In the present study, digital models were obtained directly from an intraoral scanner. Emphasis on evaluating a complete virtual workflow was recently implemented by three studies [26–28] Brown et al. [26] concluded that 3-D printed models acquired directly from intraoral scans provided clinically acceptable models and should be considered as a viable option for clinical applications. Luqmani et al. [28] assessed the validity of digital PAR scoring by comparing manual PAR scoring using conventional models and a PAR ruler with automated digital scoring for both scanned-in models and intraoral scanning (indirect and direct digital models, respectively). The authors concluded that automated digital PAR scoring was valid and that there were no significant differences between direct and indirect digital model scores.

However, to our knowledge, the digital non-automated PAR index scoring tool of the Ortho Analyzer software has not been previously validated. Therefore, the purpose of this study was to assess the validity and reproducibility of digital scoring of the PAR index and its components on digital models using this software, compared with conventional manual scoring on printed model equivalents.

2. Materials and Methods

2.1. Sample Size Calculation

A sample size calculation was performed using the formula given by Walter et al. [29] For a minimum acceptable reliability (intra-class correlation (ICC)) of 0.80, an expected reliability of 0.96, with a power of 80% and a significance of 0.05, a sample of 12 subjects was needed. It was decided to extend the sample to 15 subjects.

2.2. Setting

The study was conducted at the Section of Orthodontics, School of Dentistry and Oral Health, Aarhus University, Denmark. This type of study is exempt from ethics approval in Denmark (Health Research Ethics Committee-Central Jutland, Denmark, case no. 1-10-72-1-20).

2.3. Sample Collection

The study sample consisted of 15 consecutive patient records (the first record being randomly chosen) selected from the archives, according to the following inclusion criteria: (1) patients had undergone orthodontic treatment with full fixed appliances at the postgraduate orthodontic clinic between 2016 and 2018; and (2) digital models before and after treatment were available. No restrictions were applied with regards to age, initial malocclusion and end-of-treatment results.

The digital models for both treatment stages; pre-treatment (T0) and post-treatment (T1), had been directly generated by a TRIOS intraoral scanner (3Shape, Copenhagen, Denmark) as stereolithographic (STL) files, imported and analyzed through Ortho Analyzer software (3Shape, Copenhagen, Denmark). Subsequently, 30 digital models were printed, to generate 15 model equivalents for each stage, by means of model design software (Objet Studio, Stratasys, Eden Prairie, MN, USA) and a 3-D printing machine (Polyjet prototyping technique; Objet30 Dental prime, Stratasys, Eden Prairie, MN, USA), in the same laboratory and with the same technique.

2.4. Measurements

The PAR scoring was performed at T0 and T1 by two methods: (1) digitally, on the direct digital models using a built-in feature of the Ortho Analyzer software (Figure 1); and (2) manually, on the printed model equivalents using a digital caliper (Orthopli, Philadelphia, PA, USA), measured to the nearest 0.01 mm with an orthodontic tip accuracy of 0.001, except for overjet and overbite, which were measured with a conventional ruler. Two operators (AG and SG), previously trained and calibrated in the use of both techniques, performed all the measurements independently. Reproducibility was determined by repeated measurements on all models by both methods and by both raters at a one-week interval and under identical circumstances.

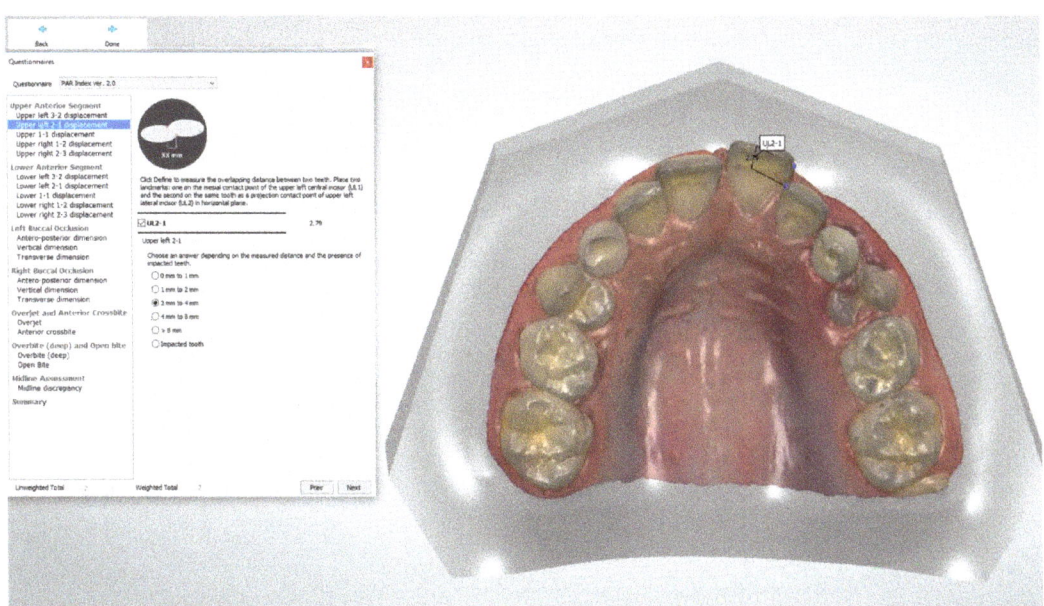

Figure 1. Peer Assessment Rating (PAR) index scoring using Ortho Analyzer software. Anterior component scoring contact point displacement between teeth 21 and 22.

The PAR scoring was performed using the UK weighting system according to Richmond et al. [7] and included five components, scoring various occlusal traits which constitute malocclusion: anterior segment, posterior segment, overjet, overbite, and centerline (Table 1). The scores of the traits were summed and multiplied by their weight. The component-weighted PAR scores were summed to constitute the total weighted PAR score. Essential information about each case was considered, such as impacted teeth, missing or extracted teeth, plans for any prosthetic replacements, and restorative work previously carried out that affected the malocclusion.

Table 1. The PAR index components and scoring.

	PAR Component	Assessment	Scoring	Weighting
1	Anterior [†]	Contact point displacement	0–4	× 1
		Impacted incisors/canines	5	
2	Posterior [‡]	Sagittal occlusion	0–2	× 1
		Vertical occlusion	0–1	
		Transverse occlusion	0–4	
3	Overjet [§]	Overjet	0–4	× 6
		Anterior crossbite	0–4	
4	Overbite [¶]	Overbite	0–3	× 2
		Open bite	0–4	
5	Centerline	Deviation from dental midline	0–2	× 4
	Total		Unweighted PAR score	Weighted PAR score

[†] Measured from the mesial contact point of canine on one side to the mesial contact point of canine on the opposite side (upper and lower arches) and recorded in millimeters as the shortest distance between contact points of adjacent teeth and parallel to the occlusal plane. [‡] Measured from the distal contact point of canine to the mesial contact point of permanent molar or last molar (right and left sides). [§] Measured as the largest horizontal distance parallel to the occlusal plane from the labial incisor edge of the most prominent upper incisor to the labial surface of the corresponding lower incisor. [¶] Recorded as the largest vertical overlap or open bite between upper incisors and lower incisors.

2.5. Statistical Analyses

Data collection and management were performed by means of the Research Electronic Data Capture (REDCap) tool hosted at Aarhus University [30,31]. Statistical analyses were carried out with Stata software (Release 16, StataCorp. 2019, College Station, TX, USA).

Descriptive statistics were used to analyze the total PAR scores at different time points, between raters and methods used. Paired sample t-tests were used to compare PAR scoring between both methods and raters at a significance level of <0.05. Both methods were assessed by ICC for intra- and inter-rater reproducibility. Intra- and inter-rater variability were determined by calculation of the error of the method according to Dahlberg's formula [32]. The agreement between the digital and manual scoring methods performed by the two raters was determined by a scatter plot and Bland-Altman plots.

3. Results

3.1. Validity

Paired-sample t-tests showed no significant differences in the mean total PAR scores and in the PAR components between both methods (Tables 2 and 3). The scatter plot (Figure 2a) and Bland-Altman plots (Figure 2b) illustrate agreement of the measurements conducted with both methods.

Table 2. Intra-rater variability (error of the method and Minimum Standard Deviation (MSD)) and reproducibility (ICC) according to time point and method, for both raters. Paired sample t-tests comparing both methods.

PAR Index Scoring and Timepoint		Scoring Method	Rater I						Rater II					
			Mean (SD) [a]	Err. Method *,[a]	MSD [a]	ICC	[95% CI]		p-Value (Paired t-Test)	Mean (SD) [a]	Err. Method *,[a]	MSD [a]	ICC	[95% CI]		p-Value (Paired t-Test)
T0	Total PAR	Manual	29.5 (10.1)	0.9	10.1	0.99	0.99	1.00	0.16	30.5 (10.7)	1.4	10.1	0.99	0.98	1.00	0.74
		Digital	30.2 (10.5)	0.9	10.1	1.00	0.99	1.00		30.4 (10.4)	0.6	10.3	1.00	0.99	1.00	
T1		Manual	1.1 (1.4)	0.2	1.4	0.99	0.99	1.00	0.72	1.2 (1.3)	0.4	1.2	0.95	0.84	0.98	0.49
		Digital	1.2 (1.3)	0.2	1.1	0.98	0.94	0.99		1.0 (0.9)	0.2	1.0	0.98	0.95	0.99	
T0	Lower anterior	Manual	4.1 (4.0)	0.5	4.0	0.99	0.99	1.00	0.12	4.4 (4.2)	0.6	4.1	0.99	0.97	1.00	0.60
		Digital	4.4 (3.6)	0.2	3.5	1.00	0.99	1.00		4.5 (3.7)	0.4	3.7	0.99	0.98	1.00	
T1		Manual	0.3 (0.6)	0.0	0.6	1.00	-	-	0.16	0.3 (0.6)	0.0	0.6	1.00	-	-	0.16
		Digital	0.1 (0.3)	0.0	0.4	1.00	-	-		0.1 (0.3)	0.0	0.4	1.00	-	-	
T0	Upper anterior	Manual	6.1 (2.8)	0.6	2.6	0.97	0.92	0.99	0.45	6.3 (2.8)	0.7	2.6	0.98	0.93	0.99	0.50
		Digital	6.3 (2.8)	0.7	2.6	0.96	0.89	0.99		6.4 (2.7)	0.6	2.6	0.98	0.95	0.99	
T1		Manual	0.2 (0.4)	0.0	0.4	1.00	-	-	0.19	0.2 (0.4)	0.0	0.4	1.00	-	-	0.19
		Digital	0.3 (0.5)	0.1	0.5	1.00	-	-		0.3 (0.5)	0.1	0.5	1.00	-	-	
T0	Posterior	Manual	1.3 (1.5)	0.4	1.4	0.97	0.91	0.99	0.16	1.4 (1.5)	0.0	1.5	1.00	-	-	0.33
		Digital	1.5 (1.6)	0.0	1.6	1.00	-	-		1.5 (1.6)	0.0	1.6	1.00	-	-	
T1		Manual	0.2 (0.6)	0.2	0.6	0.95	0.84	0.98	0.67	0.2 (0.6)	0.0	0.6	1.00	-	-	-
		Digital	0.3 (0.6)	0.0	1.5	1.00	-	-		0.3 (0.6)	0.0	0.6	1.00	-	-	
T0	Overjet	Manual	12.0 (7.5)	0.0	7.5	1.00	-	-	-	12.0 (7.5)	0.0	7.5	1.00	-	-	-
		Digital	12.0 (7.5)	0.0	7.5	1.00	-	-		12.0 (7.5)	0.0	7.5	1.00	-	-	
T1		Manual	0.0 (0.0)	0.0	0.0	**	-	-	-	0.0 (0.0)	0.0	0.0	-	-	-	-
		Digital	0.0 (0.0)	0.0	0.0	**	-	-		0.0 (0.0)	0.0	0.0	-	-	-	
T0	Overbite	Manual	3.1 (1.8)	0.0	1.8	1.00	-	-	0.33	2.9 (1.9)	0.5	1.8	0.96	0.89	0.99	1.00
		Digital	3.0 (1.8)	0.4	1.8	0.98	0.94	0.99		2.9 (1.8)	0.0	1.8	1.00	-	-	
T1		Manual	0.3 (0.7)	0.5	0.7	1.00	-	-	-	0.3 (0.7)	0.0	0.7	1.00	-	-	-
		Digital	0.3 (0.7)	0.5	0.7	1.00	-	-		0.3 (0.7)	0.4	0.5	1.00	-	-	

Table 2. Cont.

PAR Index Scoring and Timepoint	Scoring Method	Rater I						Rater II					
		Mean (SD) [a]	Err. Method *,[a]	MSD [a]	ICC	[95% CI]	p-Value (Paired t-Test)	Mean (SD) [a]	Err. Method *,[a]	MSD [a]	ICC	[95% CI]	p-Value (Paired t-Test)
T0 Centerline	Manual	2.1 (3.0)	0.0	3.0	1.00	1.00 1.00	0.33	2.1 (3.0)	0.0	3.0	1.00	1.00 1.00	0.33
	Digital	2.0 (2.7)	0.8	2.6	0.96	0.89 0.99		1.9 (2.6)	0.0	2.6	1.00	- -	
T1 Centerline	Manual	0.0 (0.0)	0.0	0.0	**	-	-	0.0 (0.0)	0.0	0.0	-	-	-
	Digital	0.0 (0.0)	0.0	0.0	**	-		0.0 (0.0)	0.0	0.0	-	-	

* Error of the method according to Dahlberg's formula. ** ICC could not be calculated as all the scores for overjet and centerline were = 0. [a] Expressed in score points unit.

Table 3. Inter-rater variability (error of the method and Minimum Standard Deviation (MSD)) (using the second measurements) and reproducibility (ICC) according to time point and method. Paired sample t-tests comparing both raters.

PAR Index Scoring and Timepoint	Scoring Method	Rater I	Rater II		Rater I vs. II			
		Mean (SD) [a]	Mean (SD) [a]	Err. Method [a],*	MSD [a]	ICC	[95% CI]	p-Value (Paired t-Test)
Total PAR T0	Manual	29.6 (10.0)	30.3 (9.72)	1.8	10.3	0.99	1.00	0.20
	Digital	30.2 (10.2)	30.4 (10.2)	0.8	10.6	1.00	1.00	0.55
Total PAR T1	Manual	1.1 (1.4)	1.1 (1.4)	0.2	1.2	0.99	0.99	1.00
	Digital	1.1 (1.2)	1.0 (1.0)	0.4	1.0	0.98	0.99	0.26
Lower anterior T0	Manual	4.1 (4.0)	4.5 (4.4)	0.6	4.0	0.99	1.00	0.06
	Digital	4.4 (3.6)	4.5 (3.7)	0.7	3.5	0.99	0.99	0.64
Lower anterior T1	Manual	0.3 (0.6)	0.3 (0.4)	0.0	0.6	1.00	-	-
	Digital	0.0 (0.1)	0.1 (0.2)	0.0	0.3	1.00	-	-
Upper anterior T0	Manual	6.1 (2.8)	6.3 (2.8)	0.5	2.8	0.99	1.00	0.33
	Digital	6.4 (2.8)	6.4 (2.7)	0.6	2.7	0.99	1.00	0.38
Upper anterior T1	Manual	0.1 (0.3)	0.1 (0.2)	0.3	0.3	1.00	0.94	-
	Digital	0.4 (0.7)	0.1 (0.3)	0.6	0.3	1.00	0.96	-

Table 3. Cont.

PAR Index Scoring and Timepoint		Scoring Method	Rater I	Rater II			Rater I vs. II			
			Mean (SD) [a]	Mean (SD) [a]	Err. Method [a,*]	MSD [a]	ICC	[95% CI]		p-Value (Paired t-Test)
Posterior	T0	Manual	1.3 (1.4)	1.4 (1.5)	0.4	1.4	0.98	0.93	0.99	0.58
		Digital	1.5 (1.6)	1.5 (1.6)	0.0	1.6	1.00	-	-	-
	T1	Manual	0.2 (0.6)	0.2 (0.6)	0.0	0.6	0.99	0.96	0.99	0.33
		Digital	0.3 (0.6)	0.2 (0.6)	0.2	0.6	0.95	0.84	0.98	0.33
Overjet	T0	Manual	12 (7.5)	12 (7.5)	0.0	7.5	1.00	-	-	-
		Digital	12 (7.5)	12 (7.5)	0.0	7.5	1.00	-	-	-
	T1	Manual	0.0 (0.0)	0.0 (0.0)	0.0	0.0	** -	-	-	-
		Digital	0.0 (0.0)	0.0 (0.0)	0.0	0.0	** -	-	-	-
Overbite	T0	Manual	3.1 (1.8)	3.1 (1.8)	0.4	1.8	0.99	0.97	1.00	0.16
		Digital	3.1 (1.8)	2.9 (1.8)	0.4	1.8	0.97	0.92	0.99	0.67
	T1	Manual	0.3 (0.7)	0.3 (0.7)	0.0	0.5	1.00	-	-	-
		Digital	0.3 (0.7)	0.3 (0.7)	0.0	0.5	1.00	-	-	-
Centerline	T0	Manual	2.1 (3.0)	2.1 (3.0)	0.0	3.0	1.00	-	-	-
		Digital	2.1 (3.0)	1.8 (2.5)	0.8	2.6	0.99	0.97	1.00	0.33
	T1	Manual	0.0 (0.0)	0.0 (0.0)	0.0	0.0	** -	-	-	-
		Digital	0.0 (0.0)	0.0 (0.0)	0.0	0.0	** -	-	-	-

* Error of the method according to Dahlberg's formula, using the second measurements. ** ICC could not be calculated as all the scores for overjet and centerline were = 0. [a] Expressed in score points unit.

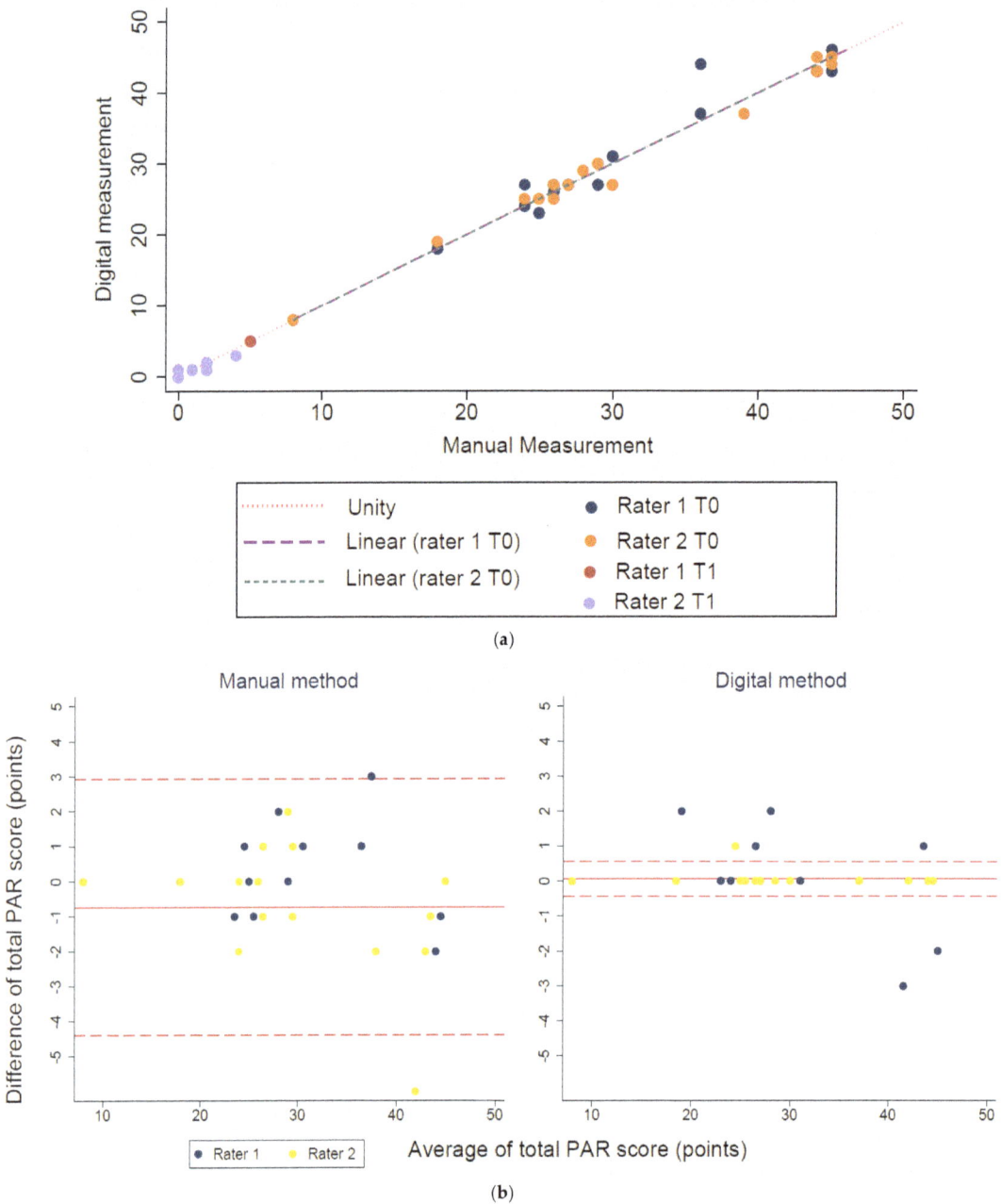

Figure 2. (**a**) Scatter plot of the total weighted PAR scores measured by both digital and manual methods and both raters, with a line of unity; (**b**) Bland-Altman plots: inter-rater agreement for the total PAR scores measured by the digital and manual PAR scoring methods at T0.

3.2. Reproducibility

ICC for the total PAR scores and the PAR components at both time points and for both methods fell in the 0.95–1.00 range for intra- and inter-rater reproducibility (Tables 2 and 3). All error-of-the-method values for the total PAR score and its components were smaller than the associated minimum standard deviation.

4. Discussion

Orthodontic model analysis is a prerequisite for diagnosis, evaluation of treatment need, treatment planning and analysis of treatment outcome. The present study assessed the validity and reproducibility of PAR index scoring for digital models and their printed model equivalents.

Digitization of plaster models (scanned-in) was introduced in the 1990s [33]. The advantages of digital models include the absence of physical storage requirements, instant accessibility, and no risk of breakage or wear [22,34]. The analysis of scanned-in models is as valid as that for plaster models [24]. However, over the last ten years, technology has evolved drastically, offering high image resolution of digital models and upgraded platforms needed for their analyses. Hence, intraoral scanning has gained popularity worldwide. Several studies have confirmed the accuracy of direct digital models to be as accurate as that of plaster models. Consequently, direct digital models are used as an alternative to conventional impression techniques and materials [35,36]. In the present study, we used the direct digital model technique.

Numerous intraoral scanners and software were developed over the last decade, with various diagnostic tools. In the present study, Ortho Analyzer software was used for scoring the digital models, and a digital caliper was used for scoring the printed models. Analyzing digital models can be associated with some concerns. The main concern with the use of digital software is, in fact, adjusting the visualization of a 3-D object on a two-dimensional screen. An appropriate evaluation requires a correct model orientation. For instance, in this study, cross bites were difficult to visualize, and rotation of the model was required to fully comprehend the magnitude of the cross bite. This problem was also reported by Stevens et al. [12]. In addition, segmentation of the dental crowns, which is an inevitable step to create a virtual setup before carrying out the scoring, is time-consuming. To ensure accurate tooth displacement measures, one should pay attention when placing the points, parallel to the occlusal plane, rotating the model adequately to facilitate good visualization of the contact points.

Another concern when dental measurements are performed on printed models, is the consideration of the printing technique and the model base design. Two studies [26,27] evaluated the accuracy of printed models acquired from intraoral scans. Brown et al. [26] compared plaster models with printed models using two types of 3-D printing techniques and concluded that both digital light processing (DLP) and polyjet printers produced clinically acceptable models. Camardella et al. [27] compared 3-D printed models with different base designs using two types of printing techniques and concluded that 3-D printed models from intraoral scans created with the polyjet printing technique were accurate, regardless of the model base design. By contrast, 3-D printed models with a horseshoe-shaped base design printed with a stereolithography printer showed a significant transversal (intra-arch distances) contraction, and a horseshoe-shaped base with a posterior connection bar was accurate compared with printed models with a regular base. Therefore, in the present study, a polyjet printing technique and regular model base designs were used to ensure accuracy.

Luqmani et al. [28] compared automated PAR scoring of direct and indirect digital models (CS 3600 software; Carestream Dental, Stuttgart, Germany) with manual scoring of plaster models using the PAR ruler. The authors found that manual PAR scoring was the most time-efficient, whereas indirect digital model scoring was the least time-efficient. The latter had minor dental cast faults that led to time-consuming software adjustments. However, automated scoring was more efficient than the software scoring used by Mayers et al. [23], which required operators to identify each relevant landmark. Hence, indirect scoring depends on the quality of the dental casts and can be time-consuming, depending on the software used. In the present study, PAR scoring was not possible as the software used (Ortho Analyzer) does not have the feature of automated scoring.

In the present study, the slightly higher reproducibility of PAR scoring for the digital method was not significant, with both methods proving to be highly reproducible. The high reproducibility of the manual method coincides with the results of Richmond et al. [7] The reproducibility and variability of the direct digital method were similar to the findings described by Luqmani et al. [28]. Furthermore, the limited variability between both methods demonstrated the high validity of the digital method compared with the conventional manual method, used as the gold standard.

5. Conclusions

PAR scoring on digital models using a software showed excellent reproducibility and presented good validity compared with manual scoring, considered as the gold standard.

Author Contributions: Conceptualization, A.G. and S.G.; Data curation, A.G.; Formal analysis, A.G.; Funding acquisition, M.A.C.; Supervision, P.M.C. and M.A.C.; Validation, A.G. and S.G.; Writing—original draft, A.G.; Writing—review & editing, A.G., S.G., M.D., P.M.C. and M.A.C. All authors have read and agreed to the published version of the manuscript.

Funding: This research was funded by Aarhus University Forskingsfond (AUFF), grant number 2432

Data Availability Statement: The data presented in this study are available on request from the corresponding author.

Acknowledgments: The authors express their gratitude to Dirk Leonhardt for his assistance in printing the models.

Conflicts of Interest: The authors declare no conflict of interest. The funders had no role in the design of the study; in the collection, analyses, or interpretation of data; in the writing of the manuscript, or in the decision to publish the results.

References

1. Gottlieb, E.L. Grading your orthodontic treatment results. *J. Clin. Orthod.* **1975**, *9*, 155–161.
2. Pangrazio-Kulbersh, V.; Kaczynski, R.; Shunock, M. Early treatment outcome assessed by the Peer Assessment Rating index. *Am. J. Orthod. Dentofac. Orthop.* **1999**, *115*, 544–550. [CrossRef]
3. Summers, C.J. The occlusal index: A system for identifying and scoring occlusal disorders. *Am. J. Orthod.* **1971**, *59*, 552–567. [CrossRef]
4. Brook, P.H.; Shaw, W.C. The development of an index of orthodontic treatment priority. *Eur. J. Orthod.* **1989**, *11*, 309–320. [CrossRef]
5. Daniels, C.; Richmond, S. The development of the index of complexity, outcome and need (ICON). *J. Orthod.* **2000**, *27*, 149–162. [CrossRef] [PubMed]
6. Casko, J.S.; Vaden, J.L.; Kokich, V.G.; Damone, J.; James, R.D.; Cangialosi, T.J.; Riolo, M.L.; Owens, S.E., Jr.; Bills, E.D. Objective grading system for dental casts and panoramic radiographs. American Board of Orthodontics. *Am. J. Orthod. Dentofacial Orthop.* **1998**, *114*, 589–599. [CrossRef]
7. Richmond, S.; Shaw, W.C.; O'Brien, K.D.; Buchanan, I.B.; Jones, R.; Stephens, C.D.; Roberts, C.T.; Andrews, M. The development of the PAR Index (Peer Assessment Rating): Reliability and validity. *Eur. J. Orthod.* **1992**, *14*, 125–139. [CrossRef] [PubMed]
8. Cons, N.C.; Jenny, J.; Kohout, F.J.; Songpaisan, Y.; Jotikastira, D. Utility of the dental aesthetic index in industrialized and developing countries. *J. Public Health Dent.* **1989**, *49*, 163–166. [CrossRef] [PubMed]
9. Richmond, S.; Shaw, W.C.; Roberts, C.T.; Andrews, M. The PAR Index (Peer Assessment Rating): Methods to determine outcome of orthodontic treatment in terms of improvement and standards. *Eur. J. Orthod.* **1992**, *14*, 180–187. [CrossRef]
10. DeGuzman, L.; Bahiraei, D.; Vig, K.W.; Vig, P.S.; Weyant, R.J.; O'Brien, K. The validation of the Peer Assessment Rating index for malocclusion severity and treatment difficulty. *Am. J. Orthod. Dentofac. Orthop.* **1995**, *107*, 172–176. [CrossRef]
11. Firestone, A.R.; Beck, F.M.; Beglin, F.M.; Vig, K.W. Evaluation of the peer assessment rating (PAR) index as an index of orthodontic treatment need. *Am. J. Orthod. Dentofac. Orthop.* **2002**, *122*, 463–469. [CrossRef]
12. Stevens, D.R.; Flores-Mir, C.; Nebbe, B.; Raboud, D.W.; Heo, G.; Major, P.W. Validity, reliability, and reproducibility of plaster vs digital study models: Comparison of peer assessment rating and Bolton analysis and their constituent measurements. *Am. J. Orthod. Dentofac. Orthop.* **2006**, *129*, 794–803. [CrossRef] [PubMed]

13. Zilberman, O.; Huggare, J.A.; Parikakis, K.A. Evaluation of the validity of tooth size and arch width measurements using conventional and three-dimensional virtual orthodontic models. *Angle Orthod.* **2003**, *73*, 301–306. [CrossRef] [PubMed]
14. Bichara, L.M.; Aragon, M.L.; Brandao, G.A.; Normando, D. Factors influencing orthodontic treatment time for non-surgical Class III malocclusion. *J. Appl. Oral Sci.* **2016**, *24*, 431–436. [CrossRef]
15. Chalabi, O.; Preston, C.B.; Al-Jewair, T.S.; Tabbaa, S. A comparison of orthodontic treatment outcomes using the Objective Grading System (OGS) and the Peer Assessment Rating (PAR) index. *Aust. Orthod. J.* **2015**, *31*, 157–164. [PubMed]
16. Dyken, R.A.; Sadowsky, P.L.; Hurst, D. Orthodontic outcomes assessment using the peer assessment rating index. *Angle Orthod.* **2001**, *71*, 164–169. [CrossRef]
17. Fink, D.F.; Smith, R.J. The duration of orthodontic treatment. *Am. J. Orthod. Dentofac. Orthop.* **1992**, *102*, 45–51. [CrossRef]
18. Ormiston, J.P.; Huang, G.J.; Little, R.M.; Decker, J.D.; Seuk, G.D. Retrospective analysis of long-term stable and unstable orthodontic treatment outcomes. *Am. J. Orthod. Dentofac. Orthop.* **2005**, *128*, 568–574. [CrossRef]
19. Pavlow, S.S.; McGorray, S.P.; Taylor, M.G.; Dolce, C.; King, G.J.; Wheeler, T.T. Effect of early treatment on stability of occlusion in patients with Class II malocclusion. *Am. J. Orthod. Dentofac. Orthop.* **2008**, *133*, 235–244. [CrossRef]
20. Garino, F.; Garino, G.B. Comparison of dental arch measurements between stone and digital casts. *Am. J. Orthod. Dentofac. Orthop.* **2002**, *3*, 250–254.
21. Mullen, S.R.; Martin, C.A.; Ngan, P.; Gladwin, M. Accuracy of space analysis with emodels and plaster models. *Am. J. Orthod. Dentofac. Orthop.* **2007**, *132*, 346–352. [CrossRef]
22. Rheude, B.; Sadowsky, P.L.; Ferriera, A.; Jacobson, A. An evaluation of the use of digital study models in orthodontic diagnosis and treatment planning. *Angle Orthod.* **2005**, *75*, 300–304. [CrossRef]
23. Mayers, M.; Firestone, A.R.; Rashid, R.; Vig, K.W. Comparison of peer assessment rating (PAR) index scores of plaster and computer-based digital models. *Am. J. Orthod. Dentofac. Orthop.* **2005**, *128*, 431–434. [CrossRef]
24. Abizadeh, N.; Moles, D.R.; O'Neill, J.; Noar, J.H. Digital versus plaster study models: How accurate and reproducible are they? *J. Orthod.* **2012**, *39*, 151–159. [CrossRef] [PubMed]
25. Dalstra, M.; Melsen, B. From alginate impressions to digital virtual models: Accuracy and reproducibility. *J. Orthod.* **2009**, *36*, 36–41. [CrossRef] [PubMed]
26. Brown, G.B.; Currier, G.F.; Kadioglu, O.; Kierl, J.P. Accuracy of 3-dimensional printed dental models reconstructed from digital intraoral impressions. *Am. J. Orthod. Dentofac. Orthop.* **2018**, *154*, 733–739. [CrossRef] [PubMed]
27. Camardella, L.T.; de Vasconcellos Vilella, O.; Breuning, H. Accuracy of printed dental models made with 2 prototype technologies and different designs of model bases. *Am. J. Orthod. Dentofac. Orthop.* **2017**, *151*, 1178–1187. [CrossRef]
28. Luqmani, S.; Jones, A.; Andiappan, M.; Cobourne, M.T. A comparison of conventional vs automated digital Peer Assessment Rating scoring using the Carestream 3600 scanner and CS Model+ software system: A randomized controlled trial. *Am. J. Orthod. Dentofac. Orthop.* **2020**, *157*, 148–155.e141. [CrossRef]
29. Walter, S.D.; Eliasziw, M.; Donner, A. Sample size and optimal designs for reliability studies. *Stat. Med.* **1998**, *17*, 101–110. [CrossRef]
30. Harris, P.A.; Taylor, R.; Minor, B.L.; Elliott, V.; Fernandez, M.; O'Neal, L.; McLeod, L.; Delacqua, G.; Delacqua, F.; Kirby, J.; et al. The REDCap consortium: Building an international community of software platform partners. *J. Biomed. Inform.* **2019**, *95*, 103208. [CrossRef]
31. Harris, P.A.; Taylor, R.; Thielke, R.; Payne, J.; Gonzalez, N.; Conde, J.G. Research electronic data capture (REDCap)—A metadata-driven methodology and workflow process for providing translational research informatics support. *J. Biomed. Inform.* **2009**, *42*, 377–381. [CrossRef] [PubMed]
32. Dahlberg, G. *Statistical Methods for Medical and Biological Students*; George Allen and Unwin: London, UK, 1940.
33. Joffe, L. Current Products and Practices OrthoCAD™: Digital models for a digital era. *J. Orthod.* **2004**, *31*, 344–347. [CrossRef] [PubMed]
34. McGuinness, N.J.; Stephens, C.D. Storage of orthodontic study models in hospital units in the U.K. *Br. J. Orthod.* **1992**, *19*, 227–232. [CrossRef] [PubMed]
35. Flügge, T.V.; Schlager, S.; Nelson, K.; Nahles, S.; Metzger, M.C. Precision of intraoral digital dental impressions with iTero and extraoral digitization with the iTero and a model scanner. *Am. J. Orthod. Dentofacial Orthop.* **2013**, *144*, 471–478. [CrossRef]
36. Grünheid, T.; McCarthy, S.D.; Larson, B.E. Clinical use of a direct chairside oral scanner: An assessment of accuracy, time, and patient acceptance. *Am. J. Orthod. Dentofac. Orthop.* **2014**, *146*, 673–682. [CrossRef] [PubMed]

Article

Incisor Occlusion Affects Profile Shape Variation in Middle-Aged Adults

Georgios Kanavakis [1,2,3,*], Anna-Sofia Silvola [3,4], Demetrios Halazonetis [5], Raija Lähdesmäki [3,4] and Pertti Pirttiniemi [3,4]

[1] Department of Pediatric Oral Health and Orthodontics, UZB-University Center for Dental Medicine, University of Basel, Mattenstrasse 40, CH-4058 Basel, Switzerland
[2] Department of Orthodontics and Dentofacial Orthopedics, Tufts University School of Dental Medicine, Boston, MA 02111, USA
[3] Oral Development and Orthodontics, Research Unit of Oral Health Sciences, Medical Faculty, University of Oulu, FI-90014 Oulu, Finland; anna-sofia.silvola@oulu.fi (A.-S.S.); raija.lahdesmaki@oulu.fi (R.L.); pertti.pirttiniemi@oulu.fi (P.P.)
[4] Oral and Maxillofacial Department, Oulu University Hospital, Medical Research Center Oulu (MRC Oulu), FI-90014 Oulu, Finland
[5] Department of Orthodontics, School of Dentistry, National and Kapodistrian University of Athens, GR-11527 Athens, Greece; dhal@dhal.com
* Correspondence: georgios.kanavakis@unibas.ch; Tel.: +41-(0)-61-267-26-15; Fax: +41-(0)-61-267-25-81

Abstract: Background: The aim of this study was to assess the effect of overjet and overbite on profile shape in middle–aged individuals. Methods: The study population comprised 1754 46-year-old individuals, members of the 1966 Northern Finland Birth Cohort. Their profile images were digitized using 48 landmarks and semi-landmarks. The subsequent landmark coordinates were then transformed to shape coordinates through Procrustes Superimposition, and final data were reduced into Principal Components (PCs) of shape. Overjet and overbite values were measured manually, during a clinical examination. A multivariate regression model was developed to evaluate the effect of overjet and overbite on profile shape. Results: The first nine PCs described more than 90% of profile shape variation in the sample and were used as the shape variables in all subsequent analyses. Overjet predicted 21.3% of profile shape in the entire sample (η^2overjet = 0.213; $p < 0.001$), while the effect of overbite was weaker (η^2overbite = 0.138; $p < 0.001$). In males, the equivalent effects were 22.6% for overjet and 14% for overbite, and in females, 25.5% and 13.5%, respectively. Conclusion: Incisor occlusion has a noteworthy effect on profile shape in middle-aged adults. Its impact becomes more significant taking into consideration the large variety of genetic and environmental factors affecting soft tissue profile.

Keywords: overjet; overbite; occlusion; profile shape; adults; morphometrics

1. Introduction

1.1. Background

Facial appearance is the strongest predictor of overall attractiveness and provides cues regarding health, personality, and psychosocial traits in humans [1]. An attractive face is perceived as trustworthy, competent, and intellectual, and is, thus, an important determinant of social, romantic, and professional interactions [2,3]. Sexual dimorphism, as reflected in the presence of masculine and feminine features, as well as facial averageness and symmetry, have been associated the most with facial attractiveness [1–3]. To a greater or lesser degree, the above factors are associated with the anatomy of individual facial features, such as the lips, eyes, and chin. The morphology of the lower facial third, in particular, contributes significantly to the variation in facial appearance among humans [4]. During adolescent growth and development, the effect of sexual hormones is largely expressed on the lower third of the face, with females exhibiting fuller lips and a less pronounced chin than males [5,6]. In adulthood, although sexual dimorphism tends to decline, facial changes continue to manifest in both sexes through flattening of the lips and an increase in nose length [7,8].

Orthodontists have historically been studying the human face as well as the underlying skeletal structures in order to observe normal variation and, most importantly, be able to predict physiologic transformation due to growth or changes caused by orthodontic treatment. There is a strong correlation between hard and soft tissue facial morphology [9] and, thus, it is expected that structural skeletal changes or positional dental changes will directly impact facial appearance. While the existing literature does confirm the influence of orthodontic treatment on soft tissues [10], the magnitude of this effect as well as its chronicity are a topic of discussion. Given that the lips are affected by orthodontic tooth movement the most, there is a lot of focus on lip responses to sagittal or vertical movements of the anterior dentition. These movements are commonly described as changes in overjet and overbite, which are defined as the sagittal/horizontal and the coronal/vertical distance between the upper and lower anterior teeth, respectively.

The amount of incisor retraction or proclination, the thickness and length of the upper lip, as well as its tonicity are the main factors linked to soft tissue treatment outcomes [11–15]. However, most of the current knowledge is based on data from adolescents or young adults. With the effect of aging on facial soft tissues, their relationship to the underlying teeth is expected to change. This, however, has not been studied sufficiently despite the fact that the percentage of adults who seek orthodontic treatment for esthetic reasons continues to increase. Previous reports have shown that there is an association between traditional linear and angular soft tissue measurements to overjet and overbite in mature adults [16]. Although these measurements are easier interpreted and more often used, they do not take the entire profile into consideration. Furthermore, they are largely dependent on size and therefore do not deliver accurate shape information [17].

1.2. Aim and Hypotheses

The aim of this study was to present a thorough assessment of the effect that overjet and overbite have on profile shape in a large, homogenous group of middle-aged adults. Our main hypothesis was that overjet and overbite explain a significant amount of profile shape variation. Secondarily, we hypothesized that profile shape alone can predict the severity of overjet and overbite in the present population.

2. Materials and Methods

2.1. Study Sample

Our sample comprised 1964 middle-aged adults, who were members of the Northern Finland Birth Cohort 1966 (NFBC1966). All of these individuals were born and have been living within a 100 km radius surrounding the city of Oulu in Northern Finland. At the age of 46, they volunteered to participate in a follow-up visit that included a series of clinical examinations. A detailed description of the NFBC1966 cohort can be found elsewhere [18]. Out of the initial population, the present study only included subjects whose clinical records were complete and of acceptable diagnostic value and who did not have any craniofacial deformities, syndromes, or a history of facial reconstructive surgery. These criteria were fulfilled by 1754 individuals (799 males and 955 females) who comprised the final study population. The research protocol was approved by the Ethical Committee of the Northern Ostrobothnia Hospital District on September 2011 (EETTMK#: 74/2011), and written consent was obtained from all volunteers prior to participation.

The clinical examination providing information regarding subjects' occlusal features was performed according to a previously reported protocol [19], and facial photographs were acquired in a standardized manner, as described elsewhere [16]. During the clinical examination, overjet and overbite were measured in millimeters using a manual caliper at the maximum intercuspation position of the mandible. Overjet was measured as the horizontal distance between the right maxillary incisor and the labial surface of its antagonist.

When the antagonist tooth was more anteriorly than the maxillary incisor (e.g., mandibular prognathism), a negative value was recorded. Overbite was measured as the vertical distance between the same teeth (vertical overlap) and was recorded as negative in cases of an anterior open bite [19]. Demographic information and clinical occlusal measurements were exported to an Excel worksheet (Microsoft Excel, Microsoft ©, Richmond WA, USA), and facial profile images were imported into Viewbox 4 software (version 4.1.0.1 BETA, dHAL Software, Kifissia, Greece) for processing and digitization.

2.2. Shape Analysis

To perform digitization, a template was created using the profile image of an individual who was not included in the study population. Facial profile shape was described with two curves (upper and lower facial curvature), encompassing 48 landmarks (4 fixed and 44 sliding semi-landmarks). The entire process was carried out by one research team member (GK), as previously described [20] (Figure S1). After the digitization process was completed, semi-landmarks were allowed to slide along their respective curve between the limits set by the fixed landmarks, in order to rearrange their position according to the average shape of the entire sample. This iterative process was repeated three times until the bending energy between individual samples and the average shape was minimized, and corresponding landmarks were more homogenous to each other [21,22]. Next, a General Procrustes Analysis (GPA) was performed in order to transform landmark space coordinates into shape coordinates (Figure S2), and a Principal Component Analysis (PCA) was used for data reduction and extraction of Principal Components (PCs) describing the shape variation within the population [23].

2.3. Statistical Analyses

The association between profile shape and occlusion was evaluated with multivariate regression models, assuming that overjet and overbite were the predictor variables and the shape PCs the dependent variables. In all analyses, shape information was provided by the first nine PCs, which described more than 90% of the variation in the sample. The decision to include the first nine PCs was based on the broken stick method [24].

An additional discriminant analysis was performed in the entire sample to investigate if profile shape alone could accurately identify the severity of overjet and overbite. The results of the discriminant analysis were cross-validated with the "leave one out" method. All statistical analyses were conducted with "ViewBox 4.1" software and IBM SPSS Statistics for Windows (Version 26.0. IBM, Armonk, NY: IBM Corp., 2020). The level of statistical significance was set at 0.05.

3. Results

3.1. Error of the Method

In order to assess the error of the method, 120 randomly selected profile images were digitized again by the same operator, after a period of two weeks, and the methodology described above was repeated. Systematic error was determined through permutation tests (100,000 permutations) to calculate the Procrustes' distance between digitizations performed at those time points and was found to be not statistically significant ($p = 0.915$). Random error, related to the digitization process, was determined as a percentage of total variance in shape space, as explained by PC1-PC9. This resulted in a low random error of 4.6%.

3.2. Shape Variation

Shape variation in the present sample has been previously described in detail [20]. The first four PCs explained more than 70% of profile shape variation (PC1: 33.1%, PC2: 23.1%, PC3: 11%, and PC4: 6.7%), while the first nine PCs collectively explained more than 90% of variation. As seen in Figure 1a–d, males and females in the present sample presented a significant difference in profile shape, which was more evident in the axis of PC3 (Figure 1d). Due to this significant dimorphism in facial morphology between sexes, and because a statistically significant difference in overjet was found between sexes (Supplementary Table S1), assessments were also performed separately for males and females.

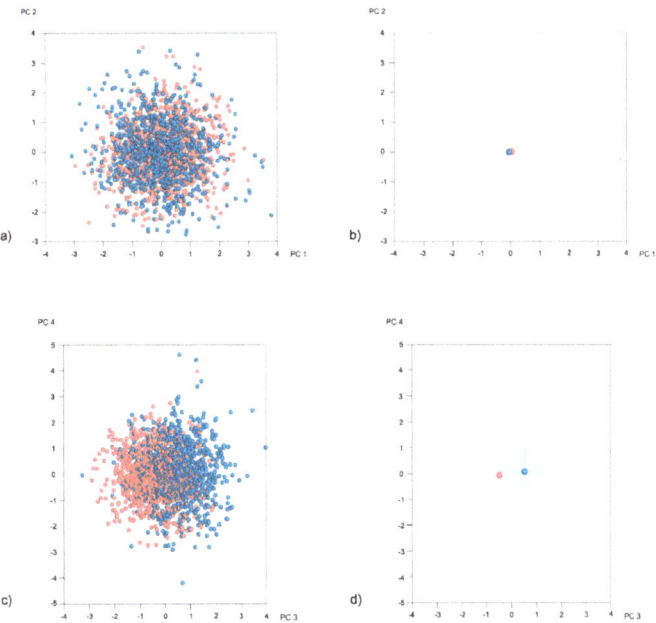

Figure 1. (**a**) Principal Component Analysis (PCA) graph displaying facial variation according to sex (in SD units), in the entire sample, as explained by PC1 (33.1%) and PC2 (23.1%) (Females: light red, Males: blue). (**b**) Average male (blue) and average female (light red) shape with respective SDs, as described by PC1 and PC2. (**c**) PCA graph displaying facial variation according to sex (in SD units), in the entire sample, as explained by PC3 (11%) and PC2 (6.7%) (Females: light red, Males: blue). (**d**) Average male (blue) and average female (light red) shape with respective SDs, as described by PC3 and PC4.

3.3. Profile Shape and Anterior Occlusion

For the entire sample, the multivariate regression model showed a statistically significant but weak effect of overjet and overbite on profile shape ($\eta^2_{overjet}$ = 0.213; $p < 0.001 / \eta^2_{overbite}$ = 0.138; $p < 0.001$). The strength of the effects remained low when the association between overjet, overbite, and profile shape was assessed separately in males and females (Table 1).

Table 1. Effect of overjet and overbite on profile shape, as explained by PC1-PC9.

	N	Predictor	η^2	p-Value
Entire Sample	1754	Overjet	0.213	<0.001
		Overbite	0.138	
Males	799	Overjet	0.226	
		Overbite	0.140	
Females	955	Overjet	0.255	
		Overbite	0.135	

In order to explore if these effects were associated with facial changes explained by specific PCs, between-subjects' effect sizes were also assessed and are presented in Supplementary Table S2. However, they did not reveal any PCs that were more significantly related to overjet and overbite values. These individual effects on the first four PCs (explaining more than 70% variation) are also displayed in Figure 2.

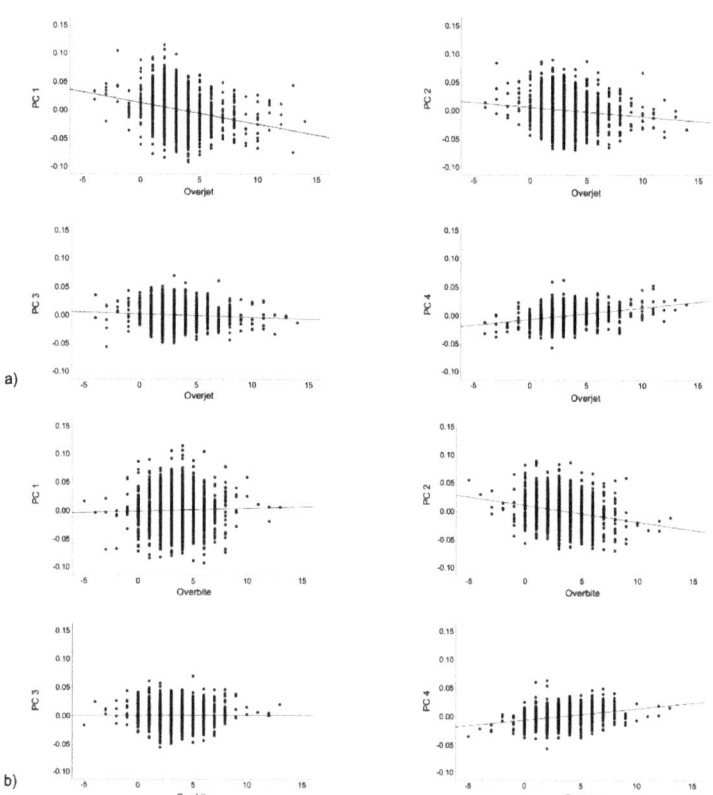

Figure 2. Association between overjet (**a**) and overbite (**b**) and the first primary PCs, explaining >70% of the sample variability.

In order to visualize profile shape as related to overjet and overbite, the shape information provided by the PCs was used to create profile morphings, representing extreme negative and extreme positive overjet and overbite values (Figure 3). Upon observation of these morphings, it is evident that maximal positive overjet values were associated with a convex profile, a pronounced upper lip, a deep mentolabial sulcus, and a retruded mandible. Subjects with negative overjet values presented a retrusive upper lip, a straighter profile, and a shallow labiomental sulcus. According to the amount and direction of shape variation depicted in the upper-middle morphing on Figure 3, differences in profile shape were primarily related to changes in the position of the upper lip. Extreme positive overbite values (deep bites) were associated with a reduced vertical dimension of the lower facial third and a deep mentolabial sulcus, while negative overbite (open bites) presented with an increased lower facial third and a straight profile. Shape variation, as related to overbite values, was mainly a result of lower lip projection and straightening of the mentolabial curve.

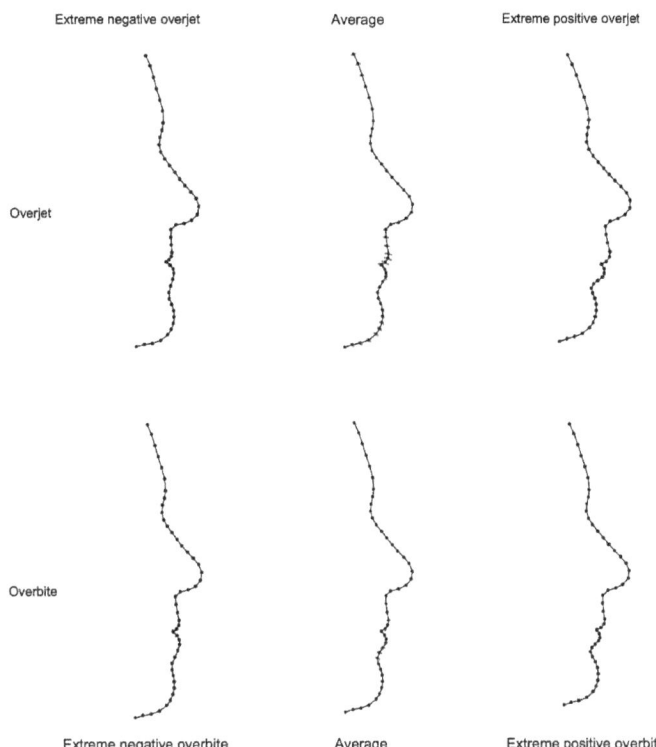

Figure 3. Profile morphings according to overjet (top row) and overbite (bottom row). The middle column depicts the average facial shape of the entire sample, as well as the amount and direction of variation at each profile landmark (blue: positive, red: negative), as explained by overjet (top row) and overbite (bottom row) values. On each row, the images left and right of the average present profile shapes of extreme overjet (top) and overbite (bottom) values.

The finding of a weak but statistically significant effect of overjet and overbite on profile shape indicates a significant association but a low predictive value for these factors. In order to further assess this relationship, a discriminant analysis with cross validation was conducted to determine if profile shape could predict the severity of overjet or overbite of a subject within the sample. For the purpose of this analysis, the sample was divided into groups according to the severity of overjet and overbite, as presented in Table 2. The results show that profile shape was not able to accurately predict if an individual presented with extreme (positive or negative) values of overjet or overbite. There was a tendency of subjects being classified on the basis of their profile as having a normal overjet and overbite, confirming the weak effect of the occlusal variables on profile shape.

Table 2. Discriminant analysis of the predictive value of profile shape on severity of overjet and overbite.

Predictors			N	Predicted Group			Predictive Percentage
				Negative	Normal	Excessive	
PC1—PC9	Overjet groups	Negative (≤0 mm)	64	3	61	0	4.7%
		Normal (1–5 mm)	1530	4	1509	17	98.6%
		Excessive (>5 mm)	160	0	144	16	10.0%
	Overbite groups	Negative (≤0 mm)	92	1	91	0	1.1%
		Normal (1–5 mm)	1454	2	1440	12	99.0%
		Excessive (>5 mm)	208	0	193	15	7.2%

4. Discussion

This investigation assesses the amount of profile shape variation explained by overbite and overjet in a large population of middle-aged adults who all had the same exact age and ethnic identity. Due to these baseline characteristics, environmental and ethnic effects are less likely to have had an effect on the results.

The clinical importance of the study lies in that there are unique facial features seen in more mature adults, primarily a flattening of the lips and a larger nose projection [23,25], which significantly differentiate their appearance to the one of younger individuals. In recent years, there has been a steep increase in adults seeking orthodontic care, primarily to address their esthetic concerns. However, due to the aging process, the esthetic principles that are used for the treatment of adolescents and young adults mostly do not apply to middle–aged adults.

Here, we show the effect of overjet and overbite on the profile shape of middle-aged individuals. Overjet alone predicted 21.3% of profile shape variation in the entire sample, while the effect of overbite was 13.8%. These results allow us to accept our main study hypothesis. Similar findings were revealed when males and females were examined separately. Statistically these effects were significant but weak. Thus, as an isolated observation this is not in line with the notion that occlusion strongly affects facial profile, which is well-documented in growing individuals and young adults [26]. However, considering that facial profile is influenced by a large variety of factors, including the skeletal pattern and the genetically determined characteristics of the soft tissues, the present findings have a meaningful biological significance. They show that anterior occlusion, although primarily determined by tooth relationships, has a broader contribution to facial appearance. Halazonetis [9] conducted a similar study associating dentoskeletal structures to soft tissue profile shape in growing individuals and reported that the former were able to predict approximately 50% of shape variation. From a biological point of view, the dentoskeletal structures used as predictors in that study would certainly be expected to have had a larger impact on facial profile compared to overjet and overbite alone. However, overjet and overbite are also related to the overall skeletal pattern, with hyperdivergent individuals, for example, presenting greater percentages of anterior open bites. This association between skeletal pattern and incisor occlusion might partly explain their impact on facial profile. It can be speculated that if in this study we had also included more dentoskeletal variables in our analyses, we would have probably found a larger effect. However, our aim was to focus on the relationship of the anterior dentition, it being the main feature contributing to smile esthetics and to the successful outcome of orthodontic treatment.

Moreno et al. also explored profile variability in adult populations by investigating subjects with moderate to severe Class II and Class III malocclusions [27,28]. Both of these studies used cephalometric images of non-growing individuals and performed a principal component analysis to identify patterns of craniofacial morphology. In the Class

II sample [27], including subjects with an overjet greater than 4 mm, they showed that 33% variation was explained by PCs related to overjet. In the Class III sample [28], including subjects with a negative overjet, approximately 34% of the phenotypic variation was explained by PCs related to incisor relationship. Both of these studies only examined cases with severe malocclusions and included a broad age spectrum of non-growing individuals, ranging between 16 and 60 years. Due to these differences, they are not directly comparable to the present study evaluating a large sample from the general population at 46 years of age. However, it is evident that the relationship of the anterior teeth described a similar percentage of phenotypic variability to the one reported here. The difference may be attributed to the fact that Moreno et al. only included cases with malocclusions.

Our results imply that it would be incorrect to undervalue the importance of obtaining optimal incisor occlusion in the treatment of older orthodontic patients. Indeed, overjet and overbite might not have a strong effect on the shape of the entire profile, but they do affect the position of the lips [11,16,29,30]. The profile morphings created in regard to overjet and overbite values of the present study population show that the largest variability in profile shape was related to the position of the upper lip (Figure 3). This finding is in agreement with the literature supporting that orthodontic repositioning of the anterior dentition has a measurable effect on the lips. Primarily in non-growing patients, where the effect of growth decreases significantly, the lips are likely the only facial structures that orthodontic treatment can impact. As presented here and in previous reports [11,16], this is particularly true for the upper lip.

In order to conduct a thorough assessment of our study aim, a discriminant analysis was also performed to reverse our initial assumption and evaluate the predictive value of profile pictures in determining anterior occlusal relationships. Interestingly, in our sample, facial profile alone was not able to predict overjet or overbite, even in extreme cases; only 10% of cases with an overjet larger than 5 mm could be correctly identified using the shape information provided by the shape PCs. This question has not been adequately addressed in the current literature. There is one study by Staudt and Kiliaridis [31] exploring the relationship between soft tissue profile and severity of Class III malocclusion in adults, showing that angular measurements on profile images may predict the underlying skeletal pattern but only in moderate to severe cases. However, their study is not comparable to the present one, because the sample only comprised individuals with a previous diagnosis of Class III malocclusion and thus was not representative of the general population. In our sample, the prevalence of negative overjet was low (64 out of 1754) and there were only a few cases with an overjet smaller than -2 mm (12 out of 64). The low predictive value, as shown here, of the entire profile shape even in severe overjet and overbite cases also implies that although there might be a significant impact of anterior occlusion on soft tissue profile, this impact is not strong enough to create a distinct phenotypic differentiation between individuals.

5. Conclusions

This study shows that overjet and overbite have a weak but significant impact on facial profile in middle-aged adults of Northern European descent. The upper lip displayed the largest amount of variation as related to severity of overjet. Overbite differences had a marginal effect on overall profile shape. These findings need to be interpreted within the context of our study population, which represented the general population of the particular geographic region and did not comprise individuals seeking orthodontic care. In addition, it was shown that profile shape was not able to predict anterior occlusion, and this was also evident in severe cases of excessive overjet and overbite values.

Supplementary Materials: The following are available online at https://www.mdpi.com/2077-038 3/10/4/800/s1, Table S1: Comparison between males and females in overjet and overbite. Table S2: Between-subjects effect of overjet and overbite on profile shape variation, as explained by PC1-PC9. Figure S1: Schematic of the digitization process. Figure S2: Procrustes Superimposition.

Author Contributions: Conceptualization, G.K., R.L. and P.P.; Data curation, G.K. and A.-S.S.; Formal analysis, G.K.; Investigation, G.K.; Methodology, G.K., D.H.; Resources, A.-S.S., R.L., and P.P.; Software, D.H.; Supervision, P.P.; Validation, G.K., D.H., R.L. and P.P.; Visualization, G.K. and D.H.; Writing—original draft, G.K.; Writing—review and editing, G.K., A.-S.S., D.H., R.L. and P.P. All authors have read and agreed to the published version of the manuscript.

Funding: NFBC1966 received financial support from University of Oulu Grant no. 24000692, Oulu University Hospital Grant no. 24301140, ERDF European Regional Development Fund Grant no. 539/2010 A31592.

Institutional Review Board Statement: The study was conducted according to the guidelines of the Declaration of Helsinki, and approved by the Ethical Committee of the Northern Ostrobothnia Hospital District on September 2011 (EETTMK#: 74/2011).

Informed Consent Statement: Written informed consent was obtained from all subjects involved in the study.

Data Availability Statement: NFBC data are available from the University of Oulu, Infrastructure for Population Studies. Permission to use the data can be applied for research purposes via electronic material request portal. In the use of data, we follow the EU general data protection regulation (679/2016) and Finnish Data Protection Act. The use of personal data is based on cohort participant's written informed consent at his or her latest follow–up study, which may cause limitations to its use. Please contact NFBC project center (NFBCprojectcenter@oulu.fi) and visit the cohort website (www.oulu.fi/nfbc (accessed on 16 February 2021)) for more information.

Acknowledgments: We thank all cohort members and researchers who participated in the 46-years study. We also wish to acknowledge the work of the NFBC project center.

Conflicts of Interest: Demetrios Halazonetis owns stock in dHAL Software, the company that markets Viewbox 4. The other authors declare no conflict of interest.

References

1. Little, A.C.; Jones, B.C.; DeBruine, L.M. Facial attractiveness: Evolutionary based research. *Philos. Trans. R. Soc. Lond. B Biol. Sci.* **2011**, *366*, 1638–1659. [CrossRef]
2. Grammer, K.; Fink, B.; Moller, A.P.; Thornhill, R. Darwinian aesthetics: Sexual selection and the biology of beauty. *Biol. Rev.* **2003**, *78*, 385–407. [CrossRef]
3. Gangestad, S.W.; Scheyd, G.J.; Scheyd, G.J. The Evolution of Human Physical Attractiveness. *Annu. Rev. Anthropol.* **2005**, *34*, 523–548. [CrossRef]
4. Claes, P.; Roosenboom, J.; White, J.D.; Swigut, T.; Sero, D.; Li, J.; Lee, M.K.; Zaidi, A.; Mattern, B.C.; Liebowitz, C.; et al. Genome-wide mapping of global-to-local genetic effects on human facial shape. *Nat. Genet.* **2018**, 1–16. [CrossRef]
5. Probst, F.; Bobst, C.; Lobmaier, J.S. Testosterone-to-oestradiol ratio is associated with female facial attractiveness. *Q. J. Ex. Psychol.* **2015**, *69*, 89–99. [CrossRef] [PubMed]
6. Penton-Voak, I.S.; Chen, J.Y. High salivary testosterone is linked to masculine male facial appearance in humans. *Evol. Hum. Behav.* **2004**, *25*, 229–241. [CrossRef]
7. Windhager, S.; Mitteroecker, P.; Rupi, I.; Lauc, T.; Polašek, O.; Schaefer, K. Facial aging trajectories: A common shape pattern in male and female faces is disrupted after menopause. *Am. J. Phys. Anthropol.* **2019**, *172*, 1–11. [CrossRef] [PubMed]
8. Shaw, R.B.; Kahn, D.M. Aging of the Mandible and Its Aesthetic Implications. *Plast. Reconstr. Surg.* **2010**, *125*, 332–342. [CrossRef]
9. Halazonetis, D.J. Morphometric correlation between facial soft-tissue profile shape and skeletal pattern in children and adolescents. *Am. J. Orthod. Dentofacial Orthop.* **2007**, *132*, 450–457. [CrossRef]
10. Konstantonis, D.; Vasileiou, D.; Papageorgiou, S.N.; Eliades, T. Soft tissue changes following extraction vs. nonextraction orthodontic fixed appliance treatment: A systematic review and meta-analysis. *Eur. J. Oral Sci.* **2018**, *126*, 167–179. [CrossRef]
11. Alkadhi, R.M.; Finkelman, M.D.; Trotman, C.A.; Kanavakis, G. The role of lip thickness in upper lip response to sagittal change of incisor position. *Orthod. Craniofac. Res.* **2019**, *22*, 53–57. [CrossRef] [PubMed]
12. Rains, M.D.; Nanda, R. Soft-tissue changes associated with maxillary incisor retraction. *Am. J. Orthod.* **1982**, *81*, 481–488. [CrossRef]
13. Talass, M.F.; Tollaae, L.; Baker, R.C. Soft-tissue profile changes resulting from retraction of maxillary incisors. *Am. J. Orthod. Dentofacial Orthop.* **1987**, *91*, 385–394. [CrossRef]
14. Kuhn, M.; Markic, G.; Doulis, I.; Göllner, P.; Patcas, R.; Hänggi, M.P. Effect of different incisor movements on the soft tissue profile measured in reference to a rough-surfaced palatal implant. *Am. J. Orthod. Dentofacial Orthop.* **2016**, *149*, 349–357. [CrossRef]
15. Yogosawa, F. Predicting soft tissue profile changes concurrent with orthodontic treatment. *Angle Orthod.* **1990**, *60*, 199–206.
16. Kanavakis, G.; Krooks, L.; Lähdesmäki, R.; Pirttiniemi, P. Influence of overjet and overbite on soft tissue profile in mature adults: A cross-sectional population study. *Am. J. Orthod. Dentofacial Orthop.* **2019**, *155*, 57–63.e3. [CrossRef]

7. Adams, D.C.; Rohlf, J.F.; Slice, D.E. A field comes of age: Geometric morphometrics in the 21st century. *Hystrix Ital. J. Mammal.* **2013**, *24*, 1–8.
8. University of Oulu: Northern Finland Birth Cohort 1966. University of Oulu. Available online: http://urn.fi/urn:nbn:fi:att:bc1e5408-980e-4a62-b899-43bec3755243 (accessed on 14 February 2021).
9. Krooks, L.; Pirttiniemi, P.; Kanavakis, G.; Lähdesmäki, R. Prevalence of malocclusion traits and orthodontic treatment in a Finnish adult population. *Acta Odontol. Scan.* **2016**, *74*, 362–367. [CrossRef]
10. Kanavakis, G.; Silvola, A.-S.; Halazonetis, D.; Lähdesmäki, R.; Pirttiniemi, P. Facial shape variation in middle-aged northern Europeans. *Eur. J. Orthod.* **2021**. [CrossRef]
11. Bookstein, F.L. Landmark methods for forms without landmarks: Morphometrics of group differences in outline shape. *Med. Image Anal.* **1997**, *1*, 225–243. [CrossRef]
12. Rohlf, F.J.; Slice, D. Extensions of the Procrustes Method for the Optimal Superimposition of Landmarks. *Syst. Zool.* **1990**, *39*, 40. [CrossRef]
13. Behrents, R. *Growth in the Aging Craniofacial Skelton*; Craniofacial Growth Series; Center of Human Growth and Development University of Michigan: An Arbor, MI, USA, 1985.
14. Peres-Neto, P.; Jackson, D.; Somers, K. How many principal components? Stopping rules for determining the number of non-trivial axes revisited. *Comput. Stat. Data Anal.* **2005**, *49*, 974–997. [CrossRef]
15. Robertson, J.M.; Kingsley, B.E.; Ford, G.C. Sexually Dimorphic Faciometrics in Humans from Early Adulthood to Late Middle Age: Dynamic, Declining, and Differentiated. *Evol. Psychol.* **2017**, *15*. [CrossRef] [PubMed]
16. Cozza, P.; Baccetti, T.; Franchi, L.; De Toffol, L.; McNamara, J.A. Mandibular changes produced by functional appliances in Class II malocclusion: A systematic review. *Am. J. Orthod. Dentofacial Orthop.* **2006**, *129*, 599.e1–599.e12. [CrossRef] [PubMed]
17. Moreno Uribe, L.M.; Miller, S.F. Phenotypic diversity in white adults with moderate to severe Class II malocclusion. *Am. J. Orthod. Dentofacial Orthop.* **2014**, *145*, 305–316. [CrossRef]
18. Moreno Uribe, L.M.; Vela, K.C.; Kummet, C.; Dawson, D.V.; Southard, T.E. Phenotypic diversity in white adults with moderate to severe Class III malocclusion. *Am. J. Orthod. Dentofacial Orthop.* **2013**, *144*, 32–42. [CrossRef]
19. Bittner, C.; Pancherz, H. Facial morphology and malocclusions. *Am. J. Orthod. Dentofacial Orthop.* **1990**, *97*, 308–315. [CrossRef]
20. Arnett, G.W.; Bergman, R.T. Facial keys to orthodontic diagnosis and treatment planning—Part II. *Am. J. Orthod. Dentofacial Orthop.* **2012**, *103*, 395–411. [CrossRef]
21. Staudt, C.B.; Kiliaridis, S. A nonradiographic approach to detect Class III skeletal discrepancies. *Am. J. Orthod. Dentofacial Orthop.* **2009**, *136*, 52–58. [CrossRef]

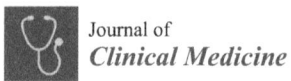

Article

Skeletal Changes in Growing Cleft Patients with Class III Malocclusion Treated with Bone Anchored Maxillary Protraction—A 3.5-Year Follow-Up

Ralph M. Steegman [1], Annemarlien Faye Klein Meulekamp [1], Arjan Dieters [1], Johan Jansma [2], Wicher J. van der Meer [1] and Yijin Ren [3],*

1. Department of Orthodontics, University of Groningen, University Medical Center Groningen, 9713 GZ Groningen, The Netherlands; r.m.steegman@umcg.nl (R.M.S.); a.f.klein.meulekamp@umcg.nl (A.F.K.M.); j.a.dieters@umcg.nl (A.D.); w.j.van.der.meer@umcg.nl (W.J.v.d.M.)
2. Department of Oral Maxillofacial Surgery, University of Groningen, University Medical Center Groningen, 9713 GZ Groningen, The Netherlands; j.jansma@umcg.nl
3. Department of Orthodontics, W.J. Kolff Institute, University of Groningen, University Medical Center Groningen, 9713 GZ Groningen, The Netherlands
* Correspondence: y.ren@umcg.nl

Abstract: This prospective controlled trial aimed to evaluate the skeletal effect of 3.5-years bone anchored maxillary protraction (BAMP) in growing cleft subjects with a Class III malocclusion. Subjects and Method: Nineteen cleft patients (11.4 ± 0.7-years) were included from whom cone beam computed tomography (CBCT) scans were taken before the start of BAMP (T0), 1.5-years after (T1) and 3.5 y after (T2). Seventeen age- and malocclusion-matched, untreated cleft subjects with cephalograms available at T0 and T2 served as the control group. Three dimensional skeletal changes were measured qualitatively and quantitatively on CBCT scans. Two dimensional measurements were made on cephalograms. Results: Significant positive effects have been observed on the zygomaticomaxillary complex. Specifically, the A-point showed a displacement of 2.7 mm ± 0.9 mm from T0 to T2 ($p < 0.05$). A displacement of 3.8 mm ± 1.2 mm was observed in the zygoma regions ($p < 0.05$). On the cephalograms significant differences at T2 were observed between the BAMP and the control subjects in Wits, gonial angle, and overjet ($p < 0.05$), all in favor of the treatment of Class III malocclusion. The changes taking place in the two consecutive periods (ΔT1-T0, ΔT2-T1) did not differ, indicating that not only were the positive results from the first 1.5-years maintained, but continuous orthopedic effects were also achieved in the following 2-years. Conclusions: In conclusion, findings from the present prospective study with a 3.5-years follow-up provide the first evidence to support BAMP as an effective and reliable treatment option for growing cleft subjects with mild to moderate Class III malocclusion up to 15-years old.

Keywords: bone anchored; maxillofacial protraction; color mapping; 3D superimposition; cleft; orthodontics; class III malocclusion; CBCT; orthopedic therapy

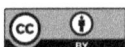

1. Introduction

Children born with cleft lip and palate (CLP) are usually characterized by a Class III malocclusion, which is primarily the result of maxillary deficiency. Maxillary deficiency in growing subjects, when left untreated, can lead to severe functional, aesthetic, breathing and psychological problems [1–6]. Important treatment goals in cleft patients are to establish a normal dental occlusion and to correct the skeletal discrepancy for psychological and functional well-being [7–10].

Currently, the most common orthopedic treatment in both cleft and non-cleft patients with a Class III malocclusion is facemask therapy (FM) with or without rapid maxillary expansion (RME). This tooth-borne treatment modality, often used in patients with early deciduous or early mixed dentition [11,12], has been reported to have undesirable side effects such as dentoalveolar compensation and a clockwise rotation of the mandible [13,14]. These side effects are caused by the induced orthopedic force, which is not transferred directly to the circum-maxillary sutures, but directly or partially on the dentition.

Bone anchored maxillary protraction (BAMP) is an increasingly used treatment modality in cleft patients with Class III malocclusion and can be started in the late mixed- or early permanent-dentition [15]. Previous studies reported positive outcomes on 1.5-years BAMP-treatment in growing CLP subjects with Class III malocclusion. Significant orthopedic changes were observed in the maxillary and zygomatic areas, in addition to the favorable dentofacial aesthetic changes [16,17]. A unique advantage of BAMP, compared to other conventional treatment modalities for Class III malocclusion, is that it transfers forces from bony structures directly onto the sutural sites of the zygomaticomaxillary complex. With this, the treatment effect achieved is mainly skeletal orthopedic with minimal undesirable dental compensation [18]. Additional advantages of BAMP over FM are the continuous light forces used rather than heavy intermittent forces and the lower degree of burden for the patient in terms of compliance. However, it remains to be seen whether the positive results of the first 1.5-years will persist, and whether more orthopedic gains can be achieved when patients reach the end of their growth spurt.

As BAMP treatment is a relatively new technique, little is known about its long-term clinical effects. To date, no results of BAMP treatment in cleft subjects longer than 1.5 y have been reported in literature. The aim of this prospective controlled trial is to investigate the 3D skeletal effect after 3.5 y of BAMP treatment in growing cleft patients using cone beam computed tomography (CBCT) scans.

2. Subjects and Methods

2.1. Trial Registration and Ethical Approval

This prospective controlled trial is registered at The Netherlands National Trial Registration (TC 6559) and at the Clinical Study Register of the University Medical Center Groningen (201700423). Ethical approval has been granted by the Ethics Committee at the UMCG (METc 2018/318).

2.2. Treatment and Control Subjects

A power analysis on the minimal number of subjects needed to detect a difference between the BAMP and the control group at T2 (3.5 y), with a power of 80% and $p < 0.05$, showed that 11 participants were needed to detect a difference on A-point Region of Interest (ROI) from CBCT surface models, and 17 participants to detect a difference on ANB angle from cephalograms. Therefore, the minimal number of subjects per group was set at 17 for the present study. Twenty-three consecutively treated cleft patients were included in the study. All 23 patients have undergone a series of interdisciplinary treatments at the University Medical Center Groningen (UMCG) in the Netherlands under the same set of protocols. Orthodontic treatment was performed by the same orthodontist (Y.R.) for all subjects at the Department of Orthodontics. Bollard bone plates were inserted by the same oral surgeon (J.J.) at the Department of Oral and Maxillofacial Surgery. The inclusion criteria were the same as in our previous study [16], namely: (1) either a complete unilateral cleft lip, palate, or both; (2) either a sagittal overjet between +2 and −5 mm, an ANB angle $<0°$, or both, or a Wits <0 mm; (3) a secondary bone transplantation prior to BAMP; (4) no or light dental alignment in the upper arch in preparation for bone transplantation, prior to BAMP; (5) both lower permanent canines have been erupted; and (6) no forced overclosure or functional shift present. From all study subjects an informed consent was obtained.

Due to ethical reasons, no CBCT scans from untreated cleft subjects could be obtained. Instead, 2D cephalograms were included from an age- and malocclusion-matched cleft lip and palate group at T0 and T2. This control group was derived from the clinical database of the Department of Orthodontics of the UMCG. All subjects signed an informed consent for the use of their X-ray photos and clinical photos for research purposes. Inclusion criteria for the control group were the same as the BAMP group except that the eruption status of the lower permanent canines was not used as a criterion.

Of the 23 initially included cleft lip and palate patients, four had to be excluded from data analysis due to CBCT acquisition errors. The age of the 19 included study subjects was 11.4 ± 0.7 y at T0. For the control group, a total of 17 patients were included who met the inclusion criteria. The mean age of the control subjects was 10.7 ± 1.2 y at T0. With regard to the protocol of wearing the elastics, a high degree of compliance was recorded for all subjects based on self-report. In 7 patients a removable bite plate was used to temporarily remove the occlusal interference.

2.3. Bone Anchored Maxillary Protraction

According to the published protocol, four Bollard bone plates (Bollard, Tita-Link, Brussels, Belgium) were placed under general anesthesia at the age of about 11 [16,17]. Two Bollard bone plates were placed onto the zygomatic buttresses and two on the anterior part of the mandible between the lateral incisor and canine. Three weeks after the placement, maxillary protraction started with intermaxillary elastics with a force of about 150 g in the first month followed by a force of 200–250 g after 2–3 months (Figure 1). Patients were instructed to wear the elastics for 24 h per day, 7 d a week, including meals, and to replace the elastics once a day.

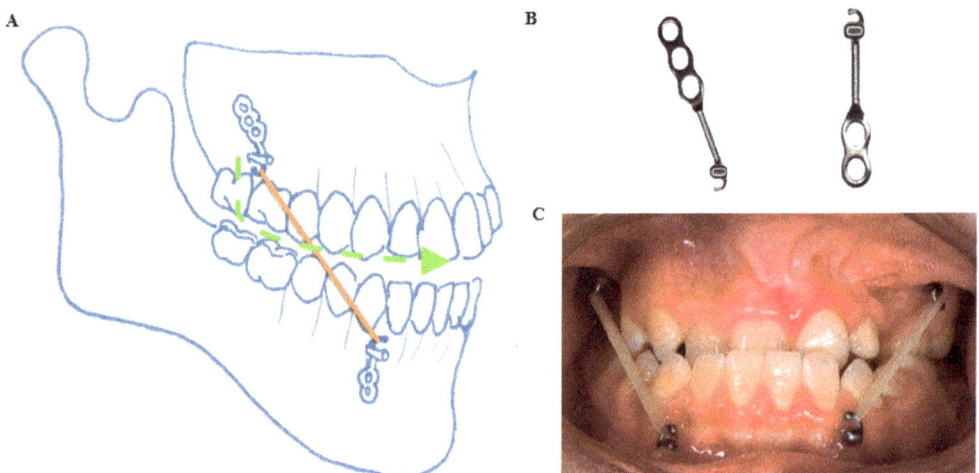

Figure 1. Bollard bone plates used in the present study for bone anchored maxillary protraction. (**A**) A schematic representation of the locations of the Bollard bone plates. (**B**) Bollard bone plates, left for the upper, right for the lower. (**C**) An intra-oral picture of bone anchored maxillary protraction with intermaxillary elastics.

2.4. CBCT Scans

All cone beam computed tomography (CBCT) scans were made by the same experienced X-ray technician (A.D.), before the start of BAMP as part of a standardized documentation for diagnostic purposes (T0), 1.5 y after BAMP (T1) and 3.5 y after BAMP treatment (T2). The exact timing of all scans was aligned as much as possible to the need for a CBCT scan for diagnostic purposes or treatment progress evaluations in order to minimize the total number of radiographs subscribed for each individual subject. All patients were positioned in the CBCT scanner in a sitting position with the Frankfurt horizontal plane (FH) parallel to the floor and positioned centrally in the field of view (FoV) using laser alignment. Subjects were instructed not to move, not to swallow and to breathe normally during the acquisition. The CBCT scans were performed using the

Planmeca ProMax 3D set at 90 kV and 20.25 mAs while using a 170 × 200 mm FoV and with an isotropic voxel size of 0.3 mm. Acquisition time was 9.0 s in all scans.

2.5. Superimposition of the CBCT 3D Surface Models

The Digital Imaging and Communications in Medicine (DICOM) data resulting from each CBCT scan were exported to specialized software (Mimics 10.01, V10.2.1.2 by Materialise Inc., HQ Leuven. Belgium) for hard tissue segmentation to create a 3D surface polygon model, saved as a stereolithography (STL) file. Three-dimensional surface models from the same subjects were imported into Geomagic (version 2013.0.1.1206, Geomagic Solutions, Rock Hill, CA, USA) for a three-dimensional superimposition and color mapping comparison between T1 and T0 and between T2 and T0. The T0 surface model served as the reference model, whereas the T1 and T2 surface models served as the test models. For superimposition, the anterior cranial base and the occipital area posterior of the foramen magnum were selected as the stable structures (Figure 2A) [19].

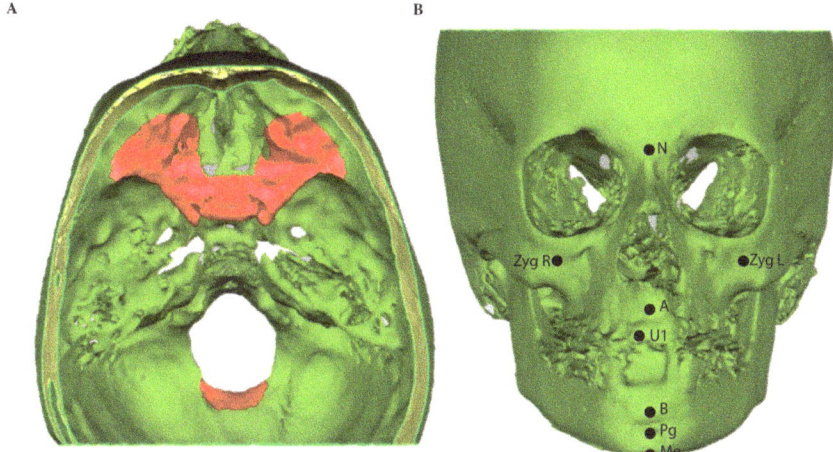

Figure 2. Stable structures used for superimposition and Regions of Interest on cone beam computed tomography (CBCT) 3D surface models. (**A**) Anterior cranial base and posterior of the foramen magnum were selected (areas indicated in red) as the stable structures for superimposition [14]. (**B**) ROIs of A-point (A), B-point (B), nasion (N), menton (Me), pogonion (Pg), right upper incisor (U1), zygoma left and right (Zyg L, Zyg R), respectively.

The predefined Regions of Interest (ROI) measurements were performed on a color map of the two superimposed surface models, namely nasion (N), the left and right zygomatic processes (Zyg), A-point, the right upper central incisors (U1), B-point, pogonion (Pg) and menton (Me) (Figure 2B). Each ROI consists of an area of 4.5 mm^2 around a pre-defined anatomical landmark containing approximately 60 polygons. Measurement outcomes are the average of these 60 included points at the respective ROIs. The superimposition was set to be stable if the deviations of the ROI at the cranial base and posterior of the foramen magnum were within the range of −0.3 and +0.3 mm, the same as the voxel size. The overall displacement of an ROI is further divided into: the horizontal component (y-axis), the vertical component (z-axis) and the transverse component (x-axis).

2.6. Tracing on Lateral Cephalograms

From all CBCT scans of the BAMP group at T0, T1 and T2, a lateral cephalogram was extracted according to an established protocol [20]. All tracings were performed in ViewBox (version 3.00 dHal software, Demetrios Halazonetis, Kifissia, Greece). Before tracing, all lateral cephalograms were set at the same scale. A standard set of cephalometric measurements was included.

2.7. Quantitative Measurements

In the BAMP subjects both 3D and 2D quantitative measurements were performed based on either the CBCT surface models or lateral cephalograms derived from the CBCT scans. All 3D measurements were carried out twice by two observers (R.S. and A.K.M.), with an interval of at least one week to reduce the risk of bias. A maximum of 15 measurements per day were conducted to prevent a possible effect of fatigue. In the control subjects only 2D quantitative measurements on the lateral cephalogram were measured. All 2D measurements were carried out twice by one observer (A.K.M.) at an interval of at least one week. The CBCT surface models or cephalograms of different subjects were randomly assigned to the observers during the measurements.

2.8. Statistics

Statistical analyses were performed with SPSS (version 23.0, IBM, Armonk, NY, USA) by one author (R.S.). Cephalometric data were tested with a Kolmogorov–Smirnov test for normal distribution. All cephalometric values were normally distributed at T0. Furthermore, 3D and 2D data were tested with a one-way ANOVA, with a Tukey's HSD post hoc test for significances. The significance level for all tests was set to $p < 0.05$. For the intra- and interclass correlation a Cronbach's alpha test was used, with a kappa of 0.81–1.00 indicating a "near perfect agreement".

3. Results

The inter-observer agreement of all 3D measurements (ICC > 0.84) and the intra-observer agreement of all 2D measurements (ICC > 0.90) were both "near perfect".

3.1. D Skeletal Changes

An illustration of skeletal changes after 1.5-years and 3.5-years BAMP treatment on a 3D color map is given in Figure 3. The zygomatic and maxillary anterior regions show more intense yellow, orange and red colors in the entire 3.5-year period (ΔT2-T0) than in the first 1.5-year period (ΔT1-T0), indicating more forward and outward displacements.

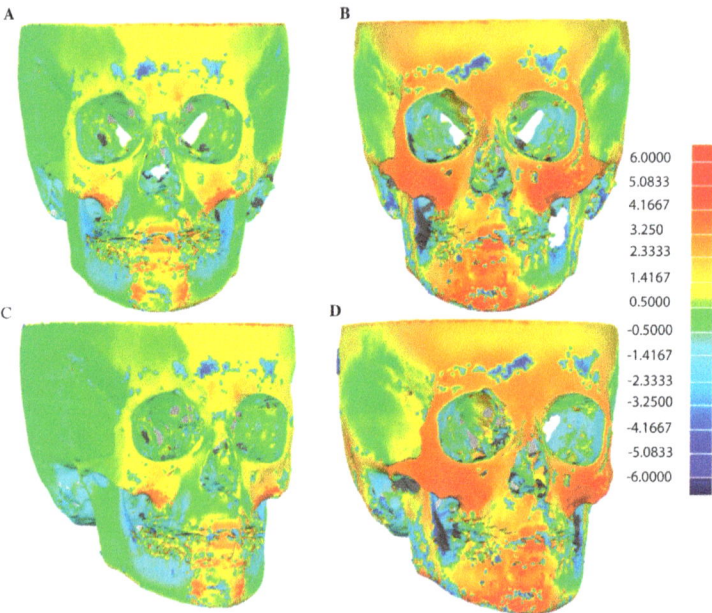

Figure 3. An example of illustration of skeletal changes on 3D colormap. (**A,C**) superimpositions of T0 and T1, (**B,D**) superimpositions of T0 and T2.

In Figure 4, skeletal changes on superimposed 3D surface models are visualized from a "median patient", namely, the patient whose displacement of A-point ROI represents the median value among all 19 subjects from the BAMP group. From a frontal and lateral view (Figure 4 A,B,E,F), forward, outward and downward displacements of the zygomatico-maxillary complex could be observed at both 1.5-years and 3.5-years, with the latter more pronounced. Similar observations could be seen from the axial views of the zygoma arches and the mandibular body (Figure 4 C,D,G,H).

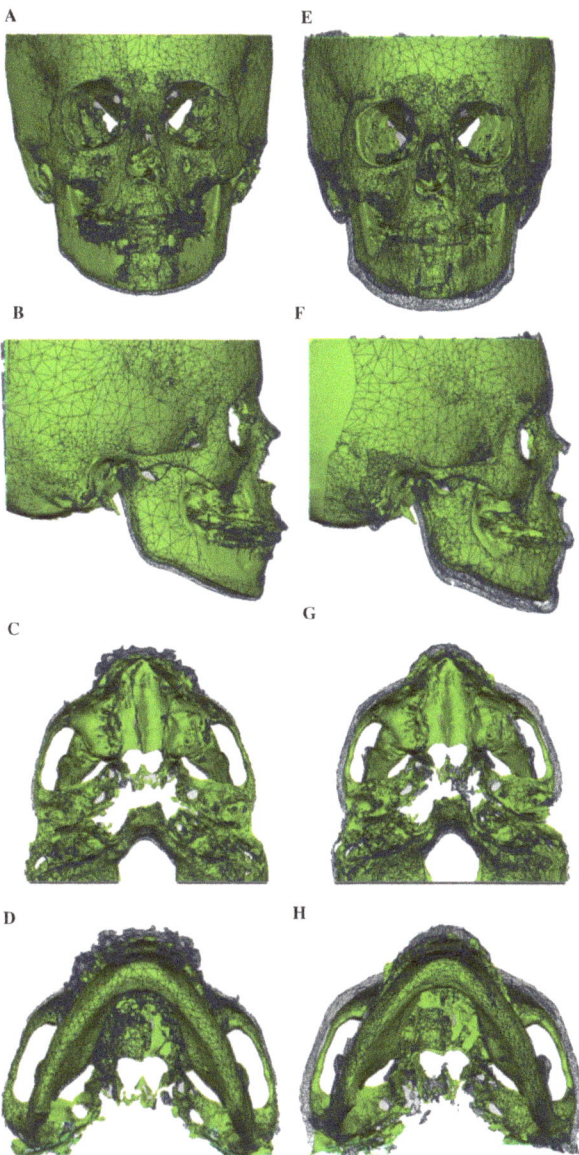

Figure 4. Skeletal changes on superimposed 3D STL surface models from a "median" patient. (**A–D**) Superimpositions of T0 and T1, (**E,F**) superimpositions of T0 and T2; (**A,E**) frontal view, (**B,F**) sagittal view, (**C,G**) axial view from the cranial base and (**D,H**) axial view from the mandible body. T0 STL surface models in green and T1 or T2 in grey mesh.

Table 1 presents the 3D quantitative data measured on the colormap. On superimposed CBCT surface models, except for the B-point and the upper incisor, all other studied ROIs showed significantly more displacements in the 3.5-year period (ΔT2-T0) than in the first 1.5-year period (ΔT1-T0) ($p < 0.05$). The significant changes at A-point and nasion at 3.5-years (2.7 mm ± 0.9 mm and 1.7 mm ± 1.1 mm, respectively) are mainly attributed to the horizontal component (2.6 mm ± 0.8 mm and 1.6 mm ± 1.1 mm, respectively), indicating forward and outward displacements ($p < 0.05$). Zygoma regions showed significant displacements in all three dimensions (horizontal, vertical and transverse) ($p < 0.05$). B-point is the only region that did not show any significant displacement at either 1.5-years or 3.5-years after BAMP treatment.

Table 1. Three-dimensional skeletal changes based on CBCT surface models.

N = 19		T1-T0	T2-T1	T2-T0
		1.5-years	2-years	3.5-years
		Mean (SD)	Mean (SD)	Mean (SD)
A	overall	1.5 ± 1.5	0.9 ± 1.7	2.7 ± 0.9 *
	horizontal	1.5 ± 1.4	0.8 ± 1.5	2.6 ± 0.8 *
	vertical	−0.2 ± 0.5	0.1 ± 0.4	−0.1 ± 0.4
B	overall	1.2 ± 1.9	1.1 ± 1.9	2.4 ± 1.2
	horizontal	1.2 ± 1.9	1.0 ± 1.9	2.3 ± 1.2
	vertical	0.1 ± 0.4	0.0 ± 0.4	0.1 ± 0.4
Zygoma left	overall	1.7 ± 0.9	2.2 ± 1.3	3.9 ± 1.3 *
	horizontal	1.3 ± 0.7	1.7 ± 1.0	3.1 ± 1.0 *
	vertical	0.4 ± 0.4	1.0 ± 0.7 #	1.4 ± 0.7 *
	transversal	1.0 ± 0.7	0.8 ± 0.8	1.6 ± 0.9 *
Zygoma right	overall	1.6 ± 1.2	2.0 ± 1.4	3.7 ± 1.1 *
	horizontal	1.2 ± 1.1	1.6 ± 1.3	3.0 ± 1.2 *
	vertical	0.4 ± 0.5	1.1 ± 0.7 #	1.5 ± 0.6 *
	transversal	0.6 ± 0.6	0.6 ± 0.5	1.2 ± 0.4 *
Zygoma overall	overall	1.7 ± 1.0	2.1 ± 1.2	3.8 ± 1.2 *
	horizontal	1.3 ± 0.9	1.6 ± 1.1	3.0 ± 0.9 *
	vertical	0.4 ± 0.4	1.0 ± 0.6 #	1.4 ± 0.7 *
	transversal	0.8 ± 0.6	0.7 ± 0.5	1.4 ± 0.7 *
Nasion	overall	0.7 ± 1.2	1.0 ± 1.1	1.7 ± 1.1 *
	horizontal	0.6 ± 1.1	1.0 ± 1.1	1.6 ± 1.1 *
	vertical	0.0 ± 0.3	0.1 ± 0.5	0.1 ± 0.3
Pogonion	overall	1.0 ± 2.0	1.3 ± 1.5	2.3 ± 1.5 *
	horizontal	1.0 ± 1.9	1.1 ± 1.4	2.0 ± 1.3
	vertical	0.2 ± 0.3	0.5 ± 0.7	0.7 ± 0.6 *
Menton	overall	1.6 ± 1.7	1.4 ± 2.0	3.1 ± 1.5 *
	horizontal	1.0 ± 1.1	0.6 ± 1.2	1.5 ± 0.8
	vertical	1.2 ± 1.4	1.3 ± 1.5	2.5 ± 1.3 *
U1	overall	2.3 ± 1.4	0.5 ± 1.6 #	2.8 ± 1.2
	horizontal	2.1 ± 1.4	0.4 ± 1.5 #	2.5 ± 1.1
	vertical	0.1 ± 0.6	−0.3 ± 0.7	−0.3 ± 1.0

The 3D surface model of T0 was set as the reference model, whereas T1 and T2 were set to be the test models. A difference is considered significant if $p < 0.05$. * indicates significant difference between ΔT2-T0 and ΔT1-T0, # indicates significant difference between ΔT2-T1 and ΔT1-T0.

Interestingly, comparisons of the changes occurring in the two consecutive observation periods only showed differences in the upper incisor with less displacement in the second 2-year period (ΔT2-T1, 0.5 mm ± 1.6 mm) than in the first 1.5-year period (ΔT1-T0, 2.3 mm ± 1.4 mm) ($p < 0.05$). The zygoma regions also showed more vertical displacement in the second period (ΔT2-T1, 1.0 mm ± 0.6 mm) than in the first period (ΔT1-T0, 0.4 mm ± 0.4 mm) ($p < 0.05$).

3.2. 2D Cephalometric Changes

All cephalometric measurements and changes in the BAMP group and the control group are presented in Table 2. In the control group the U1-palatal plane and U1-NA were significantly lower at T0 than at T2 (96.3° ± 6.9° vs. 107.9° ± 8.0°, $p < 0.001$). Consequently a significantly higher inter-incisor angle was found at T0 than at T2 (149.0° ± 9.6° vs. 138.5° ± 12.2°, $p < 0.05$). Interestingly, at T0 there were significant differences between the BAMP and control group on exactly the same three parameters ($p < 0.05$). Nevertheless, all these differences between the two groups at T0 disappeared at T2. Noteworthy, was that the significant differences observed at T2 between the BAMP and control group were in Wits (−0.4 mm ± 4.0 mm vs. −4.3 mm ± 4.7 mm) ($p < 0.05$), gonial angle (126.6° ± 7.0° vs. 133.1° ± 7.3°) ($p < 0.05$) and overjet (2.2 mm ± 2.8 mm vs. −2.6 mm ± 4.1 mm) ($p < 0.01$); all appeared to favor orthopedic treatment of Class III malocclusion. Regarding the net changes between T2 and T0, the control group showed a tendency for mild improvement in overjet and mild deterioration in ANB and Wits, all indicating a temporary dental camouflage. Over the 3.5-year period (ΔT2-T0) the most significant difference between the BAMP and control group was observed in the ANB angle (−2.2 ± 2.3 vs. 1.1 ± 2.1, $p < 0.000$), with an average improvement of 3.3°.

Table 2. Cephalometric measurements of the BAMP treated group and the control group.

	Control Group (N = 17)			Bone Anchored Maxillary Protraction Group (N = 19)					
	T0	T2	ΔT2-T0	T0	T1	T2	ΔT1-T0	ΔT2-T1	ΔT2-T0
Age	10.7 ± 1.2	14.3 ± 1.4	3.7 ± 0.7	11.4 ± 0.7	12.9 ± 0.8	15.0 ± 0.7	1.5 ± 0.4	2.1 ± 0.7	3.6 ± 0.7
SN-FH (°)	10.5 ± 4.0	8.5 ± 5.8	−2.0 ± 5.0	10.4 ± 4.2	10.4 ± 4.2	10.6 ± 3.8	0.0 ± 1.8	0.2 ± 2.7	0.2 ± 2.6
SNA (°)	75.5 ± 5.5	75.2 ± 5.1	−0.3 ± 3.5	77.1 ± 5.3	78.6 ± 5.2	78.6 ± 5.8	1.6 ± 1.5	0.0 ± 2.5	1.6 ± 2.7
SNB (°)	75.9 ± 4.5	77.8 ± 5.7	1.9 ± 3.8	78.1 ± 4.1	78.5 ± 4.1	78.5 ± 4.9	0.4 ± 2.2	0.1 ± 2.8	0.5 ± 2.2
ANB (°)	−0.4 ± 3.5	−2.6 ± 2.7	−2.2 ± 2.3	−1.0 ± 3.1	0.1 ± 3.1	0.1 ± 3.2	1.1 ± 1.7	0.1 ± 1.9	1.1 ± 2.1 @
Wits (mm)	−2.9 ± 2.8	−4.3 ± 4.7	−1.4 ± 4.9	−1.8 ± 3.4	−0.2 ± 3.4	−0.4 ± 4.0 @	1.6 ± 2.2	−0.2 ± 2.9	1.4 ± 2.9
ANS-PNS/Go-Gn (°)	27.1 ± 6.1	26.9 ± 5.1	−0.2 ± 4.4	23.9 ± 5.6	24.0 ± 6.0	23.2 ± 5.3	0.1 ± 2.0	−0.7 ± 2.9	−0.6 ± 3.1
SN/GoGn (°)	36.4 ± 7.6	35.7 ± 7.7	−0.8 ± 3.1	33.6 ± 6.0	33.6 ± 5.0	32.5 ± 5.0	−0.1 ± 2.8	−1.1 ± 3.2	−1.0 ± 4.1
Occlusal plane (°)	18.1 ± 6.2	14.7 ± 7.6	−3.3 ± 4.1	14.1 ± 5.1	12.6 ± 4.5	12.5 ± 4.6	−1.5 ± 2.6	−0.1 ± 3.2	−1.6 ± 3.0
Gonial angle (°)	133.2 ± 5.9	133.1 ± 7.3	−0.1 ± 3.7	130.0 ± 6.9	129.0 ± 6.5	126.6 ± 7.0 @	−1.0 ± 4.0	−2.4 ± 2.5	−3.4 ± 5.4
UI to Pal (°)	96.3 ± 6.9	107.9 ± 8.0 #	11.6 ± 8.9	108.1 ± 11.0 @	111.8 ± 7.5	114.5 ± 5.7	3.7 ± 8.6	2.3 ± 7.3	6.1 ± 11.2 @
UI to NA (°)	11.4 ± 8.3	23.9 ± 7.2 #	12.5 ± 7.5	19.7 ± 11.7	23.0 ± 8.7	26.8 ± 6.8	3.2 ± 7.7	3.9 ± 7.9	7.1 ± 9.9 @
LI to GoGn (°)	87.6 ± 7.0	86.6 ± 6.3	−1.0 ± 6.7	91.4 ± 8.3	89.5 ± 6.7	90.6 ± 7.3	−1.8 ± 3.8	−0.8 ± 5.3	−1.1 ± 4.2
LI to NB (°)	19.2 ± 7.6	20.2 ± 7.5	1.0 ± 7.0	22.6 ± 5.8	21.6 ± 6.3	21.5 ± 6.2	−1.0 ± 3.7	−0.1 ± 5.1	−1.1 ± 4.2
InterI angle (°)	149.0 ± 9.6	138.5 ± 12.2 #	−10.5 ± 10.6	136.2 ± 11.4 @	133.3 ± 9.6	131.6 ± 6.3	−2.8 ± 10.2	−4.7 ± 13.0	−7.5 ± 13.8
Overjet (mm)	−4.4 ± 3.1	−2.6 ± 4.1	1.8 ± 3.7	−1.3 ± 2.7	1.0 ± 3.2	2.2 ± 2.8 *@	2.3 ± 3.3	1.2 ± 2.4	3.5 ± 3.3
Overbite (mm)	3.1 ± 3.0	2.1 ± 2.8	−1.0 ± 2.7	1.3 ± 2.0	1.4 ± 1.5	1.2 ± 1.9	0.1 ± 1.6	−0.2 ± 1.7	−0.1 ± 2.4

T0 (baseline), T1 (1.5-years) and T2 (3.5-years). A difference is considered significant if $p < 0.05$. * indicates a significant difference in BAMP group between T0 and T2, or between ΔT1-T0 and ΔT2-T1; # indicates a significant difference in control group between T0 and T2; @ indicates a significant difference between control and BAMP groups at T0, T2 or ΔT2-T0.

Within the BAMP group, only one single parameter, overjet, showed significant changes between T0 and T2, from −1.3 mm ± 2.7 mm at the start of BAMP to 2.2 mm ± 2.8 mm 3.5-years after ($p < 0.05$), an average increase of 3.5 mm. Changes taking place in the two consecutive periods (ΔT1-T0 and ΔT2-T1) showed no difference in any measurements in the BAMP group.

4. Discussion

Application of BAMP treatment modality in cleft subjects is relatively new. A recent systematic review of orthopedic therapies in growing cleft patients, only included five studies using BAMP therapy with treatment durations ranging from 7.9 to 18 months [21]. To our knowledge, the present study is the first in which both 3D and 2D effects of BAMP treatment on the zygomaticomaxillary and mandibular structures were evaluated with a follow-up of 3.5-years.

Our previous study on 1.5-years of follow-up showed a significant difference between the BAMP group and untreated cleft control group in ANB angle, SNA angle, Wits and overjet ($p < 0.05$), all in favor of improvement of Class III malocclusion by BAMP therapy. [16] Here, with a follow-up of 3.5-years, the difference between the BAMP and the control group is most notable at the skeletal level as measured by the ANB angle, with an average increase of 3.3°; this is not only statistically significant but also highly clinically meaningful.

Although the upper incisor inclinations were not the same in the BAMP and control group at T0, these differences disappeared at T2. The more retroclined upper incisor in the control group to start with, became less retroclined after 3.5-years, explaining the mild improvement in negative overjet at T2 in the control group. Although the dental relationship appeared mildly improved in the control subjects, their skeletal Class III relationship had actually worsened after 3.5-years as seen in the decreased ANB and Wits.

Since the changes ΔT2-T0 in the control group can largely be considered the result of growth, the observed difference between the BAMP and control group can therefore be attributed to the effect of BAMP treatment. Had this study not included a control group, this important effect of growth would have been overlooked. That said, it is understandable that comparisons within the BAMP group at different time points were mostly statistically insignificant, as any deterioration due to normal growth would have camouflaged the positive treatment effect. The true treatment effect can only be appreciated by comparing the differences between the BAMP group and the control group over the same observation period. Nonetheless, we observed significant differences at T2 between the BAMP and control group in Wits, gonial angle and overjet, with an average change of +4.7 mm, −6.5° and +4.8 mm, respectively, all in favor of BAMP treatment of Class III malocclusion.

An important finding in the present study is that changes that occured in the two consecutive periods (ΔT1-T0 and ΔT2-T1) did not show a difference in the BAMP group in any measurements, with the exception of the upper inclination of the upper incisor. This means that not only the positive results from the first 1.5-years were maintained, but also continuous orthopedic effect was achieved in the following 2-years. In other words, treatment efficacy of BAMP therapy observed in the first period continues to the same extent in the second period. This is unexpected, as the growth potential decreases with the progress of treatment. By the end of the 3.5-year observation period, the average age of the study subjects was close to 15, typically at the tail of the growth spurt. These results seem to indicate that the optimal age to start BAMP therapy may warrant a critical evaluation. Oppositely, it can also imply that the age of 11 to 12-years is indeed the optimum, as continuous treatment benefit is ensured when the treatment has started by then. More extensive studies are needed to clarify the optimal timing.

Another important finding is that the overall displacement of the upper incisor, ΔT2-T1 is less than ΔT1-T0, indicating that most of the possible dental compensation effect occurred in the first period, as was also observed in the control group, and that any improvement in the position of the upper incisor observed in the second period is mainly due to the skeletal effect.

In the vertical dimension, a significant decrease of 6.5° in the gonial angle was observed in the BAMP group compared to the control. Such a "closing" effect of the gonial angle has been previously reported in non-cleft subjects after 1.5-years of BAMP treatment [22]. Additionally, other vertical angular measurements from the BAMP group, such as ANS-PNS/GoGn and SN/GoGn, showed a tendency for a greater decrease compared to the control group. These results point out that BAMP treatment did not cause clockwise rotation of the mandible, which is a common observation related to the treatment mechanics for Class III malocclusion [23]. BAMP therapy appears to improve the skeletal relationship by shifting the differential growth of the maxilla and mandible to a more convex direction, namely, more relative growth in the maxilla and less in the mandible. As discussed previously, BAMP therapy likely stimulates more forward growth of the maxilla by opening the palatomaxillary suture and zygomaticomaxillary suture [18,24].

However, the underlying mechanism how the relatively less growth of the mandible is realized has not been much investigated. One hypothesis could be the remodeling of the condylar head and the fossa due to the light compression force on the condyles resulting from the intermaxillary elastics, which reduces the gonial angle producing an effect of the mandible moving "backward" and "counter-clockwise", as supported by the slightly reduced occlusal plane angle (occlusal-SN) in addition to a significantly reduced gonial angle.

Large variations exist in the individual subjects regarding the effect of the treatment. For example, in the BAMP group, a displacement of A-point has been observed with a maximum of 6.5 mm and a minimum of −0.8 mm. Such a large individual variation could be caused by zygomatic suture maturation, with more favorable results reported for patients at an early stage of maturation [25]. According to Angelierri et al., the zygomaticomaxillary sutures show a high level of fusion at the chronological age of 15-years and older. However, fusion of the sutures has also been observed in younger patients [15].

Several limitations of this study need to be acknowledged. First is our choice for the control group. It would be ideal to have CBCT surface models from an untreated cleft group matched by age, gender and skeletal deformity to understand the effect of BAMP therapy at a three-dimensional level. However, ethical reasons made it impossible to include such a group. As an alternative we used two-dimensional cephalograms from a cleft group as the control. One limitation is that we could not visualize the effect of growth in 3D color mapping either during the entire observation period or in the two respective observation periods. Another limitation is the sample size of the study. Although the number of subjects in both the BAMP and the control groups was above the required minimum, they are both relatively small. Given the lack of a control group with 3D data, caution should be taken when drawing conclusions from the 3D results. The favorable changes observed in the BAMP group is a combined result of the normal growth and the orthopedic effect of the BAMP therapy throughout the entire observation period. More independent studies with a larger scope are needed to verify the findings of the current study, and more importantly, to identify predictable factors of individual characteristics for a favorable treatment outcome of BAMP therapy.

5. Conclusions

In conclusion, this prospective study with a follow-up of 3.5-years showed significant positive effects on the zygomaticomaxillary complex and in the vertical dimension of the mandible, providing the first evidence to support BAMP as an effective and reliable treatment option for growing cleft subjects with mild to moderate Class III malocclusion up to 15-years of age.

Author Contributions: Conceptualization, Y.R., R.M.S., A.F.K.M., W.J.v.d.M. and J.J.; methodology, Y.R., R.M.S. and A.F.K.M.; software, R.M.S., A.F.K.M., A.D. and W.J.v.d.M.; validation, R.M.S., A.F.K.M. and A.D.; formal analysis, R.M.S. and A.F.K.M.; investigation, Y.R., R.M.S. and A.F.K.M.; resources, Y.R. and J.J.; data curation, R.M.S. and A.F.K.M.; writing—original draft preparation, R.M.S., A.F.K.M. and Y.R.; writing—review and editing, R.M.S., A.F.K.M., Y.R., W.J.v.d.M. and J.J.; visualization, R.M.S., A.F.K.M. and A.D.; supervision, Y.R. and W.J.v.d.M.; project administration, R.M.S. and A.F.K.M.; funding acquisition, none. All authors have read and agreed to the published version of the manuscript.

Funding: The work was supported by the Department of Orthodontics of the University Medical Center Groningen, The Netherlands.

Institutional Review Board Statement: All procedures performed in studies involving human participants were in accordance with the ethical standards of the institutional and/or national research committee and with the 1964 Helsinki declaration and its later amendments or comparable ethical standards.

Informed Consent Statement: Informed consent was obtained from all individual participants included in the study.

Data Availability Statement: The data presented in this study are available on request from the corresponding author. The data are not publicly available due to privacy reasons.

Conflicts of Interest: Author Steegman declares that he has no conflict of interest. Author Klein Meulekamp declares that she has no conflict of interest. Author Dieters declares that he has no conflict of interest. Author van der Meer declares that he has no conflict of interest. Author Jansma declares that he has no conflict of interest and author Ren declares that she has no conflict of interest.

References

1. Ertaş, Ü.; Ataol, M. Evaluation of Nasal Airway Volume of Operated Unilateral Cleft Lip and Palate Patients Compared with Skeletal Class III Individuals. *Cleft Palate-Craniofacial J.* **2019**, *56*, 15–20. [CrossRef]
2. Hunt, O.; Burden, D.; Hepper, P.; Stevenson, M.; Johnston, C. Self-Reports of Psychosocial Functioning among Children and Young Adults with Cleft Lip and Palate. *Cleft Palate-Craniofacial J.* **2006**, *43*, 598–605. [CrossRef] [PubMed]
3. Muntz, H.; Wilson, M.; Park, A.; Smith, M.; Grimmer, J.F. Sleep Disordered Breathing and Obstructive Sleep Apnea in the Cleft Population. *Laryngoscope* **2008**, *118*, 348–353. [CrossRef] [PubMed]
4. Silvestre, J.; Tahiri, Y.; Paliga, J.T.; Taylor, J.A. Screening for obstructive sleep apnea in children with syndromic cleft lip and/or palate. *J. Plast. Reconstr. Aesthetic Surg.* **2014**, *67*, 1475–1480. [CrossRef] [PubMed]
5. Brouillette, R.T.; Fernbach, S.K.; Hunt, C.E. Obstructive sleep apnea in infants and children. *J. Pediatr.* **1982**, *100*, 31–40. [CrossRef]
6. Gislason, T.; Benediktsdóttir, B. Snoring, Apneic Episodes, and Nocturnal Hypoxemia Among Children 6 Months to 6 Years Old. *Chest* **1995**, *107*, 963–966. [CrossRef]
7. Havakeshian, G.; Koretsi, V.; Eliades, T.; Papageorgiou, S.N. Effect of Orthopedic Treatment for Class III Malocclusion on Upper Airways: A Systematic Review and Meta-Analysis. *J. Clin. Med.* **2020**, *9*, 3015. [CrossRef]
8. Alrejaye, N.; Gao, J.; Hatcher, D.; Oberoi, S. Effect of maxillary expansion and protraction on the oropharyngeal airway in individuals with non-syndromic cleft palate with or without cleft lip. *PLoS ONE* **2019**, *14*, e0213328. [CrossRef]
9. Jesani, A.; DiBiase, A.T.; Cobourne, M.T.; Newton, T. Perceived Changes by Peer Group of Social Impact Associated with Combined Orthodontic-Surgical Correction of Class III Malocclusion. *J. Dent.* **2014**, *42*, 1135–1142. [CrossRef]
10. Javed, O.; Bernabe, E. Oral Impacts on Quality of Life in Adult Patients with Class I, II and III Malocclusion. *Oral Health Prev. Dent.* **2016**, *14*, 27–32. [CrossRef]
11. Watkinson, S.; Harrison, J.E.; Furness, S.; Worthington, H.V. Orthodontic Treatment for Prominent Lower Front Teeth (Class III Malocclusion) in Children. *Cochrane Database Syst. Rev.* **2013**, CD003451. [CrossRef] [PubMed]
12. Buschang, P.H.; Porter, C.; Genecov, E.; Genecov, D.; Sayler, K.E. Face Mask Therapy of Preadolescents with Unilateral Cleft Lip and Palate. *Angle Orthod.* **1994**, *64*, 145–150. [CrossRef]
13. Van Hevele, J.; Nout, E.; Claeys, T.; Meyns, J.; Scheerlinck, J.; Politis, C. Bone-Anchored Maxillary Protraction to Correct a Class III Skeletal Relationship: A Multicenter Retrospective Analysis of 218 Patients. *J. Craniomaxillofac. Surg.* **2018**, *46*, 1800–1806. [CrossRef]
14. Hino, C.T.; Cevidanes, L.H.; Nguyen, T.T.; De Clerck, H.J.; Franchi, L.; McNamara, J.A. Three-Dimensional Analysis of Maxillary Changes Associated with Facemask and Rapid Maxillary Expansion Compared with Bone Anchored Maxillary Protraction. *Am. J. Orthod. Dentofacial Orthop.* **2013**, *144*, 705–714. [CrossRef] [PubMed]
15. Angelieri, F.; Franchi, L.; Cevidanes, L.H.S.; Hino, C.T.; Nguyen, T.; McNamara, J.A. Zygomaticomaxillary Suture Maturation: A Predictor of Maxillary Protraction? Part I—A Classification Method. *Orthod. Craniofac Res.* **2017**, *20*, 85–94. [CrossRef] [PubMed]
16. Ren, Y.; Steegman, R.; Dieters, A.; Jansma, J.; Stamatakis, H. Bone-Anchored Maxillary Protraction in Patients with Unilateral Complete Cleft Lip and Palate and Class III Malocclusion. *Clin. Oral. Investig.* **2019**, *23*, 2429–2441. [CrossRef]
17. Yatabe, M.; Garib, D.G.; Faco, R.A.S.; de Clerck, H.; Janson, G.; Nguyen, T.; Cevidanes, L.H.S.; Ruellas, A.C. Bone-Anchored Maxillary Protraction Therapy in Patients with Unilateral Complete Cleft Lip and Palate: 3-Dimensional Assessment of Maxillary Effects. *Am. J. Orthod. Dentofacial Orthop.* **2017**, *152*, 327–335. [CrossRef]
18. Nguyen, T.; Cevidanes, L.; Cornelis, M.A.; Heymann, G.; de Paula, L.K.; De Clerck, H. Three-Dimensional Assessment of Maxillary Changes Associated with Bone Anchored Maxillary Protraction. *Am. J. Orthod. Dentofacial Orthop.* **2011**, *140*, 790–798. [CrossRef]
19. Gkantidis, N.; Schauseil, M.; Pazera, P.; Zorkun, B.; Katsaros, C.; Ludwig, B. Evaluation of 3-Dimensional Superimposition Techniques on Various Skeletal Structures of the Head Using Surface Models. *PLoS ONE* **2015**, *10*, e0118810. [CrossRef]
20. Navarro Rde, L.; Oltramari-Navarro, P.V.; Fernandes, T.M.; Oliveira, G.F.; Conti, A.C.; Almeida, M.R.; Almeida, R.R. Comparison of Manual, Digital and Lateral CBCT Cephalometric Analyses. *J. Appl. Oral. Sci.* **2013**, *21*, 167–176. [CrossRef]
21. Ahn, H.; Kim, S.; Baek, S. Miniplate-anchored Maxillary Protraction in Adolescent Patients with Cleft Lip and Palate: A Literature Review of Study Design, Type and Protocol, and Treatment Outcomes. *Orthod. Craniofac. Res.* **2020**, ocr.12446. [CrossRef] [PubMed]
22. De Clerck, H.; Cevidanes, L.; Baccetti, T. Dentofacial Effects of Bone-Anchored Maxillary Protraction: A Controlled Study of Consecutively Treated Class III Patients. *Am. J. Orthod. Dentofacial Orthop.* **2010**, *138*, 577–581. [CrossRef] [PubMed]
23. Cordasco, G.; Matarese, G.; Rustico, L.; Fastuca, S.; Caprioglio, A.; Lindauer, S.J.; Nucera, R. Efficacy of Orthopedic Treatment with Protraction Facemask on Skeletal Class III Malocclusion: A Systematic Review and Meta-Analysis. *Orthod. Craniofac. Res.* **2014**, *17*, 133–143. [CrossRef] [PubMed]

4. Mao, J.J. Mechanobiology of Craniofacial Sutures. *J. Dent. Res.* **2002**, *81*, 810–816. [CrossRef]
5. Angelieri, F.; Ruellas, A.C.; Yatabe, M.S.; Cevidanes, L.H.S.; Franchi, L.; Toyama-Hino, C.; De Clerck, H.J.; Nguyen, T.; McNamara, J.A. Zygomaticomaxillary Suture Maturation: Part II-The Influence of Sutural Maturation on the Response to Maxillary Protraction. *Orthod. Craniofac Res.* **2017**, *20*, 152–163. [CrossRef] [PubMed]

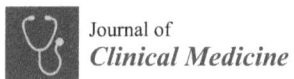 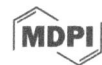

Article

Reliability and Reproducibility of Landmark Identification in Unilateral Cleft Lip and Palate Patients: Digital Lateral Vis-A-Vis CBCT-Derived 3D Cephalograms

Anuraj Singh Kochhar [1,*], Ludovica Nucci [2], Maninder Singh Sidhu [3], Mona Prabhakar [3], Vincenzo Grassia [2], Letizia Perillo [2], Gulsheen Kaur Kochhar [4], Ritasha Bhasin [5], Himanshu Dadlani [6] and Fabrizia d'Apuzzo [2]

1. Former Consultant Orthodontist Max Hospital Gurgaon, Haryana 122001, India
2. Multidisciplinary Department of Medical-Surgical and Dental Specialties, University of Campania Luigi Vanvitelli, 80138 Naples, Italy; ludovica.nucci@unicampania.it (L.N.); grassiavincenzo@libero.it (V.G.); letizia.perillo@unicampania.it (L.P.); fabrizia.dapuzzo@unicampania.it (F.d.)
3. Department of Orthodontics & Dean, Research & Development Faculty of Dental Sciences, SGT University Gurugram, Haryana 122505, India; deanresearch@sgtuniversity.org (M.S.S.); mona.prabhakar@sgtuniversity.org (M.P.)
4. Department of Pediatric & Preventive Dentistry, National Dental College & Hospital, Punjab 140507, India; gulsheenuppal@gmail.com
5. Faculty of Dentistry, University of Toronto, Toronto, ON M5G1G6, Canada; ritasha.bhasin@mail.utoronto.ca
6. Senior Consultant Department of Dentistry (Periodontology), Max Hospital, Gurgaon, Haryana 122001, India; himdent@hotmail.com
* Correspondence: anuraj_kochhar@yahoo.co.in

Citation: Kochhar, A.S.; Nucci, L.; Sidhu, M.S.; Prabhakar, M.; Grassia, V.; Perillo, L.; Kochhar, G.K.; Bhasin, R.; Dadlani, H.; d'Apuzzo, F. Reliability and Reproducibility of Landmark Identification in Unilateral Cleft Lip and Palate Patients: Digital Lateral Vis-A-Vis CBCT-Derived 3D Cephalograms. *J. Clin. Med.* 2021, 10, 535. https://doi.org/10.3390/jcm10030535

Academic Editors: Emmanuel Andrès and Gianrico Spagnuolo

Received: 3 January 2021
Accepted: 26 January 2021
Published: 2 February 2021

Publisher's Note: MDPI stays neutral with regard to jurisdictional claims in published maps and institutional affiliations.

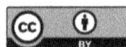

Copyright: © 2021 by the authors. Licensee MDPI, Basel, Switzerland. This article is an open access article distributed under the terms and conditions of the Creative Commons Attribution (CC BY) license (https://creativecommons.org/licenses/by/4.0/).

Abstract: Background: The aim of the retrospective observational study was to compare the precision of landmark identification and its reproducibility using cone beam computed tomography-derived 3D cephalograms and digital lateral cephalograms in unilateral cleft lip and palate patients. Methods: Cephalograms of thirty-one (31) North Indian children (18 boys and 13 girls) with a unilateral cleft lip and palate, who were recommended for orthodontic treatment, were selected. After a thorough analysis of peer-reviewed articles, 20 difficult-to-trace landmarks were selected, and their reliability and reproducibility were studied. These were subjected to landmark identification to evaluate interobserver variability; the coordinates for each point were traced separately by three different orthodontists (OB_A, OB_B, OB_C). Statistical analysis was performed using descriptive and inferential statistics with paired t-tests to compare the differences measured by the two methods. Real-scale data are presented in mean ± SD. A p-value less than 0.05 was considered as significant at a 95% confidence level. Results: When comparing, the plotting of points posterior nasal spine (PNS) ($p < 0.05$), anterior nasal spine (ANS) ($p < 0.01$), upper 1 root tip ($p < 0.05$), lower 1 root tip ($p < 0.05$), malare ($p < 0.05$), pyriforme ($p < 0.05$), porion ($p < 0.01$), and basion ($p < 0.05$) was statistically significant. Conclusion: In patients with a cleft lip and palate, the interobserver identification of cephalometric landmarks was significantly more precise and reproducible with cone beam computed tomography -derived cephalograms vis-a-vis digital lateral cephalograms.

Keywords: cleft; accuracy; unilateral cleft lip and palate; CBCT; interobserver; cephalogram

1. Introduction

Since its advent in 1931 [1], conventional cephalometry has been one of the essential diagnostic tools for analyzing orthodontic problems, maxillofacial deformities, evaluating growth, and planning treatment [2]. However, difficulty in locating imperceivable anatomic landmarks and superimposition of craniofacial structures, owing to the two-dimensional (2D) representation of three-dimensional (3D) anatomy, are amongst the limitations of traditional cephalometrics [3–5]. Young cleft lip and palate (CLP) patients usually present with a flattened cranial base, midface deficiency with a retruded maxilla and elongated mandible, anterior and/or posterior crossbites, and an increased vertical dimension, thereby making the recognition of cephalometric landmarks even more arduous [4,5].

The localization of landmarks like point A, the anterior nasal spine (ANS), and the posterior nasal spine (PNS) is challenging due to the decreased opacity resulting from the cleft [6]. The remodeling of the tooth germs in young patients, especially in the anterior contour of the maxilla, can be a possible cause for the same according to Hotz and Gnoinski [7]. According to published data, it is difficult to interpret radiographs in patients with CLP before the exfoliation of the incisors for the abovementioned problems, thus questioning the reliability of cephalometric measurements for the same [8,9].

In the present times, when imaging has been revolutionized, cone beam computed tomography (CBCT) aids in avoiding the anatomic superimpositions and problems caused by magnification, thereby permitting the evaluation of the craniofacial structures from unobstructed perspectives with minimal distortion. Three-dimensional (3D) images from CBCT scans can be rotated easily by changing the rotational axis, as convenient to the observer [2,10]. Specifically, regarding cleft patients, previous studies have advocated CBCT as an exceptional tool for the determination of bone volume [11–14], bone and root morphology, the assessment of tooth development in the vicinity of the cleft area [15–18], and soft tissue depth.

In orthodontics, cephalograms are repeatedly traced and reviewed. For impeccable treatment planning, the reliability and reproducibility of these anatomical landmarks are imperative, especially in patients with CLP where the identification of landmarks is highly challenging and, therefore, difficult to perceive and reproduce. Although the synchronal literature in the past several years has emphasized the pivotal role of CBCT to determine the reliability [19–27] of anatomic landmarks, there is a paucity of studies for the same, along with their reproducibility in CLP patients versus cephalometrics where the localization of anatomy is challenging.

A lot of studies have emphasized the difficulty in the plotting of bilateral landmarks [2,19–21], but none have been done in a compromised craniofacial morphology. To know the actual degree of midfacial retrusion along with the compromised craniofacial morphology that is usually present in cleft patients, the accuracy of landmark identification plays an important role [6,26].

Therefore, the present study was conducted to compare the reliability and reproducibility of landmark identification using two systems: CBCT-derived 3D cephalograms vis-a-vis digital lateral cephalograms in unilateral cleft lip and palate (UCLP) patients.

2. Materials and Methods

2.1. Ethical Approval

Approval for the retrospective observational study was obtained from Shree Guru Gobind Singh Tricentenary (SGT) Dental College, Hospital, and Research Institute, Budhera, Gurgaon, India (SGTDC/PPL/Com./E.C./14 August 2010) (institutional ethical committee). All records acquired from the Department of Orthodontics and Dentofacial Orthopedics from March 2011 to May 2013 were used only for research purposes, for which prior informed consent had been taken.

2.2. Methodology

Examination of records of 54 North Indian children (aged 10–14 years) with a repaired CL ± P anomaly was done. For the sample size estimation in the present study, power analysis at 80% power, a 0.5 alpha level, and an effect size of 0.8 suggested that a minimum of 21 patients were required. Records of thirty-one children (Table 1) who had primary CLP repair performed before 18 months of age, with no secondary alveolar bone grafts and no prior orthodontic/orthopedic appliance intervention (but recommended for comprehensive orthodontic treatment), were selected and designated as samples. Patients' records not fulfilling any of the above inclusion criteria or with any syndrome or mental retardation as documented in the medical history were excluded.

Table 1. Sample Characteristics.

	Boys (n = 18)			Girls (n = 13)			Total Sample (n = 31)		
	Mean	SD	Range	Mean	SD	Range	Mean	SD	Range
Age (yrs.)	12.035	0.690	10–14	12.13	0.724	10–14	12.09	0.698	10–14

Cephalograms had been acquired using PlanmecaPromax (Planmeca Co, Helsinki, Finland) in a natural head position, stabilized by ear rods. The scans were obtained at 66 kvp and 5 mA. The JPG images were obtained and transferred to the Nemoceph NX software (Visiodent, Saint-Denis, France) for calibration and analysis, which was done with a scale present on the X-ray as a 10 mm measurement marked on the cephalogram.

CBCT scans had been acquired using an i-CAT next-generation machine (Imaging Sciences International, Hatfield, PA, USA) with a field of view (fov) of 17 × 22 cm and a scan time of 26 s. The data gathered were saved in DICOM (version 1.7) format with an isometric voxel size of 0.25 mm. The DICOM images, using InVivoDental 5.0 (Anatomage, anatomy imaging software, San Jose, CA, USA), were reoriented according to Kochhar et al. [25]. According to a recent study, the precision of landmark plotting is negligibly affected by the orientation of CBCT images, but for the current study, reoriented images were utilized [2]. Once the images were reoriented, 3D reconstruction of the lateral cephalogram was done and saved as a JPG. The digitized and calibrated images from the iCAT CBCT machine were transferred in the Nemoceph software, and the X and Y coordinates were determined.

Various relevant peer-reviewed articles were considered (Table 2), 20 difficult-to-trace landmarks were then selected (Table 3), and their reliability and reproducibility were checked.

Table 2. Studies reviewed to determine difficult-to-trace landmarks.

S.No.	Author (Year)	Difficult-to-Trace Points in These Studies/Significant Findings
1.	Bongaarts CA et al., 2008 [6]	Point A, ANS, and PNS
2.	Ludlow JB et al., 2009 [21]	Anterior Posterior (AP): Point A, ANS, Point B, Go, Mandibular Incisor Tip Cephalocaudal (CC): ANS, Co, Go, Na, Or Avg AP and CC: Point A, ANS, Co, Go, Mandibular Incisor Tip, Me, Na
3.	Chien PC et al., 2009 [3]	INTER-OBSERVER RELIABILITY X Coordinate: Subspinale, ANS, Ba, Co, L1 Root, sigmoid notch Y Coordiate: Ba, co, go, L1tip, Or, Po, S, Sigmoid notch, U1 tip INTRA-OBSERVER RELIABILITY X coordinate: Ba Y coordinate: Ba, L1 tip, Me, Or, Sella, Sigmoid Notch
4.	Grauer D et al., 2010 [28]	ANS, U1tip, Point B
5.	Chang ZC et al., 2011 [29]	Intercept: S, Or, ANS, Point A, L1, L1R, Point B, Me, Go, Ba, PNS Interaction with CBCT mode: N, Gn, Me, Ba.
6.	Zamora N et al., 2012 [30]	Supraorbitale, Right zygion, PNS
7.	Katkar RA et al., 2013 [31]	Go, Na, Or, ANS and Md1 root.
8.	Durao APR et al., 2015 [32]	X coordinate: Or, Po, Go, Co, PNS Y coordinate: Co, Point B, Point A
9.	Neiva MB et al., 2016 [33]	Right Co, Gn, Left ramus point, Right and left zygomatic suture
10.	Ghoneima A et al., 2017 [34]	X coordinate: Ba, Point B, Me, U1, L1 Y coordinate: Ba, PNS.
11	Park J et al., 2019 [20]	Skeletal: Bilateral structures showed more errors than midline structures. Go was least reliable.

Point A, Point B, Anterior Nasal Spine (ANS), Condylion (Co), Posterior Nasal Spine (PNS), Gonion (Go), Mandibular Incisor Tip (L1), Maxillary incisal tip (U1), Nasion (Na), Oribitale (Or), Menton (Me), Supspinale, Sigmond notch, Porion (Po), Sella (S), Basion (Ba), Gnathion (Gn), Supraorbitale, Zygion, Zygomatic suture.

Table 3. Twenty difficult-to-trace landmarks.

S.No.	Landmark	Definition of Landmark
1.	Nasion	Intersection of the internasal suture with the nasofrontal suture in the midsagittal plane.
2.	Orbitale	Most inferior point on the infraorbital rim
3.	Supra orbitale	Most superior point on the infraorbital rim
4.	ANS	Tip of the anterior nasal spine
5.	PNS	Point along the palate immediately inferior to the pterygomaxillary fossa
6.	Point A	Deepest point of the curve of the maxilla, between the anterior nasal spine and the dental alveolus
7.	U1, root tip	Root tip of the maxillary incisor
8.	U1, crown tip	Incisal tip of the maxillary incisor
9.	L1, crown tip	Incisal tip of the mandibular incisor
10.	L1, root tip	Root tip of the mandibular incisor
11.	Malare	Most prominent anterolateral point on the zygomatic bone that lends the malar prominence to the face
12.	Pyriforme	Anterolateral margin of the nasal aperture represented by the most anteromedial point on the maxilla, forming the bony alar base
13.	Point B	The deepest midline point on the mandible between the infradentale and the pogonion
14.	Pog	Most anterior point on the midsagittal symphysis
15.	Gonion	Point along the angle of the mandible, midway between the lower border of the mandible posterior ascending ramus
16.	Porion	Most superior point of the right external auditory meatus
17.	Sella	Center of the pituitary fossa of the sphenoid bone
18.	Basion	Most inferior point on the anterior margin of the foramen magnum, at the base of the clivus
19.	MB cusp, U6	Mesio-buccal cusp of the maxillary first molar
20.	MB cusp, L6	Mesio-buccal cusp of the mandibular first molar

The digitized and calibrated images from Planmeca (a digital cephalometric machine) and iCAT CBCT were transferred to the Nemoceph software, and the X and Y coordinates were determined. The coordinates for each point were traced separately by three different orthodontists (OBA, OBB, OBC) who were designated as observers to check the variability of the points. Intra-observer differences could be due to the nature of the cephalometric landmark, the image quality, and the blurring of the anatomic structures. In contrast, inter-observer differences might be caused by variations in the observer's training and experience [35].

2.3. Blinding

For the prevention of bias, the coordinator created datasets (digital cephalogram and CBCT-generated cephalograms) that were kept in one location and renamed from 1 to 62. All the cephalogram tracings were done two times consecutively by three different observers with a minimum gap of 10 days to eliminate the observer bias in between and to check for the inter-observer variability. Once the tracing was performed, the same coordinator decoded the data into a digital and CBCT-derived cephalogram. These findings were transferred to the excel sheet and subjected to statistical analysis.

2.4. Statistical Analysis

The statistical software SPSS version 24.0 was used for the analysis, to compare the findings of the three observers. The centroid for each landmark was obtained by marking the coordinates of the mean by all three observers. For the statistical analysis, mean distance (MD), mean deviations from the centroid, and standard deviations were computed. The gold standard observed in the study was the centroid of the markings by the three observers for each landmark. The error in the detection of each landmark was represented by the mean of the distances from the centroid of the observers' markings to each observer's marking. To assess the variation in each axis of all landmarks, the mean deviation was computed. The variations among all the samples of each landmark were represented by standard deviations. To illustrate the distribution of errors over the number of samples, the standard deviations were computed for mean deviation. Statistical analysis was performed by using descriptive and inferential statistics with paired t-tests to compare the differences measured by the two methods. Real-scale data are presented in mean ± SD. A p-value less than 0.05 was considered as significant at the 95% confidence level.

Step 1: The average of the two readings for each observer was calculated separately for the digital and CBCT-derived cephalograms.

$$OBA = (Lax + Lax)/2; OBB = (LBx + LBx)/2; OBC = (LCx + LCx)/2:$$

$$OA = (Lay + Lay)/2; OB = (LBy + LBy)/2; OC = (LCy + LCy)/2$$

where x and y are the coordinates and A, B, and C are the observers.

Step 2: The centroid was calculated for both coordinates by using the formula:

$$\text{Centroid } CLx = ((OAx + OBx + OCx)/3; CLy = (OAy + OBy + OCy))/3$$

Step 3: Calculation of the distance for each observer from the centroid for all three observers.

$$DLA = \sqrt{(CLxA - OxA)^2 + (CLyA - OyA)^2},$$

$$DLB = \sqrt{(CLxB - OxB)^2 + (CLyB - OyB)^2} \text{ and}$$

$$DLC = \sqrt{(CLxC - OxC)^2 + (CLyC - OyC)^2}$$

Step 4: The mean distance was calculated with

$$MD = (DLA + DLB + DLC)/3$$

where DL is the distance of the landmark for each observer from the centroid (for observer A (OBA), B (OBB), and C (OBC)) and L is any of the 20 landmarks.

Step 5: The mean Distance was calculated for all 20 landmarks in all 20 datasets. This whole process was adopted for each landmark.

3. Results

Landmark identification is difficult, especially in patients with a cleft lip and palate. The inter-observer variability of the 20 difficult-to-trace landmarks selected presented an excellent correlation (0.988). The mean distance of the digital and CBCT-derived cephalograms was recorded for all three observers along with the overall mean of the same. A comparison of landmark identification on the digital and CBCT-derived cephalograms was also performed using the t-test, and the p-value was calculated (a p-value less than 0.05 is considered significant at the 95% confidence level and a p-value less than 0.01 is significant at the 99% confidence level). The inter-observer findings between observers (OA, OB, and OC) for the digital cephalogram and CBCT-derived cephalograms are presented in Table 4 and Figures 1 and 2. When comparing the digital cephalogram and CBCT-generated cephalograms, the plotting of points PNS ($p < 0.05$), ANS ($p < 0.01$), upper 1 root tip ($p < 0.05$), lower 1 root tip ($p < 0.05$), malare ($p < 0.05$), pyriforme ($p < 0.05$), porion ($p < 0.01$), and basion ($p < 0.05$) was statistically significant.

Table 4. Comparison of observations obtained by different observers for digital and CBCT derived cephalograms using *t* test.

| Landmarks | Comparisons (Paired *t*-Test) *p*-Value ||||||||||
| | Digital ||| CBCT ||| Digital vs CBCT ||||
	A VS B	A VS C	B VS C	A VS B	A VS C	B VS C	A	B	C	OVERALL
NASION	0.362	0.520	0.093	0.112	0.713	0.060	0.366	0.732	0.460	0.841
ORBITALE	0.191	0.417	0.861	0.119	0.133	0.773	0.972	0.481	0.184	0.910
SUPRAORBITALE	0.974	0.235	0.118	0.005	0.129	0.157	0.913	0.041	0.167	0.177
PNS	0.220	0.113	0.009	0.057	0.196	0.375	0.120	0.153	0.001	0.016 *
ANS	0.115	0.111	<0.001	0.010	0.151	0.010	0.018	0.006	<0.001	<0.001 *
POINT A	0.225	0.395	0.006	0.029	0.709	0.028	0.599	0.859	0.023	0.600
U1 ROOT TIP	0.028	0.678	0.037	0.033	0.238	0.109	0.095	0.119	0.038	0.039 *
U1 CROWNTIP	0.003	0.843	0.182	0.144	0.176	0.270	0.088	0.158	0.246	0.162
L1 CROWNTIP	0.027	0.100	0.225	0.221	0.174	0.063	0.799	0.828	0.947	0.995
L1 ROOT TIP	0.052	0.761	0.099	0.031	0.246	0.025	0.067	0.353	0.017	0.013 *
MALARE	0.384	0.226	0.001	0.028	0.027	0.317	0.277	0.004	0.635	0.043 *
PYRIFORME	0.793	0.237	0.173	0.013	0.648	0.007	0.103	0.021	0.002	0.015 *
POINT B	0.337	0.080	0.716	0.236	0.271	0.773	0.680	0.508	0.410	0.894
POG	0.003	0.568	0.014	0.097	0.496	0.164	0.074	0.678	0.040	0.069
GONION	0.323	0.337	0.120	0.061	0.643	0.039	0.127	0.143	0.149	0.136
PORION	0.352	0.041	0.028	0.318	0.455	0.962	<0.001	<0.001	0.003	<0.001 *
SELLA	0.002	0.002	0.961	0.138	0.994	0.055	0.594	0.196	0.092	0.183
BASION	0.606	0.732	0.973	0.027	0.506	0.022	0.037	0.011	0.026	0.011 *
MB, CUSP U6	0.008	0.008	0.416	0.061	0.037	0.035	0.528	0.302	0.765	0.483
MB, CUSP L6	0.012	0.576	0.036	0.523	0.280	0.153	0.403	0.219	0.112	0.436

* *p*-value < 0.05 is considered as significant.

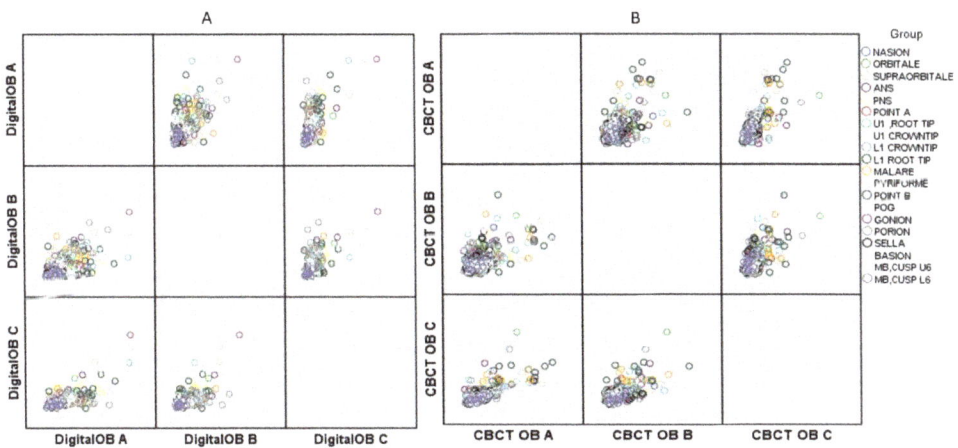

Figure 1. Graph showing associations in the observations taken by three observers in (**A**) Digital (**B**) cone beam computed tomography (CBCT).

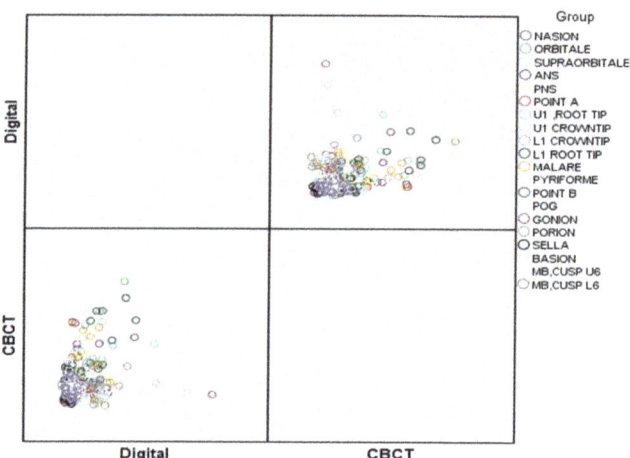

Figure 2. Inter-observer comparison of the plotting of the landmarks between the Digital and CBCT images.

4. Discussion

Cleft lip and/or palate (CL ± P) malformations are the most common congenital abnormalities in the craniofacial region and present a severe problem for health delivery systems throughout the world. Depending on the ethnicity and geographic location of the population, wide variations in the prevalence of cleft lip and palate have been reported, with higher rates amongst Asians and American Indians (one in 500 births). An isolated cleft palate is more frequently found in females than in males, at a ratio of 2:1. In contrast, there is a 2:1 male-to-female ratio for cleft lip with or without cleft palate [36].

Owing to their knowledge of the craniofacial complex and their expertise in tooth movement and dentofacial management, orthodontists' role in the cleft palate team is indispensable. Orthodontic treatment can have a dental effect, orthopedic reverberations, or both [37], but a prerequisite for successful orthodontic management is an understanding of the site, extent, and severity of the cleft-related craniofacial dysmorphology. The advancements in technology and the incorporation of novel methods aid in striving toward an accurate diagnosis. Researchers have worked diligently to achieve a micro-level accuracy in landmark identification, even comparing the efficiency in the projection of different CBCT machines [31] with a deluge of articles on the same. However, there is a paucity of data on landmark repeatability and reproducibility in the craniofacial morphologies of CL ± P patients, which is challenging to accomplish. Hence, the present study was undertaken in CL ± P patients to decipher the landmarks and verify their reproducibility so these can be applied clinically and aid in treatment planning.

The earlier studies regarding CL ± P and their analysis made use of cephalograms alone, as that was the only imaging modality available at the time. Hotz and Gnoinski [7] advised that caution should be used in the interpretation of results involving point PNS and point A, whereas Mølsted et al. [8] reported errors for the skeletal variables like point A, ANS, and PNS. The ANS and PNS points were both statistically significant in the present study.

The Nasion and Orbitale points were not significant in our study, which is in accordance with Grauer D et al. [28] who observed similar results, whereas Chang ZC et al. [29] implied that the identification error increased at the Nasion and Orbitale on the CBCT-derived cephalograms. Ludlow JB et al. [21] concluded that the Nasion and Orbitale had no significant variation in anterior–posterior (AP) measurement but had a significant variation of caudal cranial (CC) values. Moreover, Chien PC et al. [3] also presented no variation in the Nasion in inter and intra-observer variation, whereas significant inter-observer variation was perceived in the Orbitale. Lagravère MO et al. [38] concluded that the mean difference for the Nasion was not high, but the Orbitale showed a high mean difference. The landmarks of Gonion, Nasion, Orbitale, and Anterior Nasal Spine (ANS) showed the most considerable median Euclidean distances for both intra- and inter-observer measurements according to Katkar et al. 2013 [31]. According to Durao APR et al., the Gnathion (Gn) point was the least reliable landmark for orthodontists, while the Orbitale (Or) was the least reliable landmark for dentomaxillofacial radiologists [32].

The supraorbitale point presented with statistically non-significant values, however. Turhan-Haktanir N et al. [39] studied records of 399 patients on computed tomography (CT) and concluded that the presence of a double foramen/notch was higher on the right side as cephalograms are usually taken from the right. Moreover, various types of supraorbital transcranial exits were observed by Kyu LN 2019 [40], of which the frontal notch was the most common. Woo SW et al. [41] also revealed the variation and characteristics of the supraorbital foramen or notch in a Korean population based on 3D-CT images. These findings were in contrast to those of the present study.

The anterior nasal spine ($p \leq 0.05$) point was significantly variable in inter-observer tracings. Similar findings were made by Ludlow JB et al. [21], Grauer D et al. [28], McClure SR 2005 [27], and Durao APR [32], wherein the ANS showed significant variation along with point A [6,21,27], Condylion [28,32], and Gnathion [21,33]. Conventional landmarks such as points A, ANS, and PNS are challenging to mark in children with unilateral cleft lip and palate (UCLP). However, in a study by Bongaarts CA [6], no other landmarks were found to be easier to trace. Care should be taken while interpreting the results of cephalometric studies in UCLP patients, due to inter-observer tracings, digitization, and, therefore, measurement errors utilizing landmarks like points A, ANS, and PNS [6]. Chang ZC et al. [29] also showed a positive correlation, implying that the identification error increased at the ANS on the CBCT-derived cephalograms. An intraclass correlation coefficient (ICC) of more than 15% was found by Chien PC et al. [3], who showed significant variation in the inter-examiner evaluation.

Due to a significant shift from the midline in the premaxillary region of young patients, a variation in the ANS can be explained [42]. Point PNS can be influenced by a possible palatal shelf rotation from the centerline and/or a deficiency in the size of the posterior palate [42].

The posterior nasal spine ($p \leq 0.05$) presented with significant inter-observer tracings. Chang ZC et al. [29] showed an increased error in the landmark identification of the PNS. Bonagaarts CA [6] along with Ludlow JB et al. [21] and Ghoneima A [34] also presented significant variations. However, no variation in the PNS was found in a study by Chien PC et al. [3]. Lagravère MO et al. [38] also inferred the difference in the plotting of point PNS in the X-axis for both the inter- and intra-examiner evaluation.

The root tip of the maxillary and the mandibular incisor showed significant variability. These findings are in agreement with that of Chien PC et al. [3], who had a significant variation for the lower incisor root tip, but no significant finding for the upper incisor roots. Similar observations were reported by Chang ZC et al. [29], with significant findings in the root apex of the maxillary and the mandibular incisor root apex. The reason for the difficulty of root tip identification can be attributed to tooth germ moulding, unerupted teeth in the anterior part of the maxilla, and a reduced radio-opacity due to the presence of cleft [7]. Our study shows no significant finding for incisor tips. However, Grauer D et al. [28] also showed a significant variation in the maxillary incisor tip. Additionally, Ludlow JB et al. [21] and Ghoneima A [34] presented significant findings on the maxillary and mandibular incisor tips.

In the present study, the points malare and pyriforme had a significant discrepancy. These findings are in conjugation with Suri S et al. [37], who measured the asymmetry of these two points using axial and transverse CT slices and noted no significant measurement for the malare, but a significant reduction in the sagittal positioning of the pyriforme on the cleft side.

Significant variability was observed in bilateral landmarks like the porion, along with the basion. Chang ZC et al. [29] and Ghoneima A [34] showed that there was a positive regression correlation for the basion with a high variability, but no significance for the gonion, which was found to be significant in studies conducted by Ludlow JB et al. [21], Katkar RA et al. [31], and Park J et al. [20]. The variation in the porion can be attributed to the difference in opinion in localizing the point. Some authors consider the porion as a landmark in the soft tissues of the ear canal, whereas others feel it is on a bone/soft-tissue margin. A high variability was observed by Chang ZC et al. [29] and Durao APR [32]. Chien PC et al. [3] revealed a very high degree of variability for the basion for both the intra- and inter-observer evaluation, whereas the porion and gonion showed a significant variation in the Y-axis for inter-observer variability.

Since no study was available for comparing the landmark identification errors in patients with CL ± P, the comparison was made with present studies published on the general population. Many articles have been published concerning the use of CBCT in patients with a cleft lip and/or palate (CL ± P). Now, CBCT has been proven to be a better choice for assessing bone volume, deficiencies, and root development, because it provides a better image quality at a significantly lower radiation dose. However, no evidence is available, showing that CBCT is more informative than 2D concerning facial soft-tissue analysis in patients with CLP.

CBCT scans should be carried out while weighing the pros and cons. It can be regarded as a highly reliable diagnostic tool in both simple and complex cases with CLP where 3D assessment is mandatory for making the most appropriate therapeutic decision.

5. Limitations

The primary limitation can be attributed to the non-inclusion of bilateral cleft lip and palate patients, who also constitute a large proportion of patients with a cleft lip and palate. The identification of landmarks in cases of cleft lip and palate is arduous, and not all observers are able to localize the points in a similar manner. In the present study, accuracy may have been affected by the operator's skills, expertise, and exhaustion due to frequently repeated measurements. In addition, the present study was a retrospective analysis; therefore, clinical examination of the study sample could not be done and relied solely on the medical records and data.

6. Conclusions

1. The CBCT images provide a significantly more precise location of the anterior nasal spine, Point A, posterior nasal spine, pyriforme, and malare, overcoming the problem caused due to clefting in the nasomaxillary complex.
2. Bilateral landmarks like the porion, gonion, and basion were also significantly more precise in CBCT images when compared with digital cephalograms.

Author Contributions: Conceptualization, A.S.K., M.S.S., M.P., L.P. and G.K.K.; methodology, A.S.K., M.S.S., M.P., L.N., V.G. and F.d.; software, A.S.K., M.P., L.N., F.d. and L.P.; analysis, R.B.; investigation, G.K.K., F.d. and L.P.; resources, G.K.K., F.d. and L.P.; data curation, G.K.K.; writing—original draft preparation, A.S.K., M.S.S., G.K.K., R.B., L.N., F.d., L.P., V.G. and H.D.; writing—review and editing, H.D. and G.K.K.; visualization, H.D. and G.K.K.; supervision, H.D., G.K.K., F.d., V.G. and L.P.; project administration, A.S.K. All authors have read and agreed to the published version of the manuscript.

Funding: This research received no external funding.

Institutional Review Board Statement: The study was conducted according to the guidelines of the Declaration of Helsinki, and approved by the Institutional Review of SGT Dental College, Hospital, and Research Institute, Budhera, Gurgaon, India (SGTDC/PPL/Com./E.C./14Aug2010) (institutional ethical committee). Willingness to participate in the study was obtained. All records acquired from Department Orthodontics and Dentofacial Orthopedics from March 2011 to May 2013 were used only for research purposes.

Informed Consent Statement: Informed consent was obtained from all subjects involved in the study.

Data Availability Statement: The data presented in this study are available on request from the corresponding author.

Acknowledgments: The authors acknowledge Sunjay Suri, BDS, MDS, MOrth RCS (Edinburgh), DNB, DIBO, FRCDC, FACD, FICD, Professor and Director, Graduate Orthodontics, Faculty of Dentistry, University of Toronto for constant guidance and motivation.

Conflicts of Interest: The authors declare no conflict of interest.

References

1. Houston, W. The analysis of errors in orthodontic measurements. *Am. J. Orthod.* **1983**, *83*, 382–390. [CrossRef]
2. Gupta, A.; Kharbanda, O.P.; Balachandran, R.; Sardana, V.; Kalra, S.; Chaurasia, S.; Sardana, H.K. Precision of manual landmark identification between as-received and oriented volume-rendered cone-beam computed tomography images. *Am. J. Orthod. Dentofac. Orthop.* **2017**, *151*, 118–131. [CrossRef]
3. Chien, P.C.; Parks, E.; Eraso, F.; Hartsfield, J.; Roberts, W.; Ofner, S. Comparison of reliability in anatomical landmark identification using two-dimensional digital cephalometrics and three-dimensional cone beam computed tomography in vivo. *Dentomaxillofacial Radiol.* **2009**, *38*, 262–273. [CrossRef]
4. Kragskov, J.; Bosch, C.; Gyldensted, C.; Sindet-Pedersen, S. Comparison of the reliability of craniofacial anatomic landmarks based on cephalometric radiographs and three-dimensional CT scans. *Cleft Palate Craniofacial J.* **1997**, *34*, 111–116. [CrossRef] [PubMed]
5. Tulunoglu, O.; Esenlik, E.; Gulsen, A.; Tulunoglu, I. A comparison of three-dimensional and two-dimensional cephalometric evaluations of children with cleft lip and palate. *Eur. J. Dent.* **2011**, *5*, 451–458. [CrossRef] [PubMed]
6. Bongaarts, C.A.; van't Hof, M.A.; Prahl-Andersen, B.; Kuijpers-Jagtman, A.M. Identification of cephalometric landmarks in unilateral cleft lip and palate patients: Are there alternatives for Point A, ANS, and PNS? *Cleft Palate Craniofacial J.* **2008**, *45*, 81–86. [CrossRef] [PubMed]
7. Hotz, M.; Gnoinski, W. Comprehensive care of cleft lip and palate children at Zürich University: A preliminary report. *Am. J. Orthod.* **1976**, *70*, 481–504. [CrossRef]
8. Mølsted, K.; Asher-MacDade, C.; Brattström, V.; Dahl, E.; Mars, M.; McWilliam, J.; Plint, D.A.; Prahl-Andersen, B.; Semb, G.; Shaw, W.C.; et al. A six-center international study of treatment outcome in patients with clefts of lip and palate: Part Craniofacial form and soft tissue profile. *Cleft Palate Craniofacial J.* **1992**, *29*, 398–404. [CrossRef]
9. Brattström, V.; Mølsted, K.; Prahl-Andersen, B.; Semb, G.; Shaw, W.C. The Eurocleft study: Intercenter study of treatment outcome in patients with complete cleft lip and palate. Part 2: Craniofacial form and nasolabial appearance. *Cleft Palate Craniofacial J.* **2005**, *42*, 69–77. [CrossRef]
10. Kawamata, A.; Ariji, Y.; Langlais, R.P. Three-dimensional computed tomography imaging in dentistry. *Dent. Clin. N. Am.* **2000**, *44*, 395–410.
11. Garib, D.G.; Yatabe, M.S.; Ozawa, T.O.; Filho, O.G. Alveolar bone morphology in patients with bilateral complete cleft lip and palate in the mixed dentition: Cone beam computed tomography evaluation. *Cleft Palate Craniofacial J.* **2012**, *49*, 214–229. [CrossRef] [PubMed]
12. Buyuk, S.K.; Ercan, E.; Celikoglu, M.; Sekerci, A.E.; Hatipoglu, M. Evaluation of dehiscence and fenestration in adolescent patients affected by unilateral cleft lip and palate: A retrospective cone beam computed tomography study. *Angle Orthod.* **2016**, *86*, 431–436. [CrossRef] [PubMed]
13. Ercan, E.; Celikoglu, M.; Buyuk, S.K.; Sekerci, A.E. Assessment of the alveolar bone support of patients with unilateral cleft lip and palate: A cone-beam computed tomography study. *Angle Orthod.* **2015**, *85*, 1003–1008. [CrossRef] [PubMed]
14. Linderup, B.W.; Küseler, A.; Jensen, J.; Cattaneo, P.M. A novel semiautomatic technique for volumetric assessment of the alveolar bone defect using cone beam computed tomography. *Cleft Palate Craniofacial J.* **2015**, *52*, 47–55. [CrossRef]
15. Celebi, A.A.; Ucar, F.I.; Sekerci, A.E.; Caglaroglu, M.; Tan, E. Effects of cleft lip and palate on the development of permanent upper central incisors: A cone-beam computed tomography study. *Eur. J. Orthod.* **2014**, *37*, 544–549. [CrossRef]
16. Starbuck, J.M.; Ghoneima, A.; Kula, K. Facial soft-tissue asymmetry in three-dimensional cone-beam computed tomography images of children with surgically corrected unilateral clefts. *J. Craniofacial Surg.* **2014**, *25*, 476–480. [CrossRef]
17. Zhang, X.; Zhang, Y.; Yang, L.; Shen, G.; Chen, Z. Asymmetric dental development investigated by cone-beam computed tomography in patients with unilateral cleft lip and alveolus. *Cleft Palate Craniofacial J.* **2016**, *53*, 413–420. [CrossRef]
18. Zhou, W.; Li, W.; Lin, J.; Liu, D.; Xie, X.; Zhang, Z. Tooth lengths of the permanent upper incisors in patients with cleft lip and palate determined with cone beam computed tomography. *Cleft Palate Craniofacial J.* **2013**, *50*, 88–95. [CrossRef]
19. Papi, P.; Giardino, R.; Sassano, P.; Amodeo, G.; Pompa, G.; Cascone, P. Oral health related quality of life in cleft lip and palate patients rehabilitated with conventional prostheses or dental implants. *J. Int. Soc. Prev. Community Dent.* **2015**, *5*, 482–487. [CrossRef]
20. Park, J.; Baumrind, S.; Curry, S.; Carlson, S.K.; Boyd, R.L.; Oh, H. Reliability of 3D dental and skeletal landmarks on CBCT images. *Angle Orthod.* **2019**, *89*, 758–767. [CrossRef]
21. Ludlow, J.B.; Gubler, M.; Cevidanes, L.; Mol, A. Precision of cephalometric landmark identification: Cone-beam computed tomography vs conventional cephalometric views. *Am. J. Orthod. Dentofac. Orthop.* **2009**, *136*, 312.e1–312.e10. [CrossRef]

22. Kochhar, A.S.; Sidhu, M.S.; Prabhakar, M.; Bhasin, R.; Kochhar, G.K.; Dadlani, H.; Spagnuolo, G.; Mehta, V.V. Intra- and Interobserver Reliability of Bone Volume Estimation Using OsiriX Software in Patients with Cleft Lip and Palate Using Cone Beam Computed Tomography. *Dent. J.* **2021**, *9*, 14. [CrossRef] [PubMed]
23. de Oliveira, A.E.F.; Cevidanes, L.H.S.; Phillips, C.; Motta, A.; Burke, B.; Tyndall, D. Observer reliability of three-dimensional cephalo-metric landmark identification on cone-beam computerized tomography. *Oral Surg. Oral Med. Oral Pathol. Oral Radiol. Endodontol.* **2009**, *107*, 256–265. [CrossRef] [PubMed]
24. Naji, P.; Alsufyani, N.; Lagravere, M. Reliability of anatomic structures as landmarks in three-dimensional cephalometric analysis using CBCT. *Angle Orthod.* **2014**, *84*, 762–772. [CrossRef]
25. Kochhar, A.S.; Sidhu, M.S.; Prabhakar, M.; Bhasin, R.; Kochhar, G.K.; Dadlani, H.; Spagnuolo, G. Frontal and axial evaluation of craniofacial morphology in repaired unilateral cleft lip and palate patients utilizing cone beam computed tomography; an observational study. *Int. J. Environ. Res. Public Health* **2020**, *17*, 7786. [CrossRef]
26. De Grauwe, A.; Ayaz, I.; Shujaat, S.; Dimitrov, S.; Gbadegbegnon, L.; VandeVannet, B.; Jacobs, R. CBCT in orthodontics: A systematic review on justification of CBCT in a paediatric population prior to orthodontic treatment. *Eur. J. Orthod.* **2019**, *41*, 381–389. [CrossRef]
27. McClure, S.R.; Sadowsky, P.L.; Ferreira, A.; Jacobson, A. Reliability of digital versus conventional cephalometric radiology: A comparative evaluation of landmark identification error. *Semin. Orthod.* **2005**, *11*, 98–110. [CrossRef]
28. Grauer, D.; Cevidanes, L.S.H.; Styner, M.; Heulfe, I.; Harmon, E.T.; Zhu, H.; Proffit, W.R. Accuracy and landmark error calculation using cone-beam computed tomography-generated cephalograms. *Angle Orthod.* **2010**, *80*, 286–294. [CrossRef]
29. Chang, Z.C.; Hu, F.C.; Lai, E.; Yao, C.C.; Chen, M.H.; Chen, Y.J. Landmark identification errors on cone-beam computed tomography-derived cephalograms and conventional digital cephalograms. *Am. J. Orthod. Dentofac. Orthop.* **2011**, *140*, e289–e297. [CrossRef]
30. Zamora, N.; Llamas, J.; Cibrian, R.; Gandia, J.; Paredes, V. A study on the reproducibility of cephalometric landmarks when undertaking a three-dimensional (3D) cephalometric analysis. *Med. Oral Patol. Oral Cir. Bucal.* **2012**, *17*, e678–e688. [CrossRef]
31. Katkar, R.A.; Kummet, C.; Dawson, D.; Uribe, L.M.; Allareddy, V.; Finkelstein, M.; Ruprecht, A. Comparison of observer reliability of three-dimensional cephalometric landmark identification on subject images from Galileos and i-CAT cone beam CT. *Dentomaxillofacial Radiol.* **2013**, *42*, 20130059. [CrossRef] [PubMed]
32. Durão, A.P.R.; Morosolli, A.; Pittayapat, P.; Bolstad, N.; Ferreira, A.P.; Jacobs, R. Cephalometric landmark variability among orthodontists and dentomaxillofacial radiologists: A comparative study. *Imaging Sci. Dent.* **2015**, *45*, 213.
33. da Neiva, M.B.; Soares, Á.C.; Lisboa, C.d.O.; Vilella, O.d.V.; Motta, A.T. Evaluation of cephalometric landmark identification on CBCT multiplanar and 3D reconstructions. *Angle Orthod.* **2015**, *85*, 11–17. [CrossRef] [PubMed]
34. Ghoneima, A.; Cho, H.; Farouk, K.; Kula, K. Accuracy and reliability of landmark-based, surface-based and voxel-based 3D cone-beam computed tomography superimposition methods. *Orthod. Craniofacial Res.* **2017**, *20*, 227–236. [CrossRef] [PubMed]
35. Chen, Y.-J.; Chen, S.-K.; Yao, C.-C.J.; Chang, H.-F. The effects of differences in landmark identification on the cephalometric measurements in traditional versus digitized cephalometry. *Angle Orthod.* **2004**, *74*, 155–161.
36. Mossey, P.A.; Little, J.; Munger, R.G.; Dixon, M.J.; Shaw, W.C. Cleft lip and palate. *Lancet* **2009**, *374*, 1773–1785. [CrossRef]
37. Suri, S.; Utreja, A.; Khandelwal, N.; Mago, S.K. Craniofacial computerized tomography analysis of the midface of patients with repaired complete unilateral cleft lip and palate. *Am. J. Orthod. Dentofac. Orthop.* **2008**, *134*, 418–429. [CrossRef]
38. Lagravère, M.O.; Low, C.; Flores-Mir, C.; Chung, R.; Carey, J.P.; Heo, G.; Major, P.W. Intraexaminer and interexaminer reliabilities of landmark identification on digitized lateral cephalograms and formatted 3-dimensional cone-beam computerized tomography images. *Am. J. Orthod. Dentofac. Orthop.* **2010**, *137*, 598–604. [CrossRef]
39. Turhan-Haktanır, N.; Ayçiçek, A.; Haktanır, A.; Demir, Y. Variations of supraorbital foramina in living subjects evaluated with multidetector computed tomography. *Head Neck* **2008**, *30*, 1211–1215. [CrossRef]
40. Lim, N.K.; Kim, Y.H.; Kang, D.H. Precision analysis of supraorbital transcranial exits using three dimensional multidetector computed tomography. *J. Craniofacial Surg.* **2019**, *30*, 1894–1897. [CrossRef]
41. Woo, S.W.; Lee, H.J.; Nahm, F.S.; Lee, P.B.; Choi, E. Anatomic characteristics of supraorbital foramina in Korean using three-dimensional model. *Korean J. Pain* **2013**, *26*, 130–134. [CrossRef] [PubMed]
42. Atherton, J.D. A descriptive anatomy of the face in human fetuses with unilateral cleft lip and palate. *Cleft Palate Craniofacial J.* **1967**, *4*, 104–114.

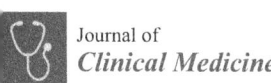

Article

Using Salivary MMP-9 to Successfully Quantify Periodontal Inflammation during Orthodontic Treatment

Ionut Luchian [1], Mihaela Moscalu [2,*], Ancuta Goriuc [3,*], Ludovica Nucci [4], Monica Tatarciuc [5], Ioana Martu [5] and Mihai Covasa [6,7]

1. Department of Periodontology, Grigore T. Popa University of Medicine and Pharmacy, 700115 Iasi, Romania; ionut.luchian@umfiasi.ro
2. Department of Preventive Medicine and Interdisciplinarity, Grigore T. Popa University of Medicine and Pharmacy, 700115 Iasi, Romania
3. Department of Biochemistry, Grigore T. Popa University of Medicine and Pharmacy, 700115 Iasi, Romania
4. Multidisciplinary Department of Medical-Surgical and Dental Specialties, University of Campania Luigi Vanvitelli, 81100 Naples, Italy; ludovica.nucci@unicampania.it
5. Department of Dental Technology, Grigore T. Popa University of Medicine and Pharmacy, 700115 Iasi, Romania; monica.tatarciuc@umfiasi.ro (M.T.); ioana.martu@umfiasi.ro (I.M.)
6. Department of Health and Human Development, Stefan cel Mare University of Suceava, 720229 Suceava, Romania; mcovasa@westernu.edu
7. Department of Basic Medical Sciences, College of Osteopathic Medicine, Western University of Health Sciences, Pomona, CA 91766, USA
* Correspondence: mihaela.moscalu@umfiasi.ro (M.M.); ancuta.goriuc@umfiasi.ro (A.G.)

Abstract: Periodontitis is one of the most common immune-mediated inflammatory conditions resulting in progressive destruction of periodontium. Metalloproteinase-9 (MMP-9), an enzyme that is involved in the degradation of gelatin and collagen and present in the gingival crevicular fluid, is markedly increased in periodontitis. The aim of the study is to evaluate the effects of periodontal treatment either alone or in combination with orthodontic treatment on MMP-9 levels. In this study, 60 individuals were subjected to periodontal treatment (PD) or periodontal treatment combined with orthodontic treatment (POD). Both periodontal and periodontal plus orthodontic treatments significantly improved clinical parameters and lowered MMP-9 levels compared to control group. However, the combination of periodontal with orthodontic treatment further improved clinical parameters and enhanced the lowering effect on MMP-9 levels compared to periodontal or control groups alone. Finally, the degree of malocclusion significantly affected the effect of the treatment on MPP-9 levels with PD treatment having the most pronounced effect. We concluded that salivary MMP-9 can serve to accurately predict the level of inflammation in affected periodontal tissues during orthodontic treatment that is also associated with the type of malocclusion, making it a viable diagnosis tool in monitoring the progression of the periodontium during orthodontic treatment.

Keywords: periodontitis; saliva; matrix metalloproteinase

1. Introduction

Periodontitis represents one of the most prevalent chronic inflammatory oral diseases. It is characterized by an inflammatory destruction of periodontal attachment complex leading to irreversible loss of bone and tooth-supporting tissue [1,2]. Among the components of periodontium lost is type I collagen, found primarily in periodontal ligament and alveolar organic matrix [3,4]. The destruction of periodontium is mediated by the plasminogen-dependent, phagocytic, osteoclastic, and matrix metalloproteinase (MMP) pathways [5,6]. The MMPs, a family of zinc and calcium-dependent proteolytic enzymes, which are secreted by immune cells in response to inflammatory stimuli, are considered the most important in mediating the degradation of the extracellular matrix [7,8] and have been recognized as important biomarkers in the early detection of several diseases [9].

Normally, these enzymes are tightly regulated and play a critical role in bone morphogenesis and tissue repair [10,11]. However, in pathological conditions such as periodontitis, these enzymes are involved in the destruction of extracellular matrix components such as collagen, elastin, fibronectin, laminin, and entactin [12,13]. This results in oral pathological processes such as the destruction of the periodontal tissue, tumor invasion, and dysfunctions of the temporomandibular joint (TMJ) [14,15]. Among these several groups of proteinases, the zinc-metalloproteinases such as matrix metallopeptidases 9 (MMP-9) contain a Zn ion in the catalytic domain. Moreover, MMP-2 and MMP-9 may have a binding domain for gelatin, inserted between the catalytic and the active domain, and this is the reason of why MMP-9 is also called gelatinase B [9]. MMP-9 or gelatinase B is primarily found in saliva and gingival crevicular fluid; it is present in dental tissues with numerous active forms, weighing 82–132 kD, and is involved in inflammation, wound healing, and tumor growth [16]. The involvement of MMP-9 both in periodontal disease and in the orthodontic periodontal reshaping has already been demonstrated by several studies [17–20]. Both in vivo and in vitro evidence show that orthodontic dental movement causes mechanical stress [21,22], which, in turn, generates biochemical and structural responses in a diversity of cell types [18,23,24]. As such, the early stage of orthodontic dental movements involves an acute inflammatory response featuring local tissular ischemia, periodontal vasodilatation, and the migration of leucocytes through the capillaries of the periodontal ligament [25]. Elevated MMPs have been associated with increased inflammation and loss of tooth-supporting tissue present in periodontal disease, while periodontal treatment decreases inflammation and lowers MMP-9 levels [23,26–28]. To determine whether MMP-9 levels can reliably predict the chronic inflammatory oral diseases, in this study, we examine the effects of periodontal treatment on salivary MMP-9 levels in patients with stabilized pre-existing periodontal history, where treatment is done either without or coupled with orthodontic treatment.

2. Materials and Methods
2.1. Subjects

The study was performed under the Institutional Review Board protocol no. 5329/2018 approved by the ethics committee of the Grigore T. Popa University of Medicine and Pharmacy, and signed informed consent was obtained from each participant in the study. The sample population included in the current research consists of consecutive patients that were selected in a 12-month interval. Sixty individuals of which 32 males and 28 females in good general health from 21 to 38-year-old were enrolled in the study. The following inclusion criteria were used: a minimum of 20 teeth in functional dentition, moderate or severe periodontitis and without periodontal treatment at the time of enrolment. Periodontal exam included the recording of periodontal pocket depths (PPD) from six sites of each tooth. The six probing sites were distributed as follows: three sites on the buccal surfaces (mesial, central, and distal) and three sites on the lingual surfaces of the teeth (mesial, central, and distal). Bleeding on probing was recorded and the sulcus bleeding index (SBI) was determined. A complete periodontal probing was performed using an electronic probe (PaOn®, Orange Dental, Biberach a. d. Riss, Baden-Würtemberg State, Germany), and data were transferred using additional software. The following exclusion criteria were applied: smoking, heavy drinkers, immunocompromised, use of anti-inflammatory drugs or other medication affecting the periodontium, use of antibiotics and steroids, and a history of systemic and infectious diseases.

The sixty patients included in the study were randomly divided in three groups as follows: group 1, a control group that included 16 (7 men, 9 women) subjects without periodontal disease and/or clinical gingival modifications; group 2, which included 22 subjects (10 men, 12 women) with periodontal disease (chronic periodontitis localized in minimum 3 teeth) who received periodontal treatment (PD); and group 3, which included 22 (11 men, 11 women) subjects with periodontal disease (chronic periodontitis localized in minimum 3 teeth), who received both periodontal and orthodontic treatment (POD). All individuals received periodontal examination and were diagnosed based on the clinical criteria established by the American Academy of Periodontology [29]. All patients underwent treatment including oral hygiene instructions. Periodontal treatment was identical for both PD and POD groups and consisted of supra- and subgingival scaling and root planning over a maximum 4-week period. The subgingival scaling was performed using the same ultrasonic device (Acteon Satelec®, Mérignac, Gironde, France), and the same type of subgingival inserts while for root planning area specific curettes (Hu-Friedy®, Chicago, IL, USA) were used. Therapeutic treatments were performed every 8 weeks starting 10 days after study commencement. For orthodontic treatment, we used metallic fixed appliances that were bonded after the periodontal status stabilized. No dropouts occurred prior or during the treatment.

2.2. Saliva Sample Collection and Analysis

Saliva was collected at two time points from patients included in PD and POD groups as follows: for the PD group, one initial baseline collection and a second collection 6 months following completion of periodontal treatment; for the POD group, one initial baseline collection and a second collection 6 months after completion of periodontal treatment and stabilization of the orthodontic treatment. The timing for the second saliva collection in the POD group was delayed compared to the PD group to allow for an evaluation of the effects of the orthodontic treatment on the inflammatory markers level once the treatment has stabilized. One baseline saliva collection was performed in the control group at the beginning of the study. All samples were collected by one investigator to ensure consistency in the protocol. Saliva was collected without stimulating its secretion from the salivary glands (i.e., paraffin gum or citric acid) in order to avoid any interference of the stimulating agent on marker release. Collection was carried out using Eppendorf tubes placed on ice; particular attention was given to contamination with blood, since MPP is also present in blood and its levels were shown to be different (i.e., higher) in blood compared to those present in the salivary fluid. Samples suspected of blood contamination were discarded. Samples were stored at $-20\ °C$ pending analysis. The levels of MMP-9 in collected saliva samples were measured via ELISA immunoassay following the manufacturer's instructions (R&D Systems Inc., Minneapolis, MN, USA) [19].

2.3. Statistical Analyses

Statistical analyses were performed using SPSS 24.0 for Windows (IBM Corporation, North Castle Drive, Armonk, NY, USA). The Kruskal–Wallis test was applied to determine the differences in MMP concentrations between groups of patients according to treatment and clinical parameters. The Newman–Keuls post hoc test was also applied for the pair analysis of two groups of patients. MMP-9 values were reported as mean values and standard deviation. The evolution of MMP-9 values was also presented in %, with the proportion being represented by the decrease of the MMP-9 value related to the value registered before the treatment. The univariate correlational analysis was performed based on the Spearman rank order correlations test. To better highlight the effect of the treatment and the degree of malocclusion, the graphs were generated using STATA 16.1 (StataCorp LLC., College Station, TX, USA). A p-value of less than 0.05 was considered statistically significant.

3. Results

3.1. Clinical Parameters

Analysis showed a significant difference before treatment between PD and control groups for PPD (4.18 ± 0.21 vs. 1.65 ± 0.14, $p < 0.0001$) and SBI (2.9 ± 0.11, vs. 0.31 ± 0.11, $p < 0.0001$) as well as between POD and control groups for the same parameters: PPD = 4.54 ± 0.17, $p < 0.0001$; SBI = 3.45 ± 0.12, $p < 0.001$. Periodontitis treatment significantly improved PPD (3.23 ± 0.19, $p < 0.01$) and SBI (2.04 ± 0.12, $p < 0.01$) while periodontitis combined with orthodontic treatment had a greater effect compared to the control group and the PD group's treatment for both clinical parameters, i.e., PPD = 2.4 ± 0.1, SBI = 2.04 ± 0.12, $p < 0.0001$ for both.

3.2. Effects of Periodontal and Combined Periodontal with Orthodontic Treatment on MMP-9 Levels

Patients with untreated periodontal disease had significantly higher levels of salivary MMP-9 compared to controls (control group: 155.6 ± 38.63 ng/mL; PD: 582.27 ± 48.2 ng/mL; POD group: 602.55 ± 64.55 ng/mL; $p < 0.0001$ for both, Figure 1). However, following intervention, periodontal treatment alone lowered MMP-9 significantly compared to the levels before treatment (17.3% reduction; $p = 0.0046$). A combination of periodontal with orthodontic treatment drastically decreased MMP-9 levels by 42.3% compared to pre-treatment levels ($p < 0.0001$). Although MMP-9 levels dropped significantly after treatment in both PD and POD groups, there was a significant difference ($p = 0.00012$) in MMP-9 levels following each of the two treatments, with the treatment for the POD group having the most significant effect in lowering MMP-9 levels compared to the PD and control groups ($p = 0.0005$) (Figure 1).

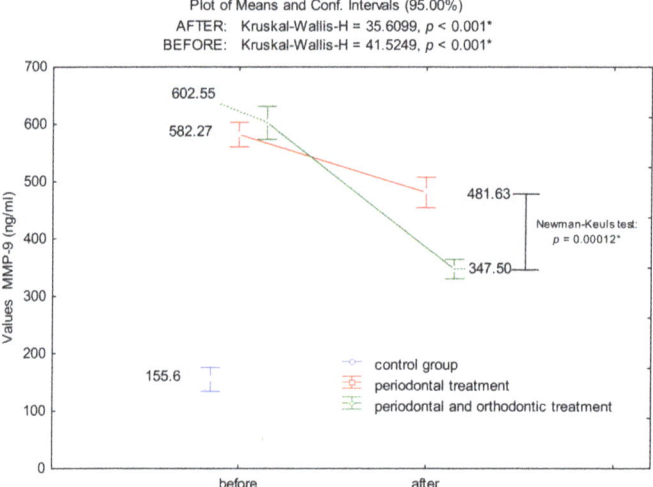

Figure 1. The means value of MMP-9 [ng/mL] in patients with periodontal disease prior and after periodontal treatment (PD) and periodontal and orthodontic treatment (POD) treatment; (*) indicates that marked effects are significant at $p < 0.05$.

3.3. The Effect of Malocclusion on MMP-9 Levels

The degree of malocclusion significantly affected salivary MMP-9 levels. Because of this, prior to treatment, patients with periodontal disease had MMP-9 values that differed significantly depending on the angle class (PD group: $p = 0.005$; POD group: $p = 0.003$); this effect was more pronounced in patients with angle class II/1 and II/2 (Figure 2). Following the PD group's treatment, MMP-9 decreased significantly compared as a function of the angle class ($p = 0.03$). The treatment in the POD group significantly lowered MMP-9 levels compared to those of the PD and control groups ($p < 0.0001$); however, there were no significant differences between the angle classes ($p = 0.176$) (Figure 2).

3.4. Correlation Between Clinical Parameters and MMP-9 Levels

Before treatment, the Spearman rank analyses showed a significant positive association between the probing pocket depth (PPD) and MMP-9 levels in POD patients ($r = 0.47$, $p = 0.03$) with no difference in the PD group ($r = 0.033$, $p = 0.88$). Following intervention, MMP-9 levels were significantly correlated with PPD in the PD group ($r = 0.33$, $p = 0.029$) but not in the POD group ($r = 0.678$, $p = 0.764$). Similarly, there was a significant correlation between SBI and MMP-9 levels before treatment in the POD group ($r = 0.47$, $p = 0.032$) but not the PD group ($r = 0.08$, $p = 0.71$). After treatment in the PD group, MMP-9 levels in the PD group were significantly correlated with SBI ($r = 0.46$, $p = 0.034$) while the treatment in POD group abrogated the correlation between SBI and MMP-9.

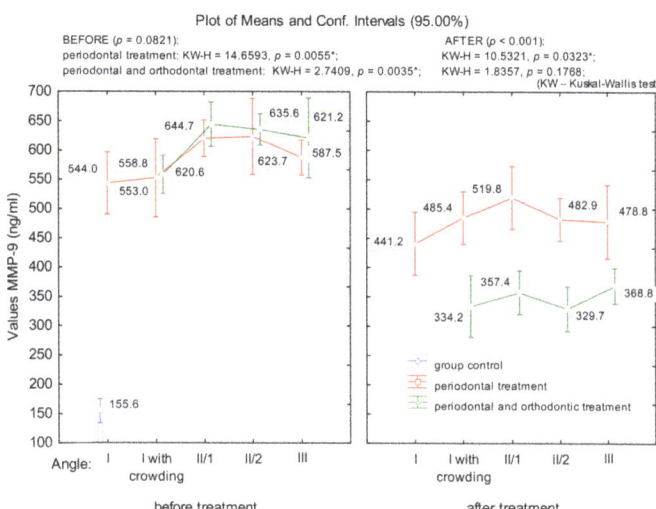

Figure 2. The means value of MMP-9 in patients with periodontal disease, in relation to angle class; (*) indicates that marked effects are significant at $p < 0.05$.

4. Discussion

The results of this study show that both periodontal and the combination of periodontal and orthodontic treatments were effective in significantly lowering MMP-9 levels compared to patients who did not receive the treatment. However, it was the combination of periodontal with orthodontic treatment that had the greatest effect on MMP-9 levels compared to periodontal or control groups alone. Furthermore, while the treatment in both the PD and POD groups significantly improved clinical parameters, the POD group treatment had the greatest effect. This improvement of clinical parameters following intervention in the PD and POD groups was positively associated with MMP-9 levels. Finally, the degree of malocclusion significantly affected the effect of the treatment on MPP-9 levels with PD treatment having the most pronounced effect.

Periodontitis is one of the most prevalent inflammatory pathology affecting nearly half of people over 30 years old [3]. It is characterized by an immune inflammatory process ultimately leading to the destruction of periodontal attachment and supporting tissue and bone resorption. Several periodontal bacteria together with microbial proteases such as metalloproteases including host-derived MMPs, all participate in the process leading to progression of periodontitis, tissue, and ligament degradation. Among them are *Aggregatibacter actinomycetemcomitans*, *Porphyromonas gingivalis*, *Treponema denticola*, and *Tannerella forsythia*; together with the host's genetics and other environmental factors, these bacteria are active contributors in the infections and inflammatory processes that result in the production of metalloproteases, including host MMPs [16,30,31]. MMP-9 is among the best studied proteinases when it comes to its role in periodontitis and its activation in infections.

In the present study, salivary MMP-9 levels were associated significantly with periodontal and orthodontic treatment and differentiated from the control group. Therefore, MMP-9 can be used with high fidelity not only as a marker of periodontal inflammation but also as a tool for assessing the effectiveness of the nonsurgical periodontal and orthodontic therapy. The increased MMPs, whether in saliva or serum samples in periodontitis, were well documented. For example, salivary as well as circulating MMP-8 and MMP-9 levels were significantly elevated in periodontitis patients [32] and reduced after periodontal treatment [19,33,34].

The use of MMPs as salivary markers for local or systemic pathologies such as CVDs, diabetes, dyslipidemia has been of interest for sometimes, but not without challenges, given their vulnerability against local inhibitors in periodontitis condition that can limit their use in systemic diseases [35]. In addition to the periodontitis group that was associated with increased MMP-9, patients who received both periodontal as well as orthodontic treatment displayed an augmentation in the inhibition of MMP-9 levels, compared with either treatment alone. To our knowledge, this is the first report demonstrating that combination of periodontal and orthodontic treatment is associated with a reduction in MMP-9 levels.

Previous work has shown increased salivary biomarkers in orthodontic treatment involving alignment with fixed appliances, which have been associated with tooth movement [36,37]. This is not surprising since there is increased osteoclast activity when orthodontic forces are applied, and MMP-9 is expressed in osteoclasts where it controls proteolysis in bone resorption. Therefore, inflammatory markers such as MMP-9 are associated with osteoclasts activity, a phenomenon present in response to orthodontic applied forces [17,38]. In vitro studies showed an increase in MMP-9 following application of orthodontic forces, an effect that is dependent on the degree of tension and compression [39]. In our study, however, we measured MMP-9 levels after orthodontic treatment was completed and patients stabilized. This resulted in a further decrease in the MMP-9 levels in patients who received orthodontic treatment after periodontitis was improved or resolved. These results are also in line with findings demonstrating that MMP-9 levels decreased significantly in patients with periodontitis with orthodontic restorations [40] and that MMP-9 levels oscillated during application of orthodontic forces and decreased as early as 24h after appliance activation [41].

Another important aspect of the study is highlighted by the findings that the MMP-9 values following the combined treatment dropped significantly more for all angle classes, with no significant differences between groups, whereas in the case of periodontal treatment MMP-9 values remain elevated in the patients who had angle classes II and III malocclusions. A comparative analysis of MMP-9 values in relation to the type of treatment and to the angle class shows that after combined periodontal and orthodontic treatment, the values of MMP-9 lowered significantly more, despite the fact that they were significantly higher before treatment.

Therefore, although at the start of the treatment patients with periodontal problems who were about to begin periodontal treatment combined with orthodontic treatment had higher values of MMP-9 (although not significant), these values dropped significantly more compared to those of patients who had only periodontal treatment. The persistence of high values of MMP-9 in patients who received only periodontal treatment, particularly in the case of those with angle classes II/2 and II/1 malocclusions, as well as those with angle class III malocclusions, is convincing and clearly demonstrates that orthodontic treatment combined with periodontal treatment significantly reduces inflammation in the affected periodontal tissues.

A complex analysis to assess changes in MMP-9 values in chronic inflammatory oral diseases could be performed using both MMP-9 levels and the type of treatment, in a clustered form. This method could lead to a significant increase in the prediction of the evolution of periodontal disease [42].

Existing literature shows that both the saliva tests and the tests performed on crevicular fluid provide valuable diagnosis information concerning the stage of the inflammation in periodontal disease. Several authors have shown that metalloproteinase-8 (MMP-8), an enzyme responsible for tissue destruction, was positively associated with periodontal disease [43–45]. Because of this, an immunochromatography assay was developed and is commercially available for assessing MMP-8 in crevicular fluid. This test can be carried out in clinical practice and has the same accuracy as a laboratory test. This facilitates testing of this particular metalloproteinase and opens new perspectives in terms of the predictability of the chosen treatment plan [46]. Currently, no similar test/assay exists for determining MMP-9 in saliva or in the crevicular fluid.

5. Conclusions

In conclusion, our results point to salivary MMP-9 as a strong candidate for quantifying inflammation in affected periodontal tissues during orthodontic treatment. It further indicates that MMP-9 can be used to accurately predict the level of inflammation associated with the type of malocclusion, which makes it a real and viable diagnosis instrument in monitoring the evolution of the periodontium during orthodontic treatment. Larger scale studies conducted on patients with various degrees of periodontitis and orthodontic treatments are needed to further establish the use of salivary MMP-9 as a predictor of inflammation following orthodontic treatment.

Author Contributions: Conceptualization, I.L., M.T., A.G., L.N. and M.C.; methodology, I.L., M.T., M.C., I.M., A.G., L.N. and M.M.; validation, M.T. and M.C.; formal analysis, M.M.; investigation, I.L., M.T., I.M. and A.G.; resources, I.L., M.T. and A.G.; data curation, M.M. and I.L.; writing—original draft preparation, I.L., L.N. and A.G.; writing—review and editing, M.T., M.C. and M.M.; visualization, I.L., A.G., M.M.; supervision, M.T. and M.C. All authors have read and agreed to the published version of the manuscript.

Funding: This research received no external funding.

Institutional Review Board Statement: The study was conducted according to the guidelines of the Declaration of Helsinki and approved by the ethics committee of the Grigore T. Popa University of Medicine and Pharmacy Iasi, Romania (number 5329/2018).

Informed Consent Statement: Informed consent was obtained from all subjects involved in the study.

Conflicts of Interest: The authors declare no conflict of interest.

References

1. Könönen, E.; Gursoy, M.; Gursoy, U.K. Periodontitis: A Multifaceted Disease of Tooth-Supporting Tissues. *J. Clin. Med.* **2019**, *8*, 1135. [CrossRef]
2. Kim, J.Y.; Kim, H.N. Changes in Inflammatory Cytokines in Saliva after Non-Surgical Periodontal Therapy: A Systematic Review and Meta-Analysis. *Int. J. Environ. Res. Public Health* **2020**, *18*, 194. [CrossRef] [PubMed]
3. Papapanou, P.N.; Susin, C. Periodontitis epidemiology: Is periodontitis under-recognized, over-diagnosed, or both? *Periodontol. 2000* **2017**, *75*, 45–51. [CrossRef] [PubMed]
4. Benjamin, R.M. Oral health: The silent epidemic. *Public Health Rep.* **2010**, *125*, 158–159. [CrossRef] [PubMed]
5. Uitto, V.J.; Overall, C.M.; McCulloch, C. Proteolytic host cell enzymes in gingival crevice fluid. *Periodontology 2000* **2003**, *31*, 77–104. [CrossRef] [PubMed]
6. Minervini, G.; Nucci, L.; Lanza, A.; Femiano, F.; Contaldo, M.; Grassia, V. Temporomandibular disc displacement with reduction treated with anterior repositioning splint: A 2-year clinical and magnetic resonance imaging (MRI) follow-up. *J. Biol. Regul. Homeost. Agents* **2020**, *34*, 151–160. [PubMed]
7. Boelen, G.J.; Boute, L.; d'Hoop, J.; EzEldeen, M.; Lambrichts, I.; Opdenakker, G. Matrix metalloproteinases and inhibitors in dentistry. *Clin. Oral. Investig.* **2019**, *23*, 2823–2835. [CrossRef]
8. Moccia, S.; Nucci, L.; Spagnuolo, C.; d'Apuzzo, F.; Piancino, M.G.; Minervini, G. Polyphenols as Potential Agents in the Management of Temporomandibular Disorders. *Appl. Sci.* **2020**, *10*, 5305. [CrossRef]
9. Laronha, H.; Caldeira, J. Structure and Function of Human Matrix Metalloproteinases. *Cells* **2020**, *9*, 1076. [CrossRef]
10. Birkedal-Hansen, H. Role of matrix metalloproteinases in human periodontal diseases. *J. Periodontol.* **1993**, *64* (Suppl. 5), 474–484.
11. Sorsa, T.; Tjaderhane, L.; Salo, T. Matrix metalloproteinases (MMPs) in oral diseases. *Oral. Dis.* **2004**, *10*, 311–318. [CrossRef] [PubMed]
12. Rathnayake, N.; Gustafsson, A.; Norhammar, A.; Kjellstrom, B.; Klinge, B.; Ryden, L.; Tervahartiala, T.; Sorsa, T.; Group, P.S. Salivary Matrix Metalloproteinase-8 and -9 and Myeloperoxidase in Relation to Coronary Heart and Periodontal Diseases: A Subgroup Report from the PAROKRANK Study (Periodontitis and Its Relation to Coronary Artery Disease). *PLoS ONE* **2015**, *10*, e0126370. [CrossRef] [PubMed]
13. Narayanan, A.S.; Page, R.C. Connective tissues of the periodontium: A summary of current work. *Coll. Relat. Res.* **1983**, *3*, 33–64. [CrossRef]

14. Aiba, T.; Akeno, N.; Kawane, T.; Okamoto, H.; Horiuchi, N. Matrix metalloproteinases-1 and -8 and TIMP-1 mRNA levels in normal and diseased human gingivae. *Eur. J. Oral. Sci.* **1996**, *104*, 562–569. [CrossRef] [PubMed]
15. Escalona, L.A.; Mastromatteo-Alberga, P.; Correnti, M. Cytokine and metalloproteinases in gingival fluid from patients with chronic periodontitis. *Investig. Clin.* **2016**, *57*, 131–142. [PubMed]
16. Sorsa, T.; Tjaderhane, L.; Konttinen, Y.T.; Lauhio, A.; Salo, T.; Lee, H.M.; Golub, L.M.; Brown, D.L.; Mantyla, P. Matrix metalloproteinases: Contribution to pathogenesis, diagnosis and treatment of periodontal inflammation. *Ann. Med.* **2006**, *38*, 306–321. [CrossRef] [PubMed]
17. Grant, M.; Wilson, J.; Rock, P.; Chapple, I. Induction of cytokines, MMP9, TIMPs, RANKL and OPG during orthodontic tooth movement. *Eur. J. Orthod.* **2013**, *35*, 644–651. [CrossRef]
18. Lahdentausta, L.S.J.; Paju, S.; Mantyla, P.; Buhlin, K.; Tervahartiala, T.; Pietiainen, M.; Alfthan, H.; Nieminen, M.S.; Sinisalo, J.; Sorsa, T.; et al. Saliva and serum biomarkers in periodontitis and coronary artery disease. *J. Clin. Periodontol.* **2018**, *45*, 1045–1055. [CrossRef]
19. Marcaccini, A.M.; Meschiari, C.A.; Zuardi, L.R.; de Sousa, T.S.; Taba, M., Jr.; Teofilo, J.M.; Jacob-Ferreira, A.L.; Tanus-Santos, J.E.; Novaes, A.B., Jr.; Gerlach, R.F. Gingival crevicular fluid levels of MMP-8, MMP-9, TIMP-2, and MPO decrease after periodontal therapy. *J. Clin. Periodontol.* **2010**, *37*, 180–190. [CrossRef]
20. Grassia, V.; D'Apuzzo, F.; Ferrulli, V.E.; Matarese, G.; Femiano, F.; Perillo, L. Dento-skeletal effects of mixed palatal expansion evaluated by postero-anterior cephalometric analysis. *Eur. J. Paediatr. Dent.* **2014**, *15*, 59–62.
21. Maspero, C.; Fama, A.; Cavagnetto, D.; Abate, A.; Farronato, M. Treatment of dental dilacerations. *J. Biol. Regul. Homeost. Agents* **2019**, *33*, 1623–1627. [PubMed]
22. Maspero, C.; Abate, A.; Cavagnetto, D.; Fama, A.; Stabilini, A.; Farronato, G.; Farronato, M. Operculectomy and spontaneous eruption of impacted second molars: A retrospective study. *J. Biol. Regul. Homeost. Agents* **2019**, *33*, 1909–1912. [PubMed]
23. Alikhani, M.; Chou, M.Y.; Khoo, E.; Alansari, S.; Kwal, R.; Elfersi, T.; Almansour, A.; Sangsuwon, C.; Al Jearah, M.; Nervina, J.M.; et al. Age-dependent biologic response to orthodontic forces. *Am. J. Orthod. Dentofac. Orthop.* **2018**, *153*, 632–644. [CrossRef] [PubMed]
24. Perinetti, G.; D'Apuzzo, F.; Contardo, L.; Primozic, J.; Rupel, K.; Perillo, L. Gingival crevicular fluid alkaline phosphate activity during the retention phase of maxillary expansion in prepubertal subjects: A split-mouth longitudinal study. *Am. J. Orthod. Dentofac. Orthop.* **2015**, *148*, 90–96. [CrossRef] [PubMed]
25. Di Domenico, M.; D'Apuzzo, F.; Feola, A.; Cito, L.; Monsurro, A.; Pierantoni, G.M.; Berrino, L.; De Rosa, A.; Polimeni, A.; Perillo, L. Cytokines and VEGF induction in orthodontic movement in animal models. *J. Biomed. Biotechnol.* **2012**, *2012*, 201689. [CrossRef]
26. Balli, U.; Keles, G.C.; Cetinkaya, B.O.; Mercan, U.; Ayas, B.; Erdogan, D. Assessment of vascular endothelial growth factor and matrix metalloproteinase-9 in the periodontium of rats treated with atorvastatin. *J. Periodontol.* **2014**, *85*, 178–187. [CrossRef]
27. Meschiari, C.A.; Marcaccini, A.M.; Santos Moura, B.C.; Zuardi, L.R.; Tanus-Santos, J.E.; Gerlach, R.F. Salivary MMPs, TIMPs, and MPO levels in periodontal disease patients and controls. *Clin. Chim. Acta* **2013**, *421*, 140–146. [CrossRef]
28. Goncalves, P.F.; Huang, H.; McAninley, S.; Alfant, B.; Harrison, P.; Aukhil, I.; Walker, C.; Shaddox, L.M. Periodontal treatment reduces matrix metalloproteinase levels in localized aggressive periodontitis. *J. Periodontol.* **2013**, *84*, 1801–1808. [CrossRef]
29. Greenwell, H.; Committee on Research, Science and Therapy; American Academy of Periodontology. Position paper: Guidelines for periodontal therapy. *J. Periodontol.* **2001**, *72*, 1624–1628.
30. Rathnayake, N.; Gieselmann, D.R.; Heikkinen, A.M.; Tervahartiala, T.; Sorsa, T. Salivary Diagnostics-Point-of-Care diagnostics of MMP-8 in dentistry and medicine. *Diagnostics (Basel)* **2017**, *7*, 7. [CrossRef]
31. Cobzeanu, B.M.; Costan, V.V.; Danciu, M.; Pasca, A.S.; Sulea, D.; Ungureanu, L.B.; Moscalu, M.; Cobzeanu, M.D.; Popescu, E. Environmental factors involved in genesis of retromolar—oropharynx junction cancer. *Environ. Eng. Manag. J.* **2017**, *16*, 1101–1106. [CrossRef]
32. Marcaccini, A.M.; Novaes, A.B., Jr.; Meschiari, C.A.; Souza, S.L.; Palioto, D.B.; Sorgi, C.A.; Faccioli, L.H.; Tanus-Santos, J.E.; Gerlach, R.F. Circulating matrix metalloproteinase-8 (MMP-8) and MMP-9 are increased in chronic periodontal disease and decrease after non-surgical periodontal therapy. *Clin. Chim. Acta* **2009**, *409*, 117–122. [CrossRef] [PubMed]
33. Correa, F.O.B.; Goncalves, D.; Figueredo, C.M.S.; Gustafsson, A.; Orrico, S.R.P. The Short-Term Effectiveness of Non-Surgical Treatment in Reducing Levels of Interleukin-1beta and Proteases in Gingival Crevicular Fluid from Patients with Type 2 Diabetes Mellitus and Chronic Periodontitis. *J. Periodontol.* **2008**, *79*, 2143–2150. [CrossRef] [PubMed]
34. Figueredo, C.M.; Areas, A.; Miranda, L.A.; Fischer, R.G.; Gustafsson, A. The short-term effectiveness of non-surgical treatment in reducing protease activity in gingival crevicular fluid from chronic periodontitis patients. *J. Clin. Periodontol.* **2004**, *31*, 615–619. [CrossRef]
35. Miller, C.S.; Foley, J.D.; Bailey, A.L.; Campell, C.L.; Humphries, R.L.; Christodoulides, N.; Floriano, P.N.; Simmons, G.; Bhagwandin, B.; Jacobson, J.W.; et al. Current developments in salivary diagnostics. *Biomark Med.* **2010**, *4*, 171–189. [CrossRef]
36. Kapoor, P.; Kharbanda, O.P.; Monga, N.; Miglani, R.; Kapila, S. Effect of orthodontic forces on cytokine and receptor levels in gingival crevicular fluid: A systematic review. *Prog. Orthod.* **2014**, *15*, 65. [CrossRef]
37. Saloom, H.F.; Carpenter, G.H.; Cobourne, M.T. A cross-sectional cohort study of gingival crevicular fluid biomarkers in normal-weight and obese subjects during orthodontic treatment with fixed appliances. *Angle Orthod.* **2019**, *89*, 930–935. [CrossRef]

8. Takahashi, I.; Onodera, K.; Nishimura, M.; Mitnai, H.; Sasano, Y.; Mitani, H. Expression of genes for gelatinases and tissue inhibitors of metalloproteinases in periodontal tissues during orthodontic tooth movement. *J. Mol. Histol.* **2006**, *37*, 333–342. [CrossRef]
9. Kapoor, P.; Monga, N.; Kharbanda, O.P.; Kapila, S.; Miglani, R.; Moganty, R. Effect of orthodontic forces on levels of enzymes in gingival crevicular fluid (GCF): A systematic review. *Dental. Press J. Orthod.* **2019**, *24*, 40.e1–40.e22. [CrossRef]
10. Kushlinskii, N.E.; Solovykh, E.A.; Karaoglanova, T.B.; Boyar, U.; Gershtein, E.S.; Troshin, A.A.; Maksimovskaya, L.N.; Yanushevich, O.O. Matrix metalloproteinases and inflammatory cytokines in oral fluid of patients with chronic generalized periodontitis and various construction materials. *Bull. Exp. Biol. Med.* **2012**, *153*, 72–76. [CrossRef]
11. Capelli, J., Jr.; Kantarci, A.; Haffajee, A.; Teles, R.P.; Fidel, R., Jr.; Figueredo, C.M. Matrix metalloproteinases and chemokines in the gingival crevicular fluid during orthodontic tooth movement. *Eur. J. Orthod.* **2011**, *33*, 705–711. [CrossRef] [PubMed]
12. Boiculese, L.V.; Dimitriu, G.; Moscalu, M. Nearest neighbor classification with improved weighted dissimilarity measure. *Proc. Rom. Acad. Ser. A* **2009**, *10*, 205–213.
13. Herr, A.E.; Hatch, A.V.; Throckmorton, D.J.; Tran, H.M.; Brennan, J.S.; Giannobile, W.V.; Singh, A.K. Microfluidic immunoassays as rapid saliva-based clinical diagnostics. *Proc. Natl. Acad. Sci. USA* **2007**, *104*, 5268–5273. [CrossRef] [PubMed]
14. Kinane, D.F.; Darby, I.B.; Said, S.; Luoto, H.; Sorsa, T.; Tikanoja, S.; Mantyla, P. Changes in gingival crevicular fluid matrix metalloproteinase-8 levels during periodontal treatment and maintenance. *J. Periodontal. Res.* **2003**, *38*, 400–404. [CrossRef]
15. Prescher, N.; Maier, K.; Munjal, S.K.; Sorsa, T.; Bauermeister, C.D.; Struck, F.; Netuschil, L. Rapid quantitative chairside test for active MMP-8 in gingival crevicular fluid: First clinical data. *Ann. N. Y. Acad. Sci.* **2007**, *1098*, 493–495. [CrossRef]
16. Sorsa, T.; Hernandez, M.; Leppilahti, J.; Munjal, S.; Netuschil, L.; Mantyla, P. Detection of gingival crevicular fluid MMP-8 levels with different laboratory and chair-side methods. *Oral. Dis.* **2010**, *16*, 39–45. [CrossRef]

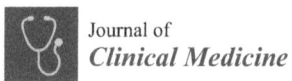

Communication

A User-Friendly Protocol for Mandibular Segmentation of CBCT Images for Superimposition and Internal Structure Analysis

Chenshuang Li [1,*], Leanne Lin [1], Zhong Zheng [2,3] and Chun-Hsi Chung [1,*]

1. Department of Orthodontics, School of Dental Medicine, University of Pennsylvania, Philadelphia, PA 19104, USA; llin21@upenn.edu
2. Division of Growth and Development, Section of Orthodontics, School of Dentistry, University of California, Los Angeles, CA 90095, USA; leozz95@ad.ucla.edu
3. Department of Surgery, David Geffen School of Medicine, University of California, Los Angeles, CA 90095, USA
* Correspondence: lichens@upenn.edu (C.L.); chunc@upenn.edu (C.-H.C.); Tel.: +1-215-898-7130 (C.-H.C)

Abstract: Background: Since cone-beam computed tomography (CBCT) technology has been widely adopted in orthodontics, multiple attempts have been made to devise techniques for mandibular segmentation and 3D superimposition. Unfortunately, as the software utilized in these methods are not specifically designed for orthodontics, complex procedures are often necessary to analyze each case. Thus, this study aimed to establish an orthodontist-friendly protocol for segmenting the mandible from CBCT images that maintains access to the internal anatomic structures. Methods: The "sculpting tool" in the Dolphin 3D Imaging software was used for segmentation. The segmented mandible images were saved as STL files for volume matching in the 3D Slicer to validate the repeatability of the current protocol and were exported as DICOM files for internal structure analysis and voxel-based superimposition. Results: The mandibles of all tested CBCT datasets were successfully segmented. The volume matching analysis showed high consistency between two independent segmentations for each mandible. The intraclass correlation coefficient (ICC) analysis on 20 additional CBCT mandibular segmentations further demonstrated the high consistency of the current protocol. Moreover, all of the anatomical structures for superimposition identified by the American Board of Orthodontics were found in the voxel-based superimposition, demonstrating the ability to conduct precise internal structure analyses with the segmented images. Conclusion: An efficient and precise protocol to segment the mandible while retaining access to the internal structures was developed on the basis of CBCT images.

Keywords: CBCT; segmentation; mandible; superimposition

Citation: Li, C.; Lin, L.; Zheng, Z.; Chung, C.-H. A User-Friendly Protocol for Mandibular Segmentation of CBCT Images for Superimposition and Internal Structure Analysis. *J. Clin. Med.* **2021**, *10*, 127. https://doi.org/10.3390/jcm10010127

Received: 6 October 2020
Accepted: 23 December 2020
Published: 1 January 2021

Publisher's Note: MDPI stays neutral with regard to jurisdictional claims in published maps and institutional affiliations.

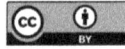

Copyright: © 2021 by the authors. Licensee MDPI, Basel, Switzerland. This article is an open access article distributed under the terms and conditions of the Creative Commons Attribution (CC BY) license (https://creativecommons.org/licenses/by/4.0/).

1. Introduction

Two-dimensional (2D) radiographs have been widely used in the field of orthodontics since 1922 [1]. At that time, when cephalometric tracing norms were established, cone-beam computed tomography (CBCT) was not available. Application of three-dimensional (3D) CBCT was first reported in 1994 [2]. As it significantly reduced radiation exposure and costs, 3D CBCT has since been broadly adopted in orthodontics after 2007 [2]. As early as 2010, Nalçaci et al. demonstrated that 3D cephalometric approaches are fairly reliable and comparable with traditional 2D cephalometry [1]. In addition, a growing body of evidence continues to demonstrate the application of CBCT in orthodontics as a front-line technology development topic [2–7]. However, the radiation exposure of cranial CBCTs is still not acceptable in most orthodontic patients, even though the dosage is dramatically reduced compared to when CBCT technology was first applied to orthodontics. To address this issue, Farronato et al. established a reliable sagittal skeletal classification system using

CBCT images with a reduced field of view [8]. Overall, both clinicians and researchers are dedicating great efforts to maximize the benefits of 3D CBCT in patient care while minimizing the radiation exposure to patients.

As the only bone that connects to the cranium by unique temporomandibular joints and exhibits variable growth and remodeling responses to orthodontic treatment, the mandible has been one of the classic and central topics for evaluating patients' growth and development and assessing the influence of orthodontic and orthopedic treatments. However, the most commonly cited method of investigating the mandible today is still 2D cephalometric radiograph-based superimposition [9]. There is no doubt that 2D image-projected 3D structure analysis not only limits the regions that can be evaluated (e.g., mandibular condyle [10], glenoid fossa [11], coronoid process, mandibular canal [12]), but also exposes the findings to inherent and unavoidable errors, such as those rooted in differences in magnification, head position, landmark identification, tracing, and reference lines and planes used for superimposition [13]. Thus, reliable 3D mandibular structure analysis technologies are in high demand, especially those that can provide valuable information previously inaccessible using 2D methods [2,3]. In particular, Kadiogly et al. stated, "Questions that were answered previously in 2D study are being asked again, and new studies are reassessing older and possibly outdated concepts with the aid of CBCT" [3].

Indeed, multiple attempts at mandibular segmentation and superimposition based on 3D CBCT imaging have been reported [13–17]. For instance, a significant amount of research into mandibular measurements has been conducted with such methods in the past few months [17–20], evidencing the high demand for 3D-based mandibular measurements. However, all of these pioneering methods utilize either open-source software such as ITK-Snap (www.itksnap.org) and 3D Slicer (www.slicer.org) or licensure-required software such as Mimics (Materialise, NV) [13–20]. Since the software packages mentioned above are not specifically designed for orthodontic applications, multiple software packages are generally necessary to analyze a single case. This issue significantly increases the complexity of usage and financial input, as well as time and labor costs for the clinicians or orthodontic researchers for mandible-related evaluations and investigations.

To overcome the technical, time-consuming, and financial challenges thus far associated with evaluations of the mandible, it is necessary to establish an efficient and precise mandibular segmentation protocol based on 3D CBCT that can (1) be performed with commonly used orthodontic imaging analysis software, (2) be easy to follow (not technique-sensitive), (3) access the internal structures, and (4) allow novel 3D and traditional 2D superimpositions.

2. Experimental Section

CBCT scans for this study were derived from preexisting clinical databases and approved by the University of Pennsylvania Institutional Review Board (IRB protocol #843611). No additional CBCT images were taken for the current study. Five CBCT scans from 3 patients were selected on the basis of the following criteria:

Patient #1: An adult female patient without craniofacial syndromes who underwent orthodontic treatment. The initial (CBCT #1, when the patient was 23 years old) and final (CBCT #2, when the patient was 25 years old) records were selected to

(1) establish the initial mandibular segmentation protocol to exclude the potential influence of gross pathologies and significant skeletal asymmetry;
(2) perform and validate the 3D voxel-based superimposition [13] with no detectable mandibular growth as determined by the American Board of Orthodontics (ABO) standard 2D landmark-based superimposition [21].

Patient #2: A late adolescent female patient diagnosed with hemifacial microsomia. The initial record (CBCT #3, when the patient was 16 years old) was selected to validate the precision and efficiency of the current protocol to segment the mandible, which presented a significant amount of asymmetry.

Patient #3: An adolescent male patient without craniofacial syndromes who underwent orthodontic treatment. The initial (CBCT #4, when the patient was 11 years old) and progress (CBCT #5, when the patient was 12 years old) records were selected to

(1) further validate the current protocol to segment the mandible;
(2) perform 3D voxel-based superimposition to determine the sensitivity of the current segmentation and superimposition protocol for detecting mandibular growth and development in the one-year interval;
(3) observe the potential growth and remodeling trends of the mandible.

CBCT DICOM files were all imported into the Dolphin 3D software (Dolphin Imaging; version 11.95 Premium, Chatsworth, CA; user license purchased by the University of Pennsylvania, School of Dental Medicine, Department of Orthodontics). The mandible was segmented from each CBCT with the following steps:

(1) In the "Orientation" module, set the facial midline as the midline of the full-volume CBCT and ensure that the cranial base structures and key ridges on the left and right sides overlap. This step is the same as the orientation setting for routine craniofacial CBCT assessments.
(2) In the "Sculpting tool" module, orient the CBCT to the right view, and sculpt the majority of the cranial and maxilla structures with the option "free form", as shown in Figure 1A,B.
(3) Orient the CBCT to the bottom view in which the borders of the condyles are clearly visible. Sculpt the visible cranial and maxillary structures, as shown in Figure 1C,D.
(4) Orient the CBCT to the right oblique view (Figure 1E), enlarge the CBCT, and change the "Seg Volumes" to identify the lower and upper density values in the appropriate range to differentiate the condyle from the surrounding structures (Figure 1F). This adjustment will produce a translucent view of the right condyle (orange arrow), glenoid fossa (yellow arrow), and remaining maxillary structures (Figure 1G). Sculpt the glenoid fossa along the inferior border and remaining maxillary structures.
(5) Repeat step 4 for the left condyle with the CBCT oriented to the left oblique view.
(6) Return to the right oblique view, in which some remaining cranial structures can be found around the left condyle (Figure 1H, yellow arrows). Sculpt them (Figure 1I).
(7) Repeat step 6 for the right condyle with the CBCT oriented to the left oblique view.
(8) The segmented mandible CBCT is ready for either "Export" as DICOM files or "Create surface," which yields an STL file (Figure 1J).

Each CBCT was segmented by the same examiner twice, with a 1-week interval in between. Each CBCT was also independently segmented by another examiner. The 3 STL files of each mandible were imported into 3D Slicer (open-source software, www.slicer.org) to evaluate intra-examiner and inter-examiner reproducibility, as well as the reliability of the current protocol using the "Model-to-Model distance" module [13]. The DICOM files of each mandible were imported into the Dolphin 3D software for voxel-based superimposition [22] using the chin and symphyseal regions [13] and internal anatomical structure analysis. To further assess the intra- and inter-examiner reliability, we used 20 additional CBCTs for mandibular segmentation by 2 individual clinicians in a blinded fashion (Figure S1). Intraclass correlation coefficient (ICC) was employed to assess the consistency of volumetric measurements on the mandibles segmented by the current protocol with IBM SPSS software (Statistical Package for Social Sciences version 26.0, Chicago, IL, USA).

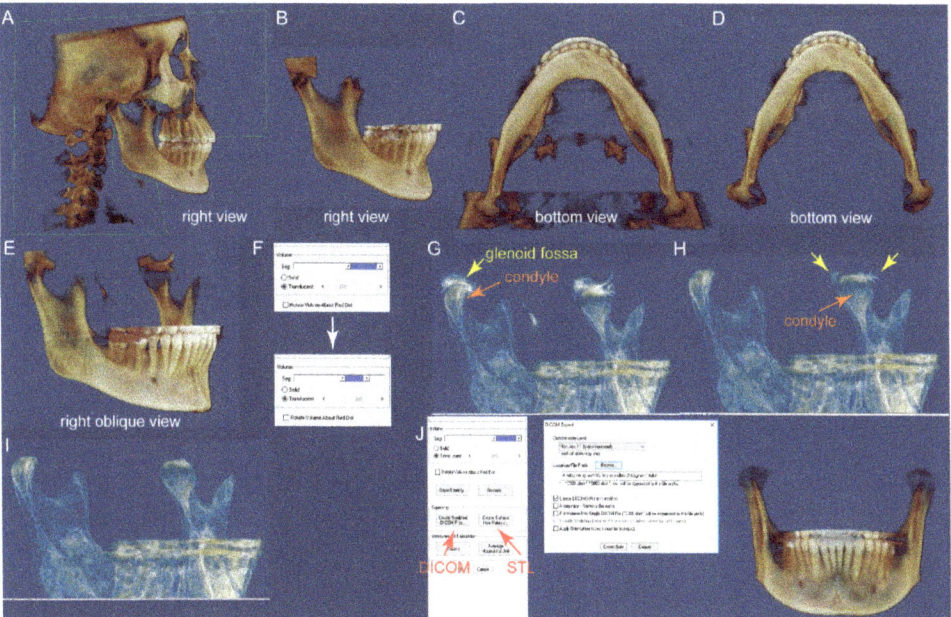

Figure 1. The flowchart of the mandible segmentation protocol by using the Dolphin 3D sculpting tool. (**A,B**) On the right view, sculpt the majority of the cranial structure and maxilla with the "free form" tool. (**C,D**) On the bottom view, the border of the condyles can clearly be seen. (**E–G**) On the right oblique view, enlarge the cone-beam computed tomography (CBCT) and change the "Seg Volumes," which will produce a translucent view of the right condyle (orange arrow), glenoid fossa (yellow arrow), and remaining maxillary structures. (**H**) After sculpting around the left condyle in the left oblique view, return to the right oblique view. Some remaining cranial structures can be found around the left condyle (yellow arrows). Sculpt them (**I**). (**J**) The segmented mandible CBCT can either be exported as DICOM files or be used to create the surface structure and saved as an STL file.

3. Results

It took less than 15 min each to complete all segmentations. The volume matching results of the two segmentations from the same clinician for each CBCT are shown in Figure 2, demonstrating intra-examiner reproducibility. Volume matching was also performed with two independent segmentations from two clinicians for each CBCT, shown in Figure 3, displaying inter-examiner reproducibility. The 3D Slicer Model-to-Model distance results showed perfect surface matching of the mandibular body, ramus, and condylar regions for all five samples in Figures 2 and 3, illustrating the reliability of the segmentation protocol described above. As no prominent landmarks could be found in the maxillary dentition to determine the segmentation border in this region, some volume differences were detected by 3D Slicer. Some slight surface differences were also observed in CBCT #1 around the lower right first molar region, which could be attributed to the metal crown-derived noise around this tooth. However, these negligible differences did not influence further analysis of the mandible. For the ICC analysis based on the segmentation of 20 mandibles by two clinicians, intra-examiner reliability (ICC = 0.998; 95% CI = 0.964–1.000) and inter-examiner reliability (ICC = 0.998; 95% CI = 0.908–1.000) were excellent.

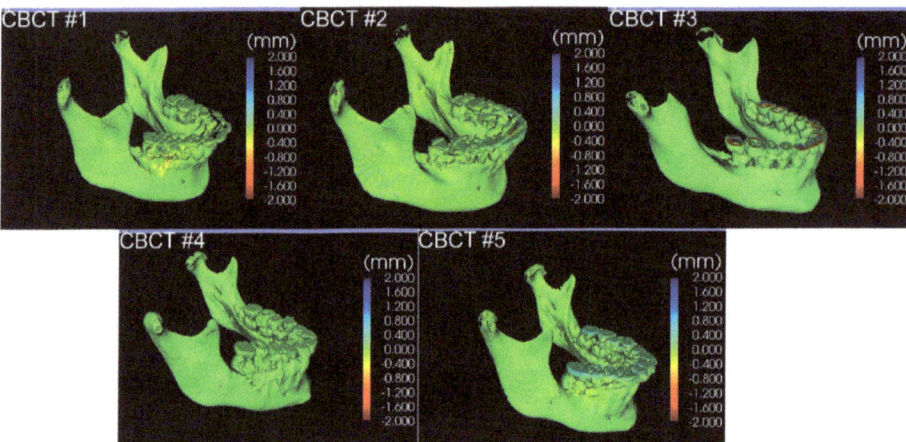

Figure 2. The model-to-model distance analysis in the 3D Slicer software for two segmentations performed by one examiner for each CBCT.

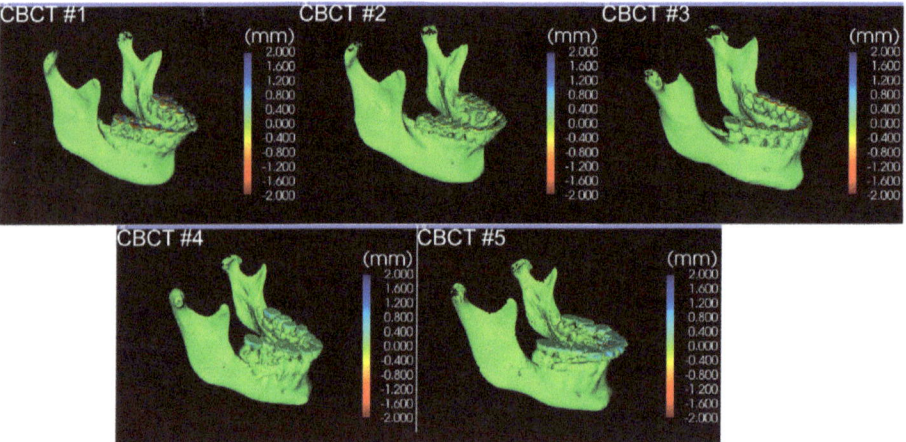

Figure 3. The model-to-model distance analysis in the 3D Slicer software for two segmentations individually performed by two examiners for each CBCT.

Comparing the panoramic radiograph images generated from the full-volume CBCT and the segmented mandible CBCT, no gross morphological differences were noted in any tested samples (Figure 4). Furthermore, the panoramic radiographs generated from the segmented mandible CBCT clearly displayed the inferior alveolar canals, tooth roots, condyles, and bone marrow (Figure 4).

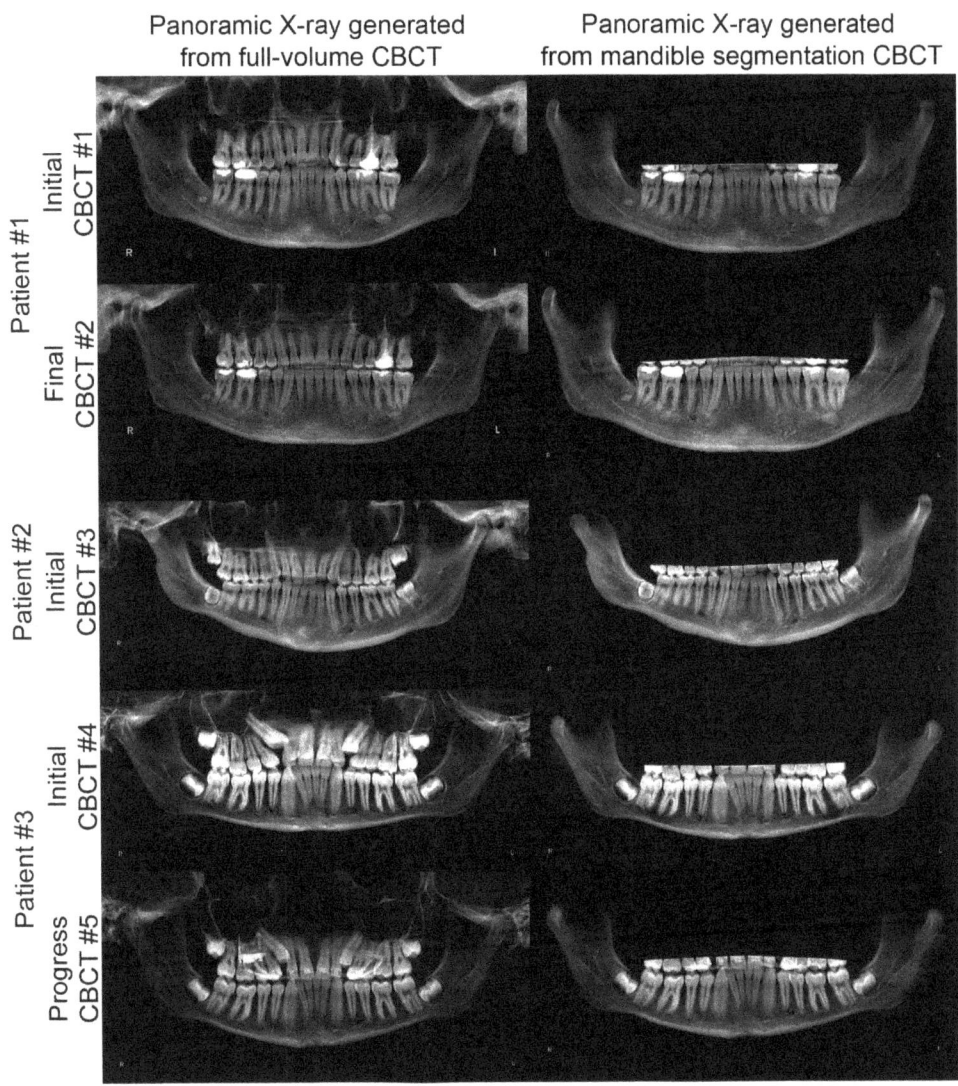

Figure 4. Comparison of the panoramic radiographs generated from the full-volume CBCT and those from the segmented mandible CBCT.

For patient #1, the Dolphin 3D voxel-based superimposition generated evenly distributed white (initial) and green (final) interval surface colors in the mandibular body and ramus regions. In contrast, only the green color was observed in the lower anterior dentition, indicating no significant change of the mandible, while there was proclination of the mandibular anterior teeth caused by orthodontic treatment (Figure 5A). To further confirm this observation, we analyzed the superimposed mandibular CBCT images in all three planes. In the sagittal slice along the facial midline, the symphyseal regions of the initial (white) and final (green) mandibles were superimposed, while the mandibular anterior teeth were more proclined in the green than in the white segment (Figure 5B). The sagittal slice in the left ramus region displayed perfectly matched white and green images (Figure 5C). The coronal slice in the retromolar region again showed completely overlapping white and green images (Figure 5D). It is worth noting that the radiopaque area on the right side of the mandible (Figure 5D, yellow arrow) and the inferior alveolar canals on both sides (Figure 5D, red arrows) were clearly seen. In the axial slices, the left inferior alveolar canal (Figure 5E, red arrow), mandibular foramen (Figure 5F, red arrows), condyles (Figure 5G, red arrows), and tips of the coronoid processes (Figure 5G, yellow arrows) were all easily located. Furthermore, all of these slices showed complete superimposition of the initial and final images at the mandibular body and ramus regions.

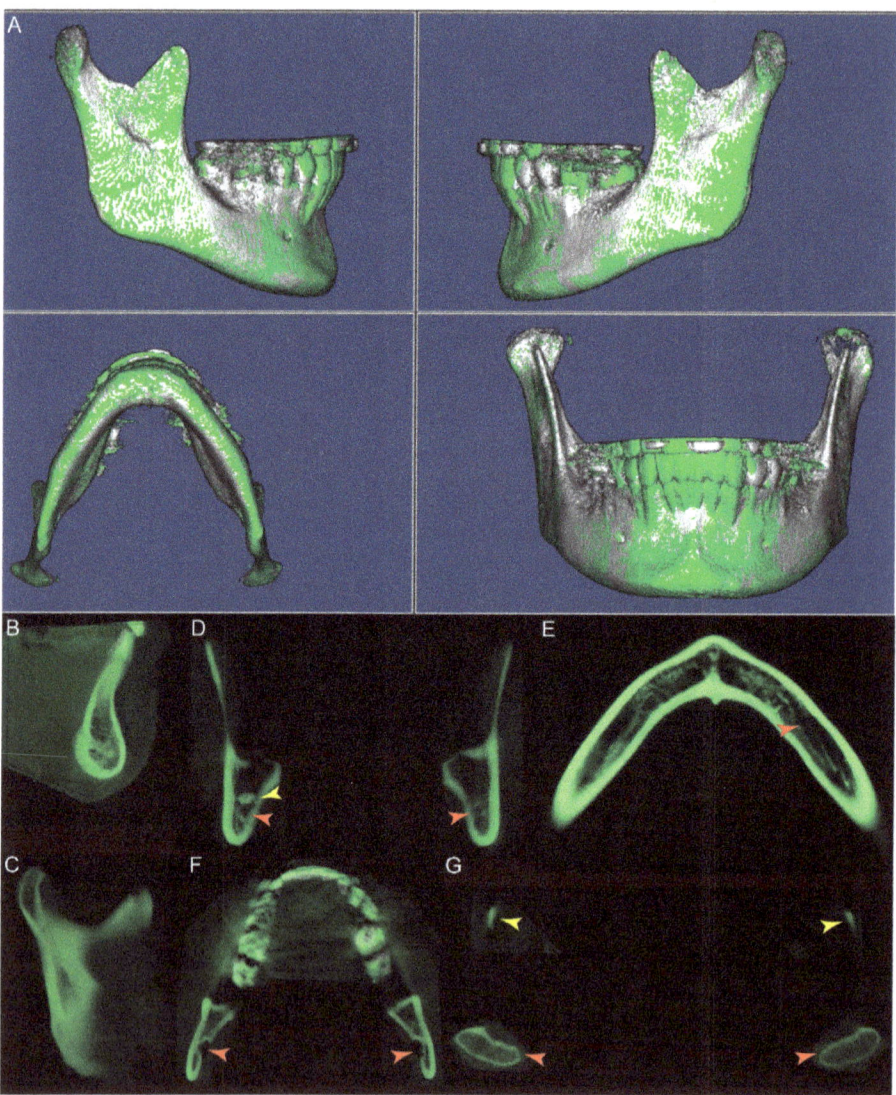

Figure 5. The Dolphin 3D voxel-based superimposition of the initial (white, CBCT #1) and final (green, CBCT #2) CBCT datasets of the mandible for patient #1. (**A**) The 3D reconstructed surface structure image of the mandible after superimposition. (**B**) Sagittal slice along the facial midline. (**C**) Sagittal slice in the left ramus region. (**D**) Coronal slice in the retromolar region. Yellow arrow: a radiopaque area on the right side of the mandible; red arrows: inferior alveolar canals. (**E**) Axial slice at the spinae mentalis level. Red arrow: left inferior alveolar canal. (**F**) Axial slice at the mandibular foramen level. Red arrows: mandibular foramen. (**G**) Axial slice at the level of the tips of the coronoid processes. Yellow arrows: coronoid process; red arrows: condyle.

Unlike the observations from patient #1, the Dolphin 3D voxel-based superimposition of patient #3 showed that the majority of the mandibular surface was green, indicating the potential growth of the mandible from the initial (white) to progress (green) time points (Figure 6A). Again, the sagittal slice along the facial midline shows superimposition of the two images at the symphyseal region (Figure 6B), while the sagittal slice in the right ramus region (Figure 6C) displays (1) superimposition of the inferior alveolar canal (red arrow), (2) resorption (blue arrow) of the anterior surface and deposition (yellow arrows) at the posterior surface of the top half of the coronoid process, (3) posterior and superior growth of the condyle, and (4) deposition (yellow arrows) at the posterior border of the ramus. For the coronal slices, in the first premolar region (Figure 6D), the mental foramen could be found and superimposed in the first premolar region (red arrows). Simultaneously, slight deposition was also noted at the buccal and inferior surfaces of the mandibular body and the inner contour of the lingual cortical plate on the right side (Figure 6D, yellow arrows). In the third molar region (Figure 6E), while the lower borders of the third molars were superimposed on both sides, deposition was found at the buccal surface of the mandibular body. For the axial slices, the slice at the root apex level (Figure 6F) showed deposition along the buccal surface of the mandibular body. In the posterior third of the mandible, both the buccal and lingual cortical plates moved buccally (Figure 6F, red arrows). The buccal movement of the buccal and lingual cortical plates in the posterior third of the mandible was also found in the axial slice at the cervical level of the teeth (Figure 6G). Finally, the axial slice at the level of the deepest portion of the mandibular notch (Figure 6H) showed (1) resorption of the anterior surface of the ramus, (2) deposition at the buccal surface of the ramus, and (3) resorption of the medial posterior surface of the condylar neck.

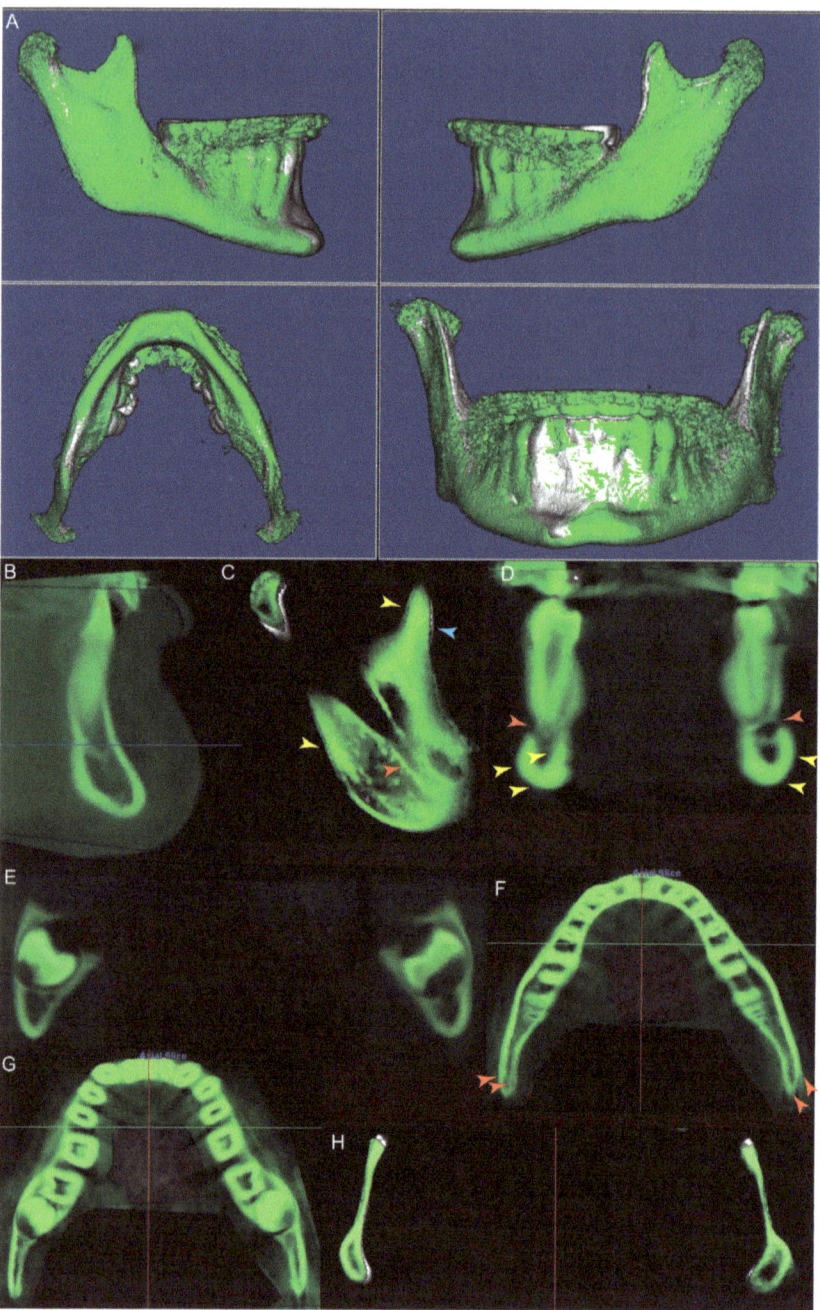

Figure 6. The Dolphin 3D voxel-based superimposition of the initial (white, CBCT #4) and progress (green, CBCT #3) CBCT datasets of the mandible for patient #3. (**A**) The 3D reconstructed surface structure image of the mandible after superimposition. (**B**) Sagittal slice along the facial midline. (**C**) Sagittal slice in the right ramus region. Red arrow: inferior alveolar canal; blue arrow: resorption; yellow arrows: deposition. (**D**) Coronal slice in the first premolar region. Yellow arrows: deposition; red arrows: mental foramen. (**E**) Coronal slice in the third molar region. (**F**) Axial slice at the root apex level. Red arrows: buccally moved cortical plates. (**G**) Axial slice at the cervical level of the teeth. (**H**) Axial slice at the level of the deepest portion of the mandibular notch.

4. Discussion

For this short Communication article, our primary aim was to establish a simple protocol to segment the mandible from a full-volume craniofacial CBCT using the "Sculpting tool" provided with the Dolphin 3D Imaging software and to evaluate the precision and reliability of this protocol. In contrast to other newly established mandibular segmentation protocols, the current protocol only involves one commonly used orthodontic imaging software, which reduces the cost, time, and energy of purchasing software, multiple-software practicing, and file transfers among different software [13–17,22].

The 3D Slicer model-to-model distance analysis demonstrates perfect volume matching of the mandibular body, ramus, and condylar regions in all five tested samples. This consistency confirms the precision and reliability of the current protocol, which is not affected by notable mandibular asymmetry, such as seen in patient #2.

We also performed superimpositions using the chin and symphyseal regions [13] with Dolphin 3D voxel-based superimposition [22]. As demonstrated by the planes of patient #1, the inner contour of the cortical plate at the lower border of the symphysis, alveolar canal, and anterior and posterior border of the ramus could all be easily located. Thus, all of the anatomical structures indicated for mandibular superimposition by the ABO can be found and superimposed using this 3D voxel-based superimposition dataset. The complete superimposition of these anatomic structures confirms the precision of the 3D voxel-based superimposition method, as previously reported [13,22], and further validates the reliability of the current mandibular segmentation protocol.

As demonstrated in the superimposition image of patient #3, we found that specifically for this patient (1) the anterior–inferior contour of the chin and the inner contour of the cortical plate at the lower border of the symphysis can be entirely superimposed for the initial and progress records, (2) there is deposition at the inferior border of the mandible at the first premolar region but not at the third molar region, and (3) the ramus demonstrates anterior border resorption and posterior border deposition. These observations align with the previously reported and accepted phenomena of mandibular growth and modeling [21].

Interestingly, some previously unreported growth trends were also found in this patient's records, such as the deposition along the buccal surface of the mandible (Figure 6A,D–G) and the lateral shift of the buccal and lingual cortical plates in the posterior third of the mandible (Figure 6F,G), indicating that the mandible may not grow posteriorly along the direction of the mandibular body. There may be a contour change during growth. Furthermore, instead of a "V"-shaped growth of the condyle, only the medial posterior resorption of the condylar neck is observed in the axial slice at the most inferior level of the mandibular notch (Figure 6H).

In fact, in the newly published article [23], by performing a longitudinal CBCT study on 25 growing skeletal class II patients, Maspero et al. found that there was significant mandibular body growth as expected, but the mandibular symphyseal angle maintained the same. This is different from what we observed in patient #3—a lateral shift of the mandible is clearly indicated in Figure 6F,G, suggesting an increasing mandibular symphyseal angle. It is worth noting that patient #3 was diagnosed as skeletal class III and had rapid maxillary expansion and facemask treatment before the progress records were taken. Thus, whether these previously unreported mandibular growth patterns resulted from a normal skeletal class III pattern of growth or from treatment requires further investigations with a larger sample size.

Using the current protocol, we could not thoroughly remove the maxillary dentition without affecting the mandibular dentition. Thus, we decided to sculpt through half of the maxillary tooth crowns. Although the remaining maxillary dentition did not appear to influence the mandible analyses, further efforts are still needed to adequately separate the maxillary and mandibular dentitions.

CBCT has also been proven to be an appropriate tool for evaluating the maxillary and mandibular bone marrow density [24–26] and condylar volume [27]. Thus, further exploring the feasibility of the current segmentation and superimposition protocol for assessing mandibular bone marrow density and tracking condyle modeling and remodeling is the next objective of our investigation.

No doubt, Dolphin 3D software is not inexpensive. However, we created this protocol based on Dolphin 3D because this software is not only routinely used in our clinic but is also widely utilized in graduate orthodontic programs. According to the PubMed database, an increasing number of researchers are employing Dolphin 3D software in their studies encompassing diverse areas of investigation, such as predicting the upper airway change in orthognathic patients [28], assisting in virtual surgical planning [29], evaluating dentoskeletal effects of rapid maxillary expansion [30], and even routine 2D tracing analysis [31]. Thus, we believe that our protocol is based on a widely used software, which minimizes the chances of imposing additional costs for clinicians and researchers who are likely to already own Dolphin 3D Imaging software.

Last but not least, the current study is a retrospective study using human data previously obtained for clinical treatment purposes. No additional radiographs were taken for the present study. Although technological developments have significantly reduced the radiation dosage associated with CBCT acquisition [2], we highly recommend that all clinical CBCTs taken should follow ALARA (as low as reasonably achievable) principles to avoid unnecessary radiation exposure to patients and clinicians [32].

In summary, a user-friendly 3D-imaging-based mandibular segmentation protocol is introduced in the current study, with five CBCT images from three patients selected to preliminarily demonstrate the feasibility of the protocol. Without a doubt, many more samples are needed to draw definitive conclusions in growth and development investigations and assess treatment efficacy. However, by disseminating our protocol in a timely manner, we hope that this sharing of knowledge can significantly benefit global collaborative efforts to achieve a more detailed understanding of how to better evaluate growth and development and ultimately improve one's ability to deliver better orthodontic clinical care.

Supplementary Materials: The following are available online at https://www.mdpi.com/2077-0383/10/1/127/s1: Figure S1: The 3D reconstructed mandibular images of the 20 samples used for intraclass correlation coefficient analysis.

Author Contributions: Conceptualization, C.L., Z.Z., and C.-H.C.; methodology, C.L. and Z.Z.; validation, L.L.; formal analysis, C.L. and L.L.; writing—original draft preparation, C.L.; writing—review and editing, Z.Z., L.L., and C.-H.C; supervision, C.-H.C.; project administration, C.L. All authors have read and agreed to the published version of the manuscript.

Funding: This research received no external funding.

Institutional Review Board Statement: The study was conducted according to the guidelines of the Declaration of Helsinki, and approved by the Institutional Review Board of University of Pennsylvania (IRB protocol #843611, date of approval: 13 July 2020).

Informed Consent Statement: Patient consent was waived as this is a retrospective study, CBCT scans for this study were derived from preexisting clinical databases. No additional CBCT images were taken for the current study. No protect health information (PHI) was used in the current study.

Data Availability Statement: The data presented in this study are contained within this article and supplementary materials.

Conflicts of Interest: The authors declare no conflict of interest.

References

1. Nalcaci, R.; Ozturk, F.; Sokucu, O. A comparison of two-dimensional radiography and three-dimensional computed tomography in angular cephalometric measurements. *Dentomaxillofacial Radiol.* **2010**, *39*, 100–106. [CrossRef] [PubMed]
2. Kula, K.; Ghoneima, A. *Cephalometry in Orthodontics: 2D and 3D*; Quintessence Pub., Co.: New Malden, UK, 2018; 202p.
3. Koerich, L.; Tufekci, E.; Lindauer, S.J. *Craniofacial 3D Imaging*; Springer: Cham, Switzerland, 2019; pp. 51–69.
4. Pan, F.; Yang, Z.; Wang, J.; Cai, R.; Liu, J.; Zhang, C.; Liao, W. Influence of orthodontic treatment with premolar extraction on the spatial position of maxillary third molars in adult patients: A retrospective cohort cone-bean computed tomography study. *BMC Oral Health* **2020**, *20*, 1–8. [CrossRef] [PubMed]

8. Pan, Y.; Wang, X.; Dai, F.; Chen, G.; Xu, T. Accuracy and reliability of maxillary digital model (MDM) superimposition in evaluating teeth movement in adults compared with CBCT maxillary superimposition. *Sci. Rep.* **2020**, *10*, 1–8. [CrossRef] [PubMed]
9. Mehta, S.; Dresner, R.; Gandhi, V.; Chen, P.-J.; Allareddy, V.; Kuo, C.-L.; Mu, J.; Yadav, S. Effect of positional errors on the accuracy of cervical vertebrae maturation assessment using CBCT and lateral cephalograms. *J. World Fed. Orthod.* **2020**, *9*, 146–154. [CrossRef]
10. Naik, M.K.; Dharmadeep, G.; Reddy, Y.M.; Cheruluri, S.; Raj, K.P.; Reddy, B.R. Three-dimensional evaluation of interradicular areas and cortical bone thickness for orthodontic miniscrew implant placement using cone-beam computed tomography. *J. Pharm. Bioallied Sci.* **2020**, *12*, 99–S104. [CrossRef]
11. Farronato, M.; Maspero, C.; Abate, A.; Grippaudo, C.; Connelly, S.T.; Tartaglia, G.M. 3D cephalometry on reduced FOV CBCT: Skeletal class assessment through AF-BF on Frankfurt plane-validity and reliability through comparison with 2D measurements. *Eur. Radiol.* **2020**, *30*, 1–8. [CrossRef]
12. Björk, A.; Skieller, V. Normal and abnormal growth of the mandible. A synthesis of longitudinal cephalometric implant studies over a period of 25 years. *Eur. J. Orthod.* **1983**, *5*, 1–46. [CrossRef]
13. Guo, X.; Yang, C.; Wang, J.; Zhao, M.; Li, Y.; Wang, L. Comparative Analysis of the Temporomandibular Joints in Patients with Chronic Periodontitis Using Cone-Beam Computed Tomography (CBCT). *Adv. Ther.* **2020**, 1–9. [CrossRef]
14. Khademi, B.; Karandish, M.; Paknahad, M.; Farmani, S. Comparison of Glenoid Fossa Morphology Between Different Sagittal Skeletal Pattern Using Cone Beam Computed Tomography. *J. Craniofacial Surg.* **2020**, *31*, e789–e792. [CrossRef]
15. Li, Y.; Li, L.; Shi, J.; Tu, J.; Niu, L.; Hu, X. Positional Changes of Mandibular Canal Before and After Decompression of Cystic Lesions in the Mandible. *J. Oral Maxillofac. Surg.* **2020**. [CrossRef]
16. Nguyen, T.; Cevidanes, L.H.S.; Franchi, L.; Ruellas, A.; Jackson, T. Three-dimensional mandibular regional superimposition in growing patients. *Am. J. Orthod. Dentofac. Orthop.* **2018**, *153*, 747–754. [CrossRef] [PubMed]
17. Giudice, A.L.; Ronsivalle, V.; Grippaudo, C.; Lucchese, A.; Muraglie, S.; Lagravère, M.O.; Isola, G. One Step before 3D Printing—Evaluation of Imaging Software Accuracy for 3-Dimensional Analysis of the Mandible: A Comparative Study Using a Surface-to-Surface Matching Technique. *Materials* **2020**, *13*, 2798. [CrossRef] [PubMed]
18. Chen, S.; Wang, L.; Li, G.; Wu, T.-H.; Diachina, S.; Tejera, B.; Kwon, J.J.; Lin, F.-C.; Lee, Y.-T.; Xu, T.; et al. Machine learning in orthodontics: Introducing a 3D auto-segmentation and auto-landmark finder of CBCT images to assess maxillary constriction in unilateral impacted canine patients. *Angle Orthod.* **2019**, *90*, 77–84. [CrossRef] [PubMed]
19. Fan, Y.; Beare, R.; Matthews, H.; Schneider, P.; Kilpatrick, N.; Clement, J.; Claes, P.; Penington, A.J.; Adamson, C. Marker-based watershed transform method for fully automatic mandibular segmentation from CBCT images. *Dentomaxillofacial Radiol.* **2019**, *48*, 20180261. [CrossRef] [PubMed]
20. Leonardi, R.M.; Aboulazm, K.; Giudice, A.L.; Ronsivalle, V.; D'Anto, V.; Lagravere, M.; Isola, G. Evaluation of mandibular changes after rapid maxillary expansion: A CBCT study in youngsters with unilateral posterior crossbite using a surface-to-surface matching technique. *Clin. Oral Investig.* **2020**. [CrossRef] [PubMed]
21. Evangelista, K.; Valladares-Neto, J.; Silva, M.A.G.; Cevidanes, L.H.S.; Ruellas, A.C.D.O. Three-dimensional assessment of mandibular asymmetry in skeletal Class I and unilateral crossbite malocclusion in 3 different age groups. *Am. J. Orthod. Dentofac. Orthop.* **2020**, *158*, 209–220. [CrossRef] [PubMed]
22. Tsukiboshi, Y.; Tanikawa, C.; Yamashiro, T. Surface-based 3-dimensional cephalometry: An objective analysis of cranio-mandibular morphology. *Am. J. Orthod. Dentofac. Orthop.* **2020**, *158*, 535–546. [CrossRef]
23. Wei, R.Y.; Atresh, A.; Ruellas, A.; Cevidanes, L.H.; Nguyen, T.; Larson, B.E.; Mangum, J.E.; Manton, D.; Schneider, P.M. Three-dimensional condylar changes from Herbst appliance and multibracket treatment: A comparison with matched Class II elastics. *Am. J. Orthod. Dentofac. Orthop.* **2020**, *158*, 505–517. [CrossRef]
24. American Board of Orthodontics Mandibular Superimposition. Available online: https://www.americanboardortho.com/orthodontic-professionals/about-board-certification/clinical-examination/certification-renewal-examinations/mail-in-cre-submission-procedure/case-report-examination/case-record-preparation/superimpositions/mandibular/ (accessed on 31 December 2020).
25. Bazina, M.; Cevidanes, L.H.S.; Ruellas, A.; Valiathan, M.; Quereshy, F.; Syed, A.; Wu, R.; Palomo, J.M. Precision and reliability of Dolphin 3-dimensional voxel-based superimposition. *Am. J. Orthod. Dentofac. Orthop.* **2018**, *153*, 599–606. [CrossRef]
26. Maspero, C.; Farronato, M.; Bellincioni, F.; Cavagnetto, D.; Abate, A. Assessing mandibular body changes in growing subjects: A comparison of CBCT and reconstructed lateral cephalogram measurements. *Sci. Rep.* **2020**, *10*, 1–12. [CrossRef]
27. Nazari, M.S.; Tallaeipoor, A.R.; Nucci, L.; Karamifar, A.A.; Jamilian, A.; Perillo, L. Evaluation of Bone Mineral Density Using Cone Beam Computed Tomography. *Stomatol. EDU J.* **2019**, *6*, 241–247. [CrossRef]
28. Çolak, M. An Evaluation of Bone Mineral Density Using Cone Beam Computed Tomography in Patients with Ectodermal Dysplasia: A Retrospective Study at a Single Center in Turkey. *Med. Sci. Monit.* **2019**, *25*, 3503–3509. [CrossRef] [PubMed]
29. Zhang, D.-Z.; Xiao, W.; Zhou, R.; Xue, L.-F.; Ma, L. Evaluation of Bone Height and Bone Mineral Density Using Cone Beam Computed Tomography After Secondary Bone Graft in Alveolar Cleft. *J. Craniofacial Surg.* **2015**, *26*, 1463–1466. [CrossRef]
30. Farronato, M.; Cavagnetto, D.; Abate, A.; Cressoni, P.; Fama, A.; Maspero, C. Assessment of condylar volume and ramus height in JIA patients with unilateral and bilateral TMJ involvement: Retrospective case-control study. *Clin. Oral Investig.* **2019**, *24*, 2635–2643. [CrossRef]

28. Elshebiny, T.; Bous, R.; Withana, T.; Morcos, S.; Valiathan, M. Accuracy of Three-Dimensional Upper Airway Prediction in Orthognathic Patients Using Dolphin Three-Dimensional Software. *J. Craniofacial Surg.* **2020**, *31*, 1098–1100. [CrossRef] [PubMed]
29. Teixeira, A.O.D.B.; Almeida, M.A.D.O.; Almeida, R.C.D.C.; Maués, C.P.; Pimentel, T.; Ribeiro, D.P.B.; De Medeiros, P.J.; Quintão, C.C.A.; Carvalho, F.D.A.R. Three-dimensional accuracy of virtual planning in orthognathic surgery. *Am. J. Orthod. Dentofac. Orthop.* **2020**, *158*, 674–683. [CrossRef] [PubMed]
30. Araújo, M.-C.; Bocato, J.-R.; Oltramari, P.-V.-P.; De Almeida, M.-R.; Conti, A.-C.-D.C.-F.; Fernandes, T.-M.-F. Tomographic evaluation of dentoskeletal effects of rapid maxillary expansion using Haas and Hyrax palatal expanders in children: A randomized clinical trial. *J. Clin. Exp. Dent.* **2020**, *12*, e922–e930. [CrossRef]
31. Kau, C.H.; Bakos, K.; Lamani, E. Quantifying changes in incisor inclination before and after orthodontic treatment in class I, II, and III malocclusions. *J. World Fed. Orthod.* **2020**, *9*, 170–174. [CrossRef]
32. Hayashi, T.; Arai, Y.; Chikui, T.; Hayashi-Sakai, S.; Honda, K.; Indo, H.; Kawai, T.; Kobayashi, K.; Murakami, S.; Nagasawa, M.; et al. Clinical guidelines for dental cone-beam computed tomography. *Oral Radiol.* **2018**, *34*, 89–104. [CrossRef]

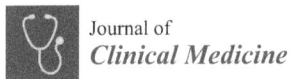

Article

3D Method for Occlusal Tooth Wear Assessment in Presence of Substantial Changes on Other Tooth Surfaces

Nikolaos Gkantidis [1,2,*], Konstantinos Dritsas [1], Christos Katsaros [1], Demetrios Halazonetis [3] and Yijin Ren [2]

[1] Department of Orthodontics and Dentofacial Orthopedics, School of Dental Medicine, University of Bern, CH-3010 Bern, Switzerland; konstantinos.dritsas@zmk.unibe.ch (K.D.); christos.katsaros@zmk.unibe.ch (C.K.)
[2] Department of Orthodontics, W.J. Kolff Institute, University Medical Center Groningen, University of Groningen, 9700RB Groningen, The Netherlands; y.ren@umcg.nl
[3] Department of Orthodontics, School of Dentistry, National and Kapodistrian University of Athens, GR-11527 Athens, Greece; dhalaz@dent.uoa.gr
* Correspondence: nikolaos.gkantidis@zmk.unibe.ch; Tel.: +41-(0)-31-632-25-91

Received: 4 November 2020; Accepted: 1 December 2020; Published: 4 December 2020

Abstract: Early diagnosis and timely management of tooth or dental material wear is imperative to avoid extensive restorations. Previous studies suggested different methods for tooth wear assessment, but no study has developed a three-dimensional (3D) superimposition technique applicable in cases where tooth surfaces, other than the occlusal, undergo extensive morphological changes. Here, we manually grinded plaster incisors and canines to simulate occlusal tooth wear of varying severity in teeth that received a wire retainer bonded on their lingual surfaces, during the assessment period. The corresponding dental casts were scanned using a surface scanner. The modified tooth crowns were best-fit approximated to the original crowns using seven 3D superimposition techniques (two reference areas with varying settings) and the gold standard technique (GS: intact adjacent teeth and alveolar processes as superimposition reference), which provided the true value. Only a specific technique (complete crown with 20% estimated overlap of meshes), which is applicable in actual clinical data, showed perfect agreement with the GS technique in all cases (median difference: −0.002, max absolute difference: 0.178 mm^3). The outcomes of the suggested and the GS technique were highly reproducible (max difference < 0.040 mm^3). The presented technique offers low cost, convenient, accurate, and risk-free tooth wear assessment.

Keywords: tooth wear; measurement method; quantitative assessment; three-dimensional imaging; surface model; three-dimensional superimposition; orthodontic retention; fixed retainers

1. Introduction

Tooth wear characterizes the superficial loss of tooth matter over time. In humans, tooth wear occurs as a consequence of normal function, parafunction, or environmental factors, such as very acidic food. The main issue of concern, when excessive tooth wear occurs, is impaired dental esthetics. However, it may also affect facial morphology and speech, impacting patients' quality of life. In recent years, the need for retaining natural teeth intact for several decades has arisen due to the increase in life expectancy. This, along with increased patient esthetic demands has designated tooth wear as an important problem that needs to be addressed [1]. Advances in the dental field, including tooth wear management, enabled teeth maintenance till late stages of life [2].

Early diagnosis is imperative for the timely management of tooth wear, to avoid subsequent problems and extensive restorations [2,3]. To facilitate tooth wear assessment, several previous studies have suggested a variety of qualitative and quantitative methods. Qualitative approaches are subjective and usually suffer from reduced precision and reproducibility [4–6]. On the contrary, certain quantitative techniques have shown adequate reproducibility, usually within the range of 15–20 µm, concerning vertical loss of tooth structure. However, the trueness of these techniques remains questionable, since studies lack a gold standard reference for comparison [7]. Other shortcomings include the high complexity of these techniques that need special equipment and expertise to be applied properly, as well as the dental impressions and physical models required. The above increase the costs, the inaccuracies, and the applicability of the techniques in actual clinical conditions [7–9].

A highly accurate three-dimensional (3D) superimposition technique has been suggested recently for occlusal tooth wear assessment using serial digital dental models [10]. Assuming that relevant software and hardware is accessible, which is realistic for a contemporary practice, this technique is applicable under regular clinical conditions. The existence of a previous dental model, obtained at a certain point in the past, is a prerequisite to apply this technique. The rapid incorporation of intraoral scanners in contemporary dentistry [11] and the use of relevant software for various applications facilitates this purpose. The aforementioned previous study [10] focused on occlusal tooth wear assessment in cases that only the occlusal tooth surfaces were subjected to changes over time, offering an accuracy of 0.033 mm^3, which corresponds to approximately 9 µm of vertical tooth loss [10]. This accuracy level is much higher than any level than might be considered clinically significant. However, other tooth surfaces might also be affected by function, pathology, or due to iatrogenic interventions [12–14]. This might complicate occlusal tooth wear assessment through serial 3D surface model superimpositions. To our knowledge, there is no study in the literature that has addressed this issue. A common instance where tooth surfaces, other than the occlusal, undergo extensive morphological changes regards the placement of bonded wire retainers. Such retainers might be bonded following orthodontic treatment, to stabilize teeth after trauma, or in periodontally compromised patients [14–17]. Thus, the purpose of the present study was to develop and validate a 3D occlusal tooth wear assessment technique, applicable when the anterior teeth crown morphology is highly altered during the testing period, in non-occlusal surfaces.

2. Experimental Section

2.1. Ethical Approval

The research project is registered and approved by the Swiss Ethical Committee of the Canton of Bern (Protocol No. 2019-00326). All experiments were performed under the relevant regulations and according to the pre-specified protocol. All participants signed an informed consent prior to the use of their data in the study.

2.2. Sample

The present sample was derived from an existing material, which was previously generated and thoroughly described [10]. In this study, sixteen dental plaster models (type IV plaster, white color, Fujirock EP Premium, GC, Leuven, Belgium) with ($n = 8$; 4 maxillary and 4 mandibular; crowding ≤ 1 mm) and without ($n = 8$; 4 maxillary and 4 mandibular; crowding: 4–10 mm) well aligned dental arches were used. These were retrieved from the archive of the Department of Orthodontics and Dentofacial Orthopedics, University of Bern, Switzerland. The models represented individuals with natural permanent dentition and no extreme morphological variation in oral structures (visual inspection).

2.3. Tooth Wear Simulation

According to a pre-specified and previously validated protocol, eighteen canines and eighteen incisors, equally distributed among the dental models described above, were manually grinded to simulate occlusal tooth wear of varying severity (approximately 0.5, 1, and 2 mm of vertical loss, respectively) [10]. Grinding was performed both symmetrically and asymmetrically, using a dental laboratory straight handpiece or a dental laboratory stone knife, to simulate a variety of normal tooth wear patterns. Additionally, for the needs of the present study, a fixed retainer that is usually bonded following orthodontic treatment or to stabilize highly mobile teeth following trauma or severe periodontally compromised teeth, was simulated in the anterior teeth. For this, a twisted white coated ligature wire (0.3 mm initial diameter, Dentaurum, Ispringen, Germany) was placed on the middle of the lingual surfaces of the test anterior teeth. A white modeling compound (Play-Doh putty, Hasbro, Pawtucket, RI, USA) was used to stabilize the wire on the teeth during scanning and simulate the bonding material placed in vivo. Both materials were selected after pilot testing that confirmed sufficient material surface acquisition by the scanner. The setting resulted in two intact teeth adjacent to each grinded tooth that received the retainer. The intact teeth and other adjacent anatomical structures that were not artificially altered, were used as superimposition reference areas to provide the gold standard (true) measurement [10,18].

2.4. 3D Model Acquisition

The dental casts of the before (T0) and after wear simulation plus retainer placement (T1) conditions, were scanned using a laboratory 3D surface scanner (stripe light/LED illumination; full dental arch accuracy <20 µm; Laboratory scanner D104a, Cendres + Métaux SA, Biel/Bienne, Switzerland). Repeated single jaw model scans with this scanner, show a distance between corresponding surfaces always smaller than 5 µm. The subsequent binary 3D Standard Tessellation Language (STL) models were imported in Viewbox 4 software (version 4.1.0.1 BETA, dHAL Software, Kifissia, Greece) to apply the methods tested in the study. Each such maxillary or mandibular full dental arch model consisted of 600.000–900.000 triangles.

2.5. Tooth Wear Volume Measurement Workflow

Following 3D superimpositions through seven test techniques and the gold standard technique, the crowns of the grinded teeth (T1) were manually segmented and compared to the segmented original crowns (T0).

For each tested tooth, the gold standard (GS) measurements were obtained through T0/T1 model superimpositions on intact adjacent teeth and alveolar processes (Figure 1a). Perfect matching is expected in these areas following a best-fit superimposition, which enables accurate occlusal tooth wear assessment [10,11,18].

Measurements were performed according to a modified, previously published protocol [10]. The first group of measurements (PC: partial crown) was obtained using part of the T0 clinical crown as superimposition reference (Figure 1b–d). This aimed to include crown areas that could be considered unaffected from occlusal wear or retainer placement. On the other hand, the complete T0 clinical crown was used as a superimposition reference for the second group (CC: complete crown) (Figure 1e). Each time, the T0/T1 3D models of each patient were superimposed using the software's implementation of the iterative closest point algorithm (ICP) [19], with predefined settings that are described below. The whole process always started from the original initial position of the models. Thus, the first step included the manual approximation of the two objects to facilitate rapid automatic registration through the ICP algorithm. For the same reason, following the manual approximation, in cases of a setting that included less than 50% estimated overlap of meshes, a partial approximation of the two models was always performed, using 100% estimated overlap of meshes, before applying the predefined setting.

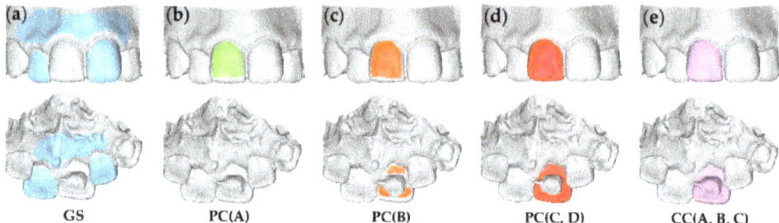

Figure 1. Reference areas used to measure tooth wear at the right maxillary permanent central incisor. (**a**) Gold standard area (GS: blue). (**b**–**d**) Partial crown areas (PC: green, orange, red). (**e**) Complete crown area (CC: purple). The upper row shows the buccal and the lower row the palatal view. The letters within the parentheses indicate the settings applied for each reference area.

Based on previous experience [10] and pilot testing, the performance of different ICP settings was assessed using the superimposition reference areas described above (Figure 1). The eight specific techniques applied in the study (combinations of ICP settings and reference areas) are listed in Table 1. The basic setting consisted of 100% estimated overlap of meshes, matching point to plane, exact nearest neighbor search, 100% point sampling, exclude overhangs, and 50 iterations. Other ICP settings were identical to the basic setting, but with user defined, 40%, or 20% estimated overlap of meshes. The user defined estimated overlap of meshes was freely chosen by the operator for each individual measurement, through an iterative process. Each time, following various adjustments of the specific setting, the user aimed to achieve the maximum overlap of the superimposed teeth and, primarily, of the adjacent intact structures. The selected value that provided the best overlap of intact structures in each case, was noted in an Excel sheet. For each reference area, the average of these values, provided the additional estimated overlap settings to be tested. It should be noted that the case-specific, user defined setting is impossible to be obtained in actual patient data, since there are no absolutely intact structures in the mouth between two time points [11]. Thus, this approach allowed the determination of a setting that might work properly, while being applicable in actual clinical conditions.

Table 1. Superimposition techniques tested in the study.

Technique	Reference Area	Estimated Overlap
GS	Adjacent intact teeth and alveolar processes	100%
PC(A)	Buccal surface	100%
PC(B)	Buccolingual surfaces without composite	User defined
PC(C)	Complete crown without composite	User defined
PC(D)	Complete crown without composite	40%
CC(A)	Complete crown	40%
CC(B)	Complete crown	User defined
CC(C)	Complete crown	20%

GS: gold standard; PC: partial crown; CC: complete crown.

The superimposed 3D tooth crown models through each technique described above, were simultaneously sliced using one (gingival) to three planes (gingival, mesial, and distal), based on a previously published protocol [10]. For each pair of teeth, the slicing planes were positioned to include the complete occlusal wear surface. At the same time care was taken to avoid significant differences between the two models at the edges of the crown parts to be sliced. This was verified though the visualization of relevant color coded distance maps. Consequently, identical filling of the holes of each occlusal part of the sliced T0 and T1 crown models was achieved (Figure 2). In certain cases, the hole created from slicing had to be split to two or more parts, through manual connection of contralateral points in sharp edges. This ensured that the edges of each hole to be filled, through the application of the software's algorithm, were located on the same plane. Thus, it ensured identical hole filling and creation of watertight T0 and T1 3D models that were matching at all parts, apart from the occlusal part that was the one to be assessed (Figure 3). Following this approach, occlusal tooth wear was defined as the difference between these two superimposed crown parts. The wear amount, expressed as volume loss of tooth structure (mm^3), that was detected through the gold standard technique, was then compared to that of the test techniques.

To assess the error of Viewbox 4 software on volumetric assessments, the volumes of ten tooth parts similar to those used for the study were measured using Viewbox 4, Artec Studio 12 Professional (Artec 3D, Luxembourg), and MeshLab 2016.12 [20] and compared. The error attributed to the used surface scanner was measured in ten teeth of various types, located on ten different models that were scanned twice. Following superimposition of the corresponding identical teeth derived from repeated scans, volumes similar to those tested in the study were calculated. Zero difference in corresponding volumes would indicate perfect superimposition of the repeated models and zero scanner error. Reproducibility of tooth wear assessment techniques was tested through repeated measurements of ten teeth, on four randomly selected models, two maxillary and two mandibular (one with and one without crowding each) by one operator, following a 1-month period.

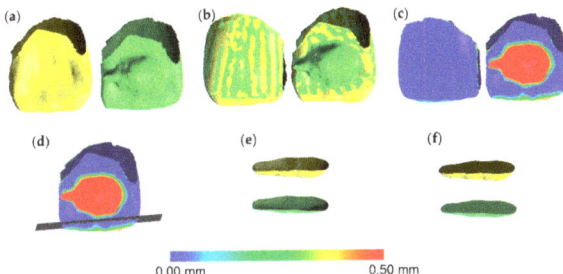

Figure 2. Tooth wear measurement process in a maxillary central incisor. (**a**) Tooth before (yellow) and after (green) tooth wear and retainer simulation. (**b**) Superimposed tooth crowns using the complete crown technique and setting C (20% estimated overlap) shown from the buccal (left) and the lingual (right) aspect. (**c**) Color coded distance map showing the tooth wear from the buccal (left) and the lingual (right) side. (**d**) Level (grey) used to simultaneously slice the two crowns. (**e**) Sliced tooth crowns. (**f**) Holes filled to create watertight models, and thus, calculate volumes.

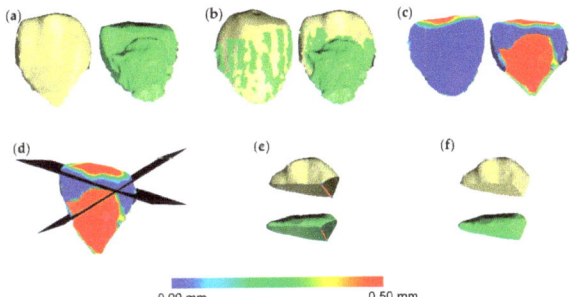

Figure 3. Tooth wear measurement process in a mandibular canine. (**a**) Tooth before (yellow) and after (green) tooth wear and retainer simulation. (**b**) Superimposed tooth crowns using the complete crown technique and setting C (20% estimated overlap) shown from the buccal (left) and the lingual (right) aspect. (**c**) Color coded distance map showing the tooth wear from the buccal (left) and the lingual (right) side. (**d**) Two levels (grey) used to simultaneously slice the two crowns. (**e**) Sliced tooth crowns with connected contralateral points (blue) in sharp edges (red line), splitting the hole in two parts to ensure identical hole filling process. (**f**) Holes filled to create watertight models, and thus, calculate volumes.

2.6. Statistical Analysis

The statistical approach followed here is comparable to that of a previous similar study [10]. Statistical analysis was carried out by using the IBM SPSS statistics for Windows (Version 26.0. IBM Corp: Armonk, NY, USA). Non-parametric statistics were applied based on abnormal distribution of the raw data of certain variables (Kolmogorov–Smirnov and Shapiro–Wilk tests).

Agreement between different techniques with the gold standard technique (trueness) regarding tooth wear, was shown in box plots. Perfect trueness is indicated by zero median value, whereas the larger the deviation from zero the lower the trueness. Within techniques, the range of deviation of individual values from the median value shows precision. Differences in trueness and precision among different techniques were tested using Friedman's test, followed, where applicable, by Wilcoxon's signed rank test for pairwise comparisons [10].

Potential effects of presence of crowding, tooth type, or tooth wear amount on the trueness and precision of each technique were explored through visual inspection of relevant plots and unpaired comparative tests within techniques [10].

Intra-operator error (reproducibility) of the gold standard and the technique of choice was assessed through Bland Altman plots, with markers set by tooth category. Any deviation from zero shows imprecision of the technique. Differences in the reproducibility of the two techniques were tested in an unpaired manner through Mann–Whitney U test [10].

For all tests, a two-sided significance test was carried out at an alpha level of 0.05. When multiple pairwise comparisons were performed, the level of significance was altered according to the Bonferroni adjustment.

3. Results

Regarding the volumetric assessment of tooth crown parts of interest, all three tested software provided identical values for all tested models. Following superimposition of corresponding single teeth, derived from repeated scans, with the CC(C) technique, the median volume difference was 0.0115 mm^3 (range: 0.0003, 0.0350 mm^3) when all differences were transformed to absolute values. The original position of the second scan was randomly altered prior to these tests. This value indicates the scanner plus the superimposition error regarding tooth wear assessment using single teeth. Repeated tooth wear measurements with the gold standard technique and the CC(C) technique of choice showed no systematic error (one sample t-test, $p > 0.05$). The amount of tooth wear and the tooth type did not seem to affect reproducibility. The outcomes of both techniques were considered highly reproducible overall and in individual measurements (max difference < 0.040 mm^3) (Figure 4). There was no difference in the reproducibility of the gold standard and the technique of choice ($p = 0.94$). The superimposition error of the gold standard technique that provided the reference measurements is shown in Figure 4a and it was on average less than 0.005 mm^3 and in all cases less than 0.020 mm^3.

There were significant differences in the trueness of the tested techniques (Friedman test: $p < 0.001$). PC(A) and PC(B) differed clearly from all other techniques. Among the rest, all techniques differed significantly to each other apart from CC(A) vs. PC(D), CC(B) vs. PC(C), CC(B) vs. CC(C), and CC(C) vs. PC(C) (Wilcoxon signed rank test: $p < 0.01$; Figure 5). Analogous differences in precision were evident among all techniques (Figure 5). The CC(C) technique was the only technique that showed perfect agreement with the GS technique in all cases (median difference: −0.002, max absolute difference: 0.178 mm^3) and is applicable in actual clinical conditions.

Tooth type did not affect the trueness of each technique (Mann–Whitney U test, $p > 0.05$). However, measurements in canines tended to be more precise compared to those of incisors (Figure 6a). Tooth alignment in the dental arches also did not affect the outcomes of any technique (Mann–Whitney U test: $p > 0.05$). Tooth wear amount did not show any significant effects (Kruskal–Wallis test, $p > 0.01$), though there was a tendency for slightly reduced trueness and precision in the group with the highest amount of tooth wear (Figure 6b).

The difference between the CC(C) technique of choice and the GS technique was always small for any tested tooth type or amount of tooth wear (Supplementary Materials Figure S1). However, there was a tendency for decreased precision in case of 2 mm vertical height loss of tooth structure (Kruskal–Wallis test, $p = 0.029$). Pairwise comparisons showed a significant difference only between the 0.5 mm and the 2 mm groups (Mann–Whitney U test, $p < 0.01$).

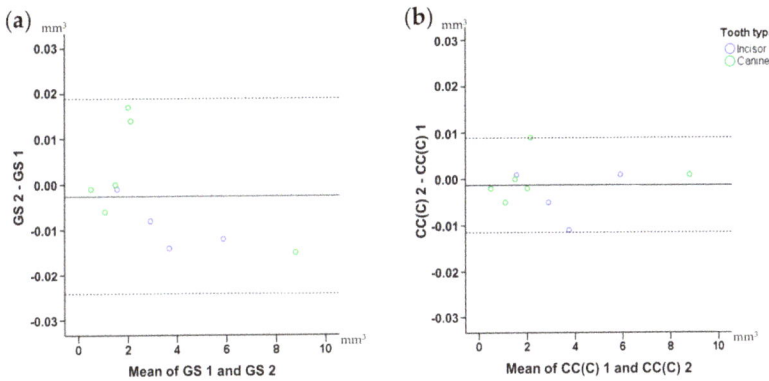

Figure 4. Bland–Altman plots showing intra-operator error on tooth wear volume measurements. (**a**) Gold standard (GS) technique. (**b**) Technique of choice: complete crown (CC) with 20% estimated overlap. The axes length represents the true range of measured tooth wear values. The continuous horizontal line shows the mean and the dashed lines the 95% confidence intervals.

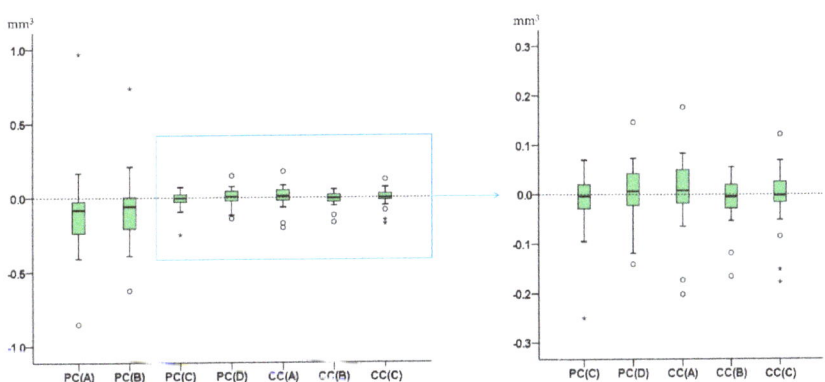

Figure 5. Box plots showing in the Y-axis the difference of each technique with the gold standard technique in tooth wear measurements. The upper limit of the black line represents the maximum value, the lower limit the minimum value, the box the interquartile range, and the horizontal black line the median value (trueness). Outliers are shown as black circles (°) or asterisks (*), in more extreme cases, with a step of 1.5 × IQR (interquartile range). Zero value (dashed horizontal line) indicates perfect agreement with the gold standard. The vertical length of each plot indicates precision. The blue box on the left image indicates the area of the graph shown in the right image in a larger scale. PC: partial crown; CC: complete crown.

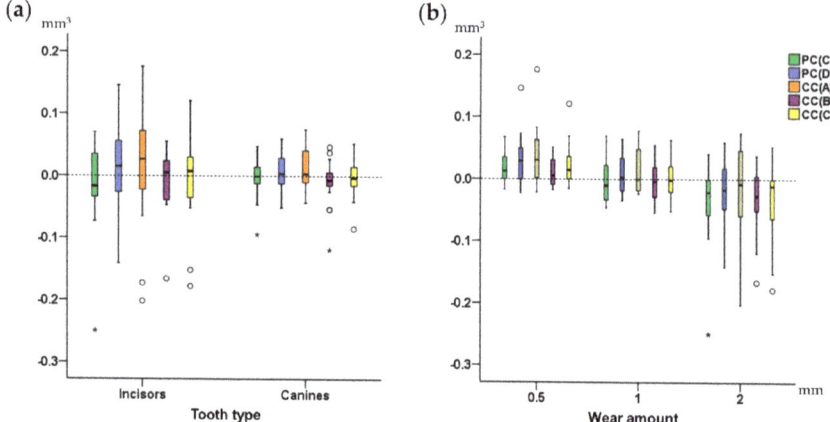

Figure 6. Box plots showing on the Y-axis the difference of each technique from the gold standard technique in tooth wear measurements, (**a**) by tooth type, and (**b**) by amount of tooth wear. The upper limit of the black line represents the maximum value, the lower limit the minimum value, the box the interquartile range, and the horizontal black line the median value (trueness). Outliers are shown as black circles or asterisks, in more extreme cases, with a step of 1.5 × IQR (interquartile range). Zero value (dashed horizontal line) indicates perfect agreement with the gold standard. The vertical length of each plot indicates precision. PC: partial crown; CC: complete crown.

4. Discussion

Additional to proper diagnosis, easily applicable methods that facilitate accurate assessment of tooth wear will support the scientific community in better understanding potential causes, acting mechanisms, and contributing factors. Material wear is also very important for materials science when conducting in vitro tests, but also to clinically test the real-life performance of materials [21,22]. Here we present a highly accurate and informative tooth wear assessment method, which is also more convenient than the already available laboratory methods. It allows the measurement and visualization of occlusal tooth wear in three dimensions of space, on patients that received a bonded wire retainer during the assessment period. To our knowledge, this is the first study that addresses this issue. The suggested method requires the existence of two serial dental models to assess wear progress over time. In the era of digitization, this is not considered a limitation, since it is expected that soon an intraoral patient scan will be an integral part of basic dental diagnostic records. Providing that the suggested superimposition method registers sufficiently serial surface models similar to those tested here, it can be used for any relevant purpose, including occlusal material wear testing.

The present method offers the opportunity for detailed assessment of changes over time, in corresponding surfaces, without the need for placing any landmarks, which might be a time-consuming and error prone process [23,24]. Apart from the clinically relevant applications, following the proper superimposition of serial 3D tooth models, which enables the accurate detection of the worn tooth part during a specific time period, this method can be combined with various other types of 3D shape analysis, such as those used for ecometrics in dental ecology [25], including dental topography methods [24]. The method works on a μm scale that is defined by its accuracy, as well as by the resolution of the applied scanning systems. For example, based on scanner resolution of the intraoral, as well as the current dental lab scanners [11], microwear analysis might not be possible, though it might be quite useful for testing certain hypotheses [26].

In a previous study we developed a similar method [10] applicable on teeth that did not undergo significant alterations in any crown surface, apart from the occlusal. Epidemiologic studies indicate that in modern humans, tooth wear, especially of the clinical crown, mainly concerns the occlusal part of the teeth due to the direct contacts with the antagonists [12,13]. Thus, the simulation model that was previously developed and applied here, represented adequately the most common clinical occurrence. However, certain patients may receive a fixed retainer at their buccal or more often at their lingual surfaces. This usually consists of a continuous wire bonded with composite resin at the middle of the respective tooth surfaces. This type of retainer is common in patients that received orthodontic treatment, but also in severe periodontally compromised patients, or in patients that required tooth stabilization following dental trauma [14,16,17]. Thus, we suspected that our previously suggested method might not perform similarly when a fixed retainer has been bonded to the test teeth during the assessed period. Indeed, after testing various possibilities for the latter case, we concluded that the complete crown with reduced estimated overlap of meshes to 20%, namely the CC(C) technique, provided the most accurate outcomes. The previous study, on intact teeth in non-occlusal surfaces, suggested an estimated overlap of meshes of 30% for optimal outcomes [10].

The present method offers a median accuracy of 0.002 mm^3, with the worst individual measurement showing a difference of 0.178 mm^3 from the gold standard measurement. The gold standard measurement always showed a precision higher than 0.020 mm^3. The scanner plus the superimposition error for single teeth measurements, using the suggested technique, was always smaller than 0.035 mm^3. Thus, even in the unfavorable scenario of extensive changes in non-occlusal surfaces, this method performs quite satisfactorily. A freeware and easy to use software (WearCompare, School of Dentistry, University of Leeds, Leeds, UK) [27] providing tooth wear measurements, following serial tooth surface model superimpositions, showed high performance when identical (duplicated) surfaces were used as superimposition references. However, when the original position of the duplicated models was altered, the software showed errors in volumetric assessment as high as 1 mm^3. Furthermore, when actual patient data were considered, it showed considerable and statistically significant differences on volumetric assessments from Geomagic Control software (3D Systems, Darmstadt, Germany), averaging 0.59 mm^3 [27]. This software uses the buccal and lingual surfaces as superimposition references to assess occlusal tooth wear. We also tested this approach both in a previous [10] and in the current study and it did not provide superior outcomes to that of the suggested techniques, which use the whole crown as superimposition reference. Furthermore, the performance of WearCompare software in presence of considerable changes in the used superimposition reference areas remains to be tested.

The current settings might also be applicable to patients that show extensive tooth wear on buccal or lingual surfaces [12,15]. In such cases, apart from the occlusal surface, another surface is highly altered over time, such as with the placement of a retainer. Following the superimposition of serial tooth models, the operator can generate color coded distance maps and confirm the applicability of the suggested technique, if the detected changes are comparable to those simulated here. For example, in cases of erosion, changes might be present on the entire tooth surface and, thus, the suggested technique might not be applicable. Finally, if the teeth are not subjected to any change between two time points, the present technique still performs a complete registration of the two surface models (Supplementary Materials Figure S2). However, this will be a rare occasion, since in living humans, minimal changes in form or in spatial relations are always expected over time. Even if there is no morphological change, two serial intraoral scans will not provide identical models [11].

In actual patients, the gingival margin area, and thus the corresponding clinical crown structures, might also change over time. However, with the present method this is not a limitation, since in case of large differences in the gingival part of the crown, the operator can select the shortest clinical crown as the superimposition reference. Then, by selecting the "exclude overhangs" option, which is included in the suggested default settings, the software ignores the part of crown that does not exist in both models. The performance of this function has been extensively applied and tested in previous studies, on various types of surface models and has always provided solid outcomes [10,11,18,28–30].

The present study simulated tooth wear amounts of approximately 0.5, 1, and 2 mm to represent variations of clinically significant loss of tooth crown parts, in terms of dental appearance. As evident in an analogous study [10], the high performance of the technique presented here was not considerably affected by tooth wear amount. Smaller amounts of occlusal tooth wear might be present in actual patients, but were not simulated here. We considered the tested range more relevant, since the ICP algorithm would perform equally well, if not better, in cases of smaller surface changes (Supplementary Materials Figures S1b, S2, and S3) [11,18,28]. Providing adequate superimposition of serial tooth models under the tested circumstances, the accuracy of the suggested method is defined by its difference from the tooth wear value obtained using the gold standard method. The amount of tooth wear that can be safely detected by the method is determined by the specified accuracy level. However, a potential improvement of the accuracy level in cases of minimal tooth wear remains to be verified by future research.

The high accuracy laboratory scanner used here to generate the surface models, has comparable accuracy to the current high end intraoral scanners, considering relatively small structures, such as single tooth crowns [11,18,31]. In the present study, we selected this scanner to eliminate the scanner error effect on the gold standard measurement, which requires a larger superimposition reference area. This measurement is feasible only with the present experimental design, where the structures adjacent to a worn tooth are intact. The true wear amount is measured through the use of these intact structures as superimposition reference. This measurement is then compared to the measurement obtained using the single tooth crown as superimposition reference. Only the latter option is feasible in actual clinical conditions, where no structure adjacent to single teeth can be considered morphologically stable over time. This is the main reason why gold standard measurements (true values) cannot be available when using actual clinical data.

So far, most methods used to measure tooth wear are based on qualitative assessments with limited precision or on complex laboratory quantitative approaches that require expertise and special equipment to be applied [7]. The presented method requires 3D tooth surface models that can nowadays be easily obtained through intraoral scanners [11]. These models can then be processed using software applications that are widely available under reasonable costs [32]. Thus, following the necessary short-term training, these methods can be potentially incorporated in a regular dental practice environment, enhancing the diagnostic ability of occlusal tooth wear, especially in cases that this is considered critical. Apart from this major advantage, the performance of this method is also comparable to, if not higher than most available methods [7]. So far, a direct comparison with other methods is not possible, since no other study has performed quantitative tooth wear assessment in teeth that underwent significant changes in surfaces other than the one tested. Among others, a significant strength of the present in vitro study is that it allowed the comparison of different techniques with a gold standard technique, which provided the true measurement. Thus, apart from reproducibility, the study tested the trueness of the measurements, which is usually a missing part from previous reports [7]. Furthermore, the present method is superior to methods that perform 2D measurements, such as the vertical loss of tooth structure, since it offers much higher amount of 3D information. In addition to the quantification of tooth volume loss, this 3D superimposition technique enables the visualization of a color coded distance map that allows a thorough quantitative and qualitative assessment of tooth wear in the 3D space. Thus, following the proper application of the suggested technique, patterns of tooth wear or any spatial differences in the tooth surfaces, can be easily identified and quantified according to the needs of each individual test.

Our research group has worked extensively in testing surface-based 3D superimposition in the craniofacial area, showing promising results in many different applications [10,11,18,28–30,33]. In the aforementioned studies, the performance of the used software and the specific algorithm has been thoroughly tested and shown highly reproducible results. Thus, the high reproducibility of the present techniques was an expected finding. Furthermore, the technique of choice consistently provided values very close to the true amount of tooth wear. The individual differences of the selected CC(C) technique from the true value were almost always smaller than 0.1 mm^3. This accuracy level is comparable to that achieved on teeth that underwent changes only at their occlusal surfaces [10]. However, the current approach consists a clinically applicable technique in a more challenging scenario, where the used tooth surfaces have been considerably changed over time.

In diagnostic accuracy studies, it is of utmost importance to assess differences between techniques or repeated measurements in each individual case and not only between group means [34]. In the latter, positive and negative differences between diverse cases can be eliminated providing the misleading impression of similar outcomes. However, it is important to have accurate measurements in each individual case, since, for example, this information might affect treatment decisions. Indeed, in the present study the mean values of all techniques were very close to each other and to the true value. However, when results of individual cases were considered, the superiority of the selected CC(C) technique became evident.

A limitation of the present study could be that only anterior teeth were thoroughly tested. This approach was followed because these teeth usually require a fixed retainer [14,16,17]. Furthermore, we also included canines in our tests, which are more round-formed teeth. Along with the present results, previous results have also shown that tooth type does not considerably affect the outcomes [10]. Thus, we expect that this technique will be also applicable on posterior teeth (Supplementary Materials Figure S3). Another limitation could be that intra-operator error was only assessed for the gold standard and the technique of choice. This was considered adequate since the two techniques showed satisfactory agreement and both provided excellent reproducibility outcomes. Furthermore, as described above, thorough error evaluation of similar techniques has been published previously and always provided favorable outcomes [10].

5. Conclusions

The present report suggests a 3D superimposition technique to assess occlusal tooth wear in anterior teeth that received a bonded wire retainer during the assessment period. Following the superimposition of serial tooth crown models, loss of tooth structure can be visualized and quantified in all dimensions of space. The technique is highly accurate, informative, and relatively easy to use, and thus, it will facilitate associated research, but it can also be easily incorporated in a clinical environment. Further work is required to verify the performance of the technique on posterior teeth and regarding smaller increments of tooth wear.

Supplementary Materials: The following are available online at http://www.mdpi.com/2077-0383/9/12/3937/s1, Figure S1: Box plots showing in the Y-axis the difference of the technique of choice (complete crown, setting C) from the gold standard technique in tooth wear measurements (a) by tooth type and (b) by amount of tooth wear, Figure S2: Superimposition of identical surface models of a maxillary incisor (left) and a mandibular canine (right). Figure S3: Tooth wear measurement in a mandibular molar with limited loss of tooth structure.

Author Contributions: Conceptualization, N.G.; methodology, N.G., K.D., C.K., D.H. and Y.R.; software, D.H.; validation, N.G. and K.D.; formal analysis, N.G.; investigation, N.G. and K.D.; resources, N.G., K.D., C.K., D.H., Y.R.; data curation, N.G. and K.D.; writing—original draft preparation, N.G. and K.D.; writing—review and editing, N.G., K.D., C.K., D.H., Y.R.; visualization, N.G. and K.D.; supervision, C.K., D.H. and Y.R.; project administration, N.G.; funding acquisition, N.G. All authors have read and agreed to the published version of the manuscript.

Funding: This research was funded by a grant from the European Orthodontic Society, in the context of the W J B Houston Scholarship Award that was granted to author N. Gkantidis.

Conflicts of Interest: D. Halazonetis owns stock in dHAL Software, the company that markets Viewbox 4. Authors N. Gkantidis, K. Dritsas, Y. Ren, and C. Katsaros declare no competing interest. The funders had no role in the design of the study; in the collection, analyses, or interpretation of data; in the writing of the manuscript, or in the decision to publish the results.

References

1. Lussi, A.; Carvalho, T.S. Erosive tooth wear: A multifactorial condition of growing concern and increasing knowledge. *Monogr. Oral Sci.* **2014**, *25*, 1–15. [PubMed]
2. Loomans, B.; Opdam, N.; Attin, T.; Bartlett, D.; Edelhoff, D.; Frankenberger, R.; Benic, G.; Ramseyer, S.; Wetselaar, P.; Sterenborg, B.; et al. Severe tooth wear: European consensus statement on management guidelines. *J. Adhes. Dent.* **2017**, *19*, 111–119. [PubMed]

3. Lee, A.; He, L.H.; Lyons, K.; Swain, M.V. Tooth wear and wear investigations in dentistry. *J. Oral Rehabil.* **2012**, *39*, 217–225. [CrossRef] [PubMed]
4. Wetselaar, P.; Faris, A.; Lobbezoo, F. A plea for the development of an universally accepted modular tooth wear evaluation system. *BMC Oral Health* **2016**, *16*, 115. [CrossRef]
5. Al-Omiri, M.K.; Sghaireen, M.G.; Alzarea, B.K.; Lynch, E. Quantification of incisal tooth wear in upper anterior teeth: Conventional vs. new method using toolmakers microscope and a three-dimensional measuring technique. *J. Dent.* **2013**, *41*, 1214–1221. [CrossRef]
6. Bartlett, D.; Ganss, C.; Lussi, A. Basic Erosive Wear Examination (BEWE): A new scoring system for scientific and clinical needs. *Clin. Oral Investig.* **2008**, *12*, S65–S68. [CrossRef]
7. Wulfman, C.; Koenig, V.; Mainjot, A.K. Wear measurement of dental tissues and materials in clinical studies: A systematic review. *Dent. Mater.* **2018**, *34*, 825–850. [CrossRef]
8. Heintze, S.D. How to qualify and validate wear simulation devices and methods. *Dent. Mater.* **2006**, *22*, 712–734. [CrossRef]
9. Rodriguez, J.M.; Bartlett, D.W. The dimensional stability of impression materials and its effect on in vitro tooth wear studies. *Dent. Mater.* **2011**, *27*, 253–258. [CrossRef]
10. Gkantidis, N.; Dritsas, K.; Ren, Y.; Halazonetis, D.; Katsaros, C. An accurate and efficient method for occlusal tooth wear assessment using 3D digital dental models. *Sci. Rep.* **2020**, *10*, 10103. [CrossRef]
11. Winkler, J.; Gkantidis, N. Trueness and precision of intraoral scanners in the maxillary dental arch: An in vivo analysis. *Sci. Rep.* **2020**, *10*, 1172. [CrossRef]
12. Teixeira, L.; Manso, M.C.; Manarte-Monteiro, P. Erosive tooth wear status of institutionalized alcoholic patients under rehabilitation therapy in the north of Portugal. *Clin. Oral Investig.* **2017**, *21*, 809–819. [CrossRef] [PubMed]
13. Awad, M.A.; El Kassas, D.; Al Harthi, L.; Abraham, S.B.; Al-Khalifa, K.S.; Khalaf, M.E.; Al Habashneh, R.; Bartlett, D. Prevalence, severity and explanatory factors of tooth wear in Arab populations. *J. Dent.* **2019**, *80*, 69–74. [CrossRef] [PubMed]
14. Iliadi, A.; Kloukos, D.; Gkantidis, N.; Katsaros, C.; Pandis, N. Failure of fixed orthodontic retainers: A systematic review. *J. Dent.* **2015**, *43*, 876–896. [CrossRef] [PubMed]
15. Bartlett, D.W.; Lussi, A.; West, N.X.; Bouchard, P.; Sanz, M.; Bourgeois, D. Prevalence of tooth wear on buccal and lingual surfaces and possible risk factors in young European adults. *J. Dent.* **2013**, *41*, 1007–1013. [CrossRef] [PubMed]
16. Gkantidis, N.; Christou, P.; Topouzelis, N. The orthodontic-periodontic interrelationship in integrated treatment challenges: A systematic review. *J. Oral Rehabil.* **2010**, *37*, 377–390. [CrossRef]
17. Kahler, B.; Hu, J.Y.; Marriot-Smith, C.S.; Heithersay, G.S. Splinting of teeth following trauma: A review and a new splinting recommendation. *Aust. Dent. J.* **2016**, *61* (Suppl. 1), 59–73. [CrossRef]
18. Henninger, E.; Vasilakos, G.; Halazonetis, D.; Gkantidis, N. The effect of regular dental cast artifacts on the 3D superimposition of serial digital maxillary dental models. *Sci. Rep.* **2019**, *9*, 10501. [CrossRef]
19. Besl, P.J.; Mckay, N.D. A Method for Registration of 3-D Shapes. *IEEE Trans. Pattern Anal. Mach. Intell.* **1992**, *14*, 239–256. [CrossRef]
20. Cignoni, P.; Callieri, M.; Corsini, M.; Dellepiane, M.; Ganovelli, F.; Ranzuglia, G. MeshLab: An Open-Source Mesh Processing Tool. In Proceedings of the Sixth Eurographics Italian Chapter Conference, Salerno, Italy, 2 July 2008; pp. 129–136.
21. Lazaridou, D.; Belli, R.; Petschelt, A.; Lohbauer, U. Are resin composites suitable replacements for amalgam? A study of two-body wear. *Clin. Oral Investig.* **2015**, *19*, 1485–1492. [CrossRef]
22. Lohbauer, U.; Reich, S. Antagonist wear of monolithic zirconia crowns after 2 years. *Clin. Oral Investig.* **2017**, *21*, 1165–1172. [CrossRef] [PubMed]
23. Gkantidis, N.; Schauseil, M.; Pazera, P.; Zorkun, B.; Katsaros, C.; Ludwig, B. Evaluation of 3-dimensional superimposition techniques on various skeletal structures of the head using surface models. *PLoS ONE* **2015**, *10*, e0118810. [CrossRef] [PubMed]
24. Berthaume, M.A.; Lazzari, V.; Guy, F. The landscape of tooth shape: Over 20 years of dental topography in primates. *Evol. Anthropol.* **2020**, *29*, 245–262. [CrossRef] [PubMed]
25. Evans, A.R. Shape descriptors as ecometrics in dental ecology. *Hystrix It. J. Mamm.* **2013**, *24*, 133–140.
26. Schmidt, C.W. On the relationship of dental microwear to dental macrowear. *Am. J. Phys. Anthr.* **2010**, *142*, 67–73. [CrossRef] [PubMed]

27. O'Toole, S.; Osnes, C.; Bartlett, D.; Keeling, A. Investigation into the validity of WearCompare, a purpose-built software to quantify erosive tooth wear progression. *Dent. Mater.* **2019**, *35*, 1408–1414. [CrossRef] [PubMed]
28. Vasilakos, G.; Schilling, R.; Halazonetis, D.; Gkantidis, N. Assessment of different techniques for 3D superimposition of serial digital maxillary dental casts on palatal structures. *Sci. Rep.* **2017**, *7*, 5838. [CrossRef]
29. Haner, S.T.; Kanavakis, G.; Matthey, F.; Gkantidis, N. Voxel-based superimposition of serial craniofacial CBCTs: Reliability, reproducibility and segmentation effect on hard-tissue outcomes. *Orthod. Craniofac. Res.* **2020**, *23*, 92–101. [CrossRef]
30. Friedli, L.; Kloukos, D.; Kanavakis, G.; Halazonetis, D.; Gkantidis, N. The effect of threshold level on bone segmentation of cranial base structures from CT and CBCT images. *Sci. Rep.* **2020**, *10*, 7361. [CrossRef]
31. Nedelcu, R.; Olsson, P.; Nyström, I.; Thor, A. Finish line distinctness and accuracy in 7 intraoral scanners versus conventional impression: An in vitro descriptive comparison. *BMC Oral Health* **2018**, *18*, 27. [CrossRef]
32. Stucki, S.; Gkantidis, N. Assessment of techniques used for superimposition of maxillary and mandibular 3D surface models to evaluate tooth movement: A systematic review. *Eur. J. Orthod.* **2020**, *42*, 559–570. [CrossRef] [PubMed]
33. Vasilakos, G.; Koniaris, A.; Wolf, M.; Halazonetis, D.; Gkantidis, N. Early anterior crossbite correction through posterior bite opening: A 3D superimposition prospective cohort study. *Eur. J. Orthod.* **2018**, *40*, 364–371. [CrossRef] [PubMed]
34. Bland, J.M.; Altman, D.G. Comparing methods of measurement: Why plotting difference against standard method is misleading. *Lancet* **1995**, *346*, 1085–1087. [CrossRef]

Publisher's Note: MDPI stays neutral with regard to jurisdictional claims in published maps and institutional affiliations.

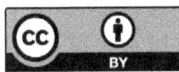

© 2020 by the authors. Licensee MDPI, Basel, Switzerland. This article is an open access article distributed under the terms and conditions of the Creative Commons Attribution (CC BY) license (http://creativecommons.org/licenses/by/4.0/).

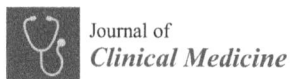

Article

Novel Sub-Clustering of Class III Skeletal Malocclusion Phenotypes in a Southern European Population Based on Proportional Measurements

Leixuri de Frutos-Valle [1], Conchita Martín [1,4], José Antonio Alarcón [2,4], Juan Carlos Palma-Fernández [1], Ricardo Ortega [3] and Alejandro Iglesias-Linares [1,4,*]

1. Section of Orthodontics, Faculty of Odontology, Complutense University, 28040 Madrid, Spain; leixuridefrutos@gmail.com (L.d.F.V.); mariacom@ucm.es or conchitamartin@mac.com (C.M.); jcarlospalma@me.com (J.C.P.-F.)
2. Section of Orthodontics, Faculty of Odontology, University of Granada, 18071 Granada, Spain; jalarcon@ugr.es
3. Section of Radiology, Faculty of Odontology, Complutense University, 28040 Madrid, Spain; ricardoortega@odon.ucm.es
4. BIOCRAN (Craniofacial Biology) Research Group, Complutense University, 28040 Madrid, Spain
* Correspondence: aleigl01@ucm.es

Received: 24 July 2020; Accepted: 16 September 2020; Published: 22 September 2020

Abstract: Current phenotypic characterizations of Class III malocclusion are influenced more by gender or ethnic origin than by raw linear skeletal measurements. The aim of the present research is to develop a Class III skeletal malocclusion sub-phenotype characterization based on proportional cranial measurements using principal component analysis and cluster analysis. Radiometric data from 212 adult subjects (115 women and 96 men) of southern European origin affected by Class III skeletal malocclusion were analyzed. A total of 120 measurements were made, 26 were proportional skeletal measurements, which were used to perform principal component analysis and subsequent cluster analysis. The remaining 94 supplementary measurements were used for a greater description of the identified clusters. Principal component analysis established eight principal components that explained 85.1% of the total variance. The first three principal components explained 51.4% of the variance and described mandibular proportions, anterior facial height proportions, and posterior–anterior cranial proportions. Cluster analysis established four phenotypic subgroups, representing 18.4% (C1), 20.75% (C2), 38.68% (C3), and 22.17% (C4) of the sample. A new sub-clustering of skeletal Class III malocclusions that avoids gender influence is provided. Our results improve clinicians' resources for Class III malocclusion and could improve the diagnostic and treatment approaches for this malocclusion.

Keywords: malocclusion; angle Class III; phenotype; principal component analysis; clustering; orthodontics

1. Introduction

Skeletal Class III malocclusions are among the most challenging malocclusions to treat, first because of the complexity of achieving an optimal treatment outcome [1–3] and second, because the clear genetic component determines the prognosis of this type of malocclusion [4–9]. Distinguishable ethnic differences have been described in this type of malocclusion, with prevalences ranging from 4.76% [10] to 31.4% [11] in Asian populations to rates below 11% in countries such as Australia (2.5%) [12], Italy (4.3%) [13], Colombia (5.8%) [14], South India (4.1%) [15], Iran (7.8%) [16], and Central Turkey (10.3%) [17]. Apart from absolute prevalence rates, clear indicators of the complexity and importance of this malocclusion are the fact that more than half the patients undergoing orthognathic surgery have skeletal Class III malocclusion and that it carries the highest need-for-correction score according to the index of the need for functional orthognathic treatment (IOFTN) [18–22]. Moreover, varying numbers and Cass III phenotypes are described, depending on the origin of the study population [23–28]. The resulting facial characteristics and skeletal structure vary according to the intrinsic features of each ethnic group with skeletal Class III malocclusion [29–32], which induces notable heterogeneity in the skeletal Class III diagnosis.

With respect to skeletal structure, differences in facial and cranial morphology have been observed between genders. Cranial measurements by gender indicate that raw linear measurements are higher in males than in females, whereas the raw values of these measurements are frequently of lower magnitude in males [29–31]. Due to these differences in total linear size, gender-related sub-phenotypic differences have been found in cases of skeletal Class III malocclusion in the same population [28,33,34].

This potential influence of gender and origin suggests that a novel diagnostic method of skeletal Class III malocclusion may be warranted, based exclusively on proportional measurements, and thus avoiding raw linear skeletal measurements. The primary aim of this study, therefore, is to design a simple and manageable clinical sub-phenotypic classification system for skeletal Class III malocclusion that will facilitate future analysis of outcome or prognostic features in Class III subjects. The aim of the present research is to characterize Class III skeletal malocclusion sub-phenotypes on the basis of proportional cranial measurements using principal component analysis and cluster analysis.

2. Experimental Section

2.1. Study Sample

A sample of 212 subjects (115 women and 96 men) of Southern European origin diagnosed with skeletal Class III malocclusion were selected. All participants were in phases IV or V of the cervical vertebral maturation stage (CVMS) [35] and, therefore, had practically completed their growth. All participants met the following inclusion criteria: molar or canine Class III malocclusion without loss of anterior space, Wits appraisal < -0.5 and/or ANB ≤ 0. The exclusion criteria were the absence of or a low-quality lateral radiograph or individuals who did not sign informed consent. The full sample selection criteria, as well as the sample size estimation, are detailed in a previous study in which the same population was used [33].

The study protocol was approved by the Institutional Ethics Committee (CE) of Complutense University of Madrid (Clinical Research Ethics Committee of the San Carlos Clinical Hospital of Madrid, reference 17/063), safeguarding the rights and interests of the people participating in the research, in accordance with the principles of the Declaration of Helsinki [36].

2.2. Measurements/Assessments: Cephalometric Measurement Selection and Analysis

The lateral cephalometric radiographs used for this study were taken as diagnostic records prior to orthodontic treatment between 1995 and 2019. Gender and ethnicity were recorded. Once all lateral radiographs were obtained, the CVMS of each patient was recorded and a single operator (L.F.-V.) imported the radiographs into Dolphin Imaging software (11.0, Dolphin Imaging and Management Solutions, Chatsworth, California) where they were calibrated.

Once calibrated, cephalometric measurements were made incorporating the respective cephalometric points. A total array of 26 proportional skeletal variables were selected for the characterization of Class III patients (Table 1) and used to obtain an n number axes model by principal component analysis and subsequent sub-phenotypic classification of clusters. In addition, 94 supplementary cephalometric measurements (7 airway, 15 soft tissue, 25 teeth, and 47 linear and angular skeletal) were used for a supplementary description of the skeletal proportional clusters and analyzed in order to complete the sub-clustering model.

Table 1. Skeletal proportional craniometric variables used in PCA.

P-A Face Height (S-Go/N-Me) (%)	Anterior Cranial Base (SN)/Length of Mand Base (Go-Pg) (%)
PFH:AFH (%)	Maxillary length (ANS-PNS)/Anterior Cranial Base (SN) (%)
S-Ar/Ar-Go (%)	Maxillary length (ANS-PNS)/Midface Length (Co-A) (%)
UFH (N-ANS/(N-ANS+ANS-Me)) (%)	Maxillary length (ANS-PNS)/Length of Mand Base (Go-Pg) (%)
LFH/TFH (ANS-Me:N-Me) (%)	Midface Length (Co-A)/Mandibular length (Co-Gn) (%)
Face Ht Ratio (N-ANS/ANS-Me) (%)	Mandibular Body Length (Go-Gn)/Mandibular length (Co-Gn) (%)
SN/GoMe (%)	Ar - A/Ar - Gn (%)
ANS-PNS/Me-Go (%)	Posterior Cranial Base (S-Ar)/Posterior Face Height (SGo) (%)
Articular Angle/SNB (%)	Ramus Height (Ar-Go)/Posterior Face Height (SGo) (%)
Saddle-Sella Angle (SN-Ar)/SNA (%)	Posterior Cranial Base (S-Ar)/Upper Face Height (N-ANS) (%)
Occ Plane to FH/FMA (MP-FH) (%)	Ramus Height (Ar-Go)/Lower Face Height (ANS-Me) (%)
Occ Plane to SN/SN - GoGn (%)	Maxillary Skeletal (A-N Perp)/Mand. Skeletal (Pg-Na Perp) (%)
Cranio-Mx Base (SN-Palatal Plane)/SN - GoGn (%)	Convexity (A-NPg)/Pg - NB (%)

2.3. Statistical Analysis

Multivariate Analysis

Principal component analysis was performed to summarize and reduce the number of proportional variables used in cephalometric analysis, minimizing any potential loss of information. The amount of information incorporated in each principal component is called variance. The more the information incorporated into a principal component, the greater the variance; and closely correlated original variables require fewer components to explain the variability in the results. Therefore, we sought a model that incorporated a few principal components and could explain a large portion of the total variance with a minimum loss of information. For this purpose, we used Varimax axis rotation with post hoc Kaiser's standardization.

Subsequently, a mixed cluster analysis (Coheris Analytics SPAD version 9.1) was performed to establish n' homogeneous sub-phenotypes of skeletal Class III malocclusion. Ward's criterion was used with the objective of achieving the lowest dispersion in the identified clusters. Subsequently, a graphical representation [37] of the defined clusters was obtained by generating the cephalometric trace closest to the nucleus of each cluster and adjusting it to the measurements of variables of each group.

The supplementary cephalometric variables, which were recorded simultaneously during cephalometric analysis, were assessed to determine their involvement in the clusters. Finally, by means of the chi-square test, the relationship between CVMS and gender with respect to the generated sub-phenotypes was established.

2.4. Method Error

Fifteen lateral cephalometric radiographs were randomly selected from the 212 participants and analysis was replicated by the main operator at a 3 week interval. A Student's t test for two-tailed paired samples was used to determine the reliability of the cephalometric measurements, establishing a p-value greater than 0.05 for all comparisons. The intraclass correlation coefficient of bidirectional mixed effects for absolute agreement (ICC) [38] and the Dahlberg formula [39] were also calculated.

3. Results

3.1. Method Error

The value of intraclass correlation coefficients was <65% in one instance (63.1% ANS − PNS/Go-Pg (%)) and <80% in two others (73.6% ANS − PNS/SN (%); 71.3% ANS − PNS/Co-A), indicating good reliability. The accuracy of measurements, as determined by the Dahlberg formula, had an error value ranging from 0 (N − ANS/ANS − Me); ANS − PNS/Me-Go) to 15.5 (Pog − NB/A − NPo).

3.2. Description of the Main Components

Principal component (PC) analysis explained 85.1% of the variance across the 8 principal axes generated in the present Class III sample (Figure 1). The first three principal components primarily described mandibular proportions (SN/GoMe; ANS − PNS/Me − Go; ASN − PNS/Go-Pg), anterior facial proportions (UFH; LFH/TFH; Face Ht Ratio) and anteroposterior cranial proportions (S − Go/N − Me; PFH:AFH), and represent more than 50% of the total variance (51.4%). In all, 21.7% of the variance was represented by the mandibular proportions in PC1: SN/GoMe; ANS − PNS/Me − Go and ASN − PNS/Go − Pg among others. PC2 accounted for 15.6% of the variance and was represented by variables that indicate facial proportions (UFH; LFH/TFH; Face Ht Ratio), while PC3 accounted for 14.1% of the variance and was represented by variables that indicate anteroposterior cranial proportions (S − Go/N − Me; PFH:AFH, Ar − Go/ANS − Me).

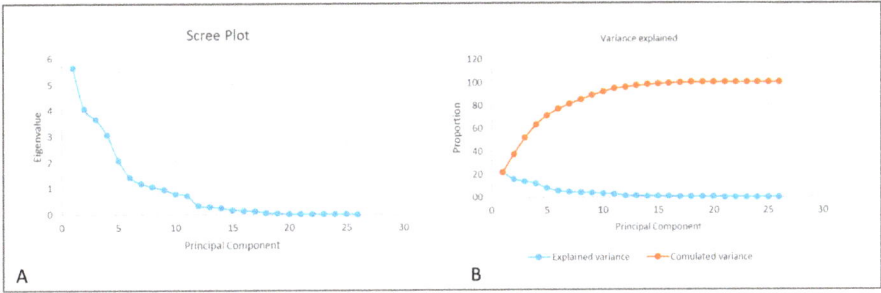

Figure 1. Scree plot of main components illustrating the eigenvalue of each main axis (**A**), the percentage of variance explained by each axis and the cumulative percentage of total variance explained (**B**). The eight main components represented 85.1% of the variance.

PC4 represented 11.7% of the total variance and was composed of proportional variables related primarily to the posterior portion of the face, including S − Ar/Ar − Go, S − Ar/S − Go, Ar − Go/S − Go and S − Ar/N − ANS. PC5 (8% of total variance) only included two variables, both of which relate to proportions of the jaw (ANS − PNS/SN and ANS − PNS/Co − A). PC6 (5.5% of total variance) was primarily composed of variables relating to the occlusal plane. PC7 represented 4.5% of the variance, and contained proportions related to mean facial length (Co − A/Co − GnM; Ar − A/Ar Gn) and the maxillary–mandibular projection (A − N Perp/Pg − N Perp). Finally, PC8 was composed of only two variables (SNB/Articular Angle, Pg − NB/A − NPo), and contributed the least to total variance (4.1%). A detailed description of the 8 main axes is provided in Table 2.

Table 2. Summary of the principal components analysis.

Principal Component	PC 1	PC 2	PC 3	PC 4	PC 5	PC 6	PC 7	PC 8
% of explained variance (a)	21.7	15.6	14.1	11.7	8.0	5.5	4.5	4.1
Cumulated % of explained variance (b)	21.7	37.3	51.4	63.1	71.1	76.5	81.8	85.1
Cephalometric variables (c)	SN/GoMe (%)	UFH (N-ANS/(N-ANS+ANS-Me)) (%)	P-A Face Height (S-Go/N-Me) (%)	S-Ar/Ar-Go (%)	Maxillary length (ANS-PNS)/Anterior Cranial Base (SN) (%)	SNA/Saddle-Sella Angle (SN-Ar) (%)	Midface Length (Co-A)/Mandibular length (Co-Gn)(%)	SNB/Articular Angle (%)
	ANS-PNS/Me-Go (%)	LFH/TFH (ANS-Me:N-Me) (%)	PFH:AFH (%)	Posterior Cranial Base (S-Ar)/Posterior Face Height (SGo) (%)	Maxillary length (ANS-PNS)/Midface Length (Co-A) (%)	Occ Plane to FH/FMA (MP-FH) (%)	Ar - A/Ar - Gn (%)	Pog - NB/Convexity (A-NPo) (%)
	Anterior Cranial Base (SN)/Length of Mand Base (Go-Pg) (%)	Face Ht Ratio (N-ANS/ANS-Me) (%)	Ramus Height (Ar-Go)/Lower Face Height (ANS-Me) (%)	Ramus Height (Ar-Go)/Posterior Face Height (SGo) (%)		Occ Plane to SN/SN – GoGn (%)	Maxillary Skeletal (A-N Perp)/Mand. Skeletal (Pg-N Perp) (%)	
	Maxillary length (ANS-PNS)/Length of Mand Base (Go-Pg) (%)	Cranio-Mx Base (SN-Palatal Plane)/SN – GoGn (%)		Posterior Cranial Base (S-Ar)/Upper Face Height (N-ANS) (%)				
	Mandibular Body Length (Go-Gn)/Mandibular length (Co-Gn) (%)							

(a) shows the variance explained by each principal component; (b) cumulative variance explained by each added principal component; (c) variables with the highest contribution in each PC.

3.3. Proportional Sub-Phenotypic Patterns

Subsequent cluster analysis defined four homogeneous sub-phenotypes of skeletal Class III malocclusion with clearly identifiable differences between them. A graphical representation of these four established clusters is detailed in Figure 2. The first proportional group (C1) includes 39 subjects, representing 18.4% of the total population. Out of all four sub-phenotypes identified, C1 was the most severe Class III skeletal malocclusion, with the largest maxillomandibular difference and the highest lower facial height. The ratios between the mandibular and maxillary measurements were the lowest among all clusters (Ar − A/Ar − Gn; Co − A/Co − Gn; ANS − PNS/Me − Go; ANS − PNS/Go − Pg). Similarly, the ratio of mandibular measurements to those of the anterior cranial base were also the lowest (SN/GoMe; SN/Go − Pg). Furthermore, individuals in C1 possessed the greatest ratio of lower facial height to total anterior facial height (ANS − Me:N − Me) (Supplementary Table S1 and Figure 2).

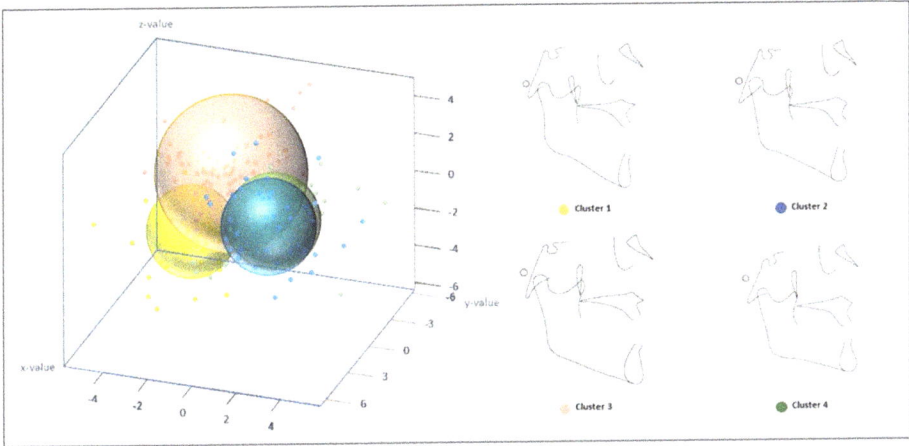

Figure 2. 3D representation of the 4 clusters resulting from the cluster analysis and proportional cluster patterns. C1 represented 18.4% of the sample, C2 represented 20.75%, C3 38.68%, and C4 22.17% of the total sample. For the rest of the description see text.

The second sub-phenotype (C2) contained 20.75% of the population, with a total of 44 subjects. C2 was characterized by a skeletal Class III malocclusion of maxillary origin with bimaxillary retrusion. This sub-phenotype had decreased angular proportions compared to those of the other groups, as was observed in the relationships between the Sella-Nassion-Point A (SNA) angle and the saddle angle (SN − Ar/SNA) as well as the Sella-Nassion-Point B (SNB) angle to the articular angle (Articular angle/SNB); this a characteristic was also observed in the additional skeletal measurements performed (Supplementary Table S1), indicating a biretrusive pattern. C2 individuals were also characterized by an increased proportion of the posterior cranial base in relation to the mandibular ramus (S − Ar/Ar − Go), while the proportion of the mandibular ramus to posterior facial height (Ar − Go/SGo) and lower anterior facial height (Ar − Go/ANS − Me) were the lowest among all groups. Therefore, C2 individuals possessed the lowest mandibular ramus height of all four groups (Supplementary Table S1). This subgroup also presented with the lowest ratio of posterior facial height to anterior facial height (PFH:AFH; S − Go/N − Me), and the occlusal plane was proportionally more inclined than the mandibular plane with respect to facial height (Occlusal plane to FH/MP − FH) in comparison to the other subgroups (Supplementary Table S1 and Figure 2).

The third proportional group (C3) was composed of the largest number of subjects in the sample (82), representing 38.68% of the sample population. C3 individuals possessed Class III malocclusions with a proportionally smaller mandibular body size compared to the that of rest of the sub-phenotypes, but this is compensated for by the total length of the mandible. Specifically, C3 individuals presented with the lowest ratio of mandibular body length to total mandibular length (Go − Gn/Co − Gn), while the ratio of both the anterior cranial base and maxillary body length to the mandibular body (SN/Go − Pg; SN/GoMe; ANS − PNS/Me − Go; ANS − PNS/Go − Pg) were the largest of the four sub-phenotypes. The C3 subgroup was also characterized by the lowest proportional relationships between the posterior cranial base and both the mandibular ramus (S − Ar/Ar − Go) and posterior facial height (S − Ar/SGo), coinciding with the fact that C3 possessed the highest posterior facial height and ramus height when compared with those of the other subgroups (Supplementary Table S1). As a result, a proportionally higher posterior facial height with respect to the anterior facial height (PFH:AFH) was observed in this subgroup (Supplementary Table S1 and Figure 2).

Lastly, 22.17% of the total sample population was classified as sub-phenotype C4, with a total of 47 subjects. C4 individuals presented with the least severe skeletal Class III malocclusion of the four sub-phenotypes, with a mandibular component, a decreased anterior facial height, and a reduced mandibular plane. C4 was characterized by the highest proportional value of the total maxillary length with respect to full mandibular length (Ar − A/Ar − Gn; Co − A/Co − Gn). In turn, the ratio of the mandibular body length to full mandibular length (Go − Gn/Co − Gn) was the highest of all groups. C4 individuals also possessed the lowest ratio of lower facial height to anterior facial height (ANS − Me:N − Me) and the highest ratio of the middle third facial height to both the anterior facial height (N − ANS/N − ANS + ANS − Me) and to the lower facial height (N − ANS/ANS − Me). As a result, C4 subjects have proportionally reduced heights in the lower third of anterior portions of the face. Furthermore, these individuals also possess the highest proportional value between posterior face height and anterior face height (S − Go/N − Me; PFH:AFH) due to the low anterior face height of C4 compared to that of the other three sub-phenotypes (Supplementary Table S1 and Figure 2).

3.4. Description of the Supplementary Variables in Each Proportional Sub-Phenotypic Cluster

For the supplementary skeletal variables, the equivalence of linear and angular measurements with respect to proportional measurements were analyzed by sub-phenotype. Measurements of soft tissue facial height corresponded to those of skeletal facial height. The longest lower third of the face (Sn'-Me') was observed in C1 and the shortest in C4. Likewise, C1 presented with the lowest retrusion of the lower lip and C4 the highest, while the highest inclination and protrusion of the lower incisor with respect to A-Pg was presented by C1 and the lowest by C4. With respect to the airway, C2 had the shortest upper airway, while C3 had the widest upper airway.

Finally, with respect to the supplementary descriptive dental variables, C1 presented with the lowest overbite and overjet, while the greatest were observed in C4. C2 was characterized by the lowest angulation of the upper incisor with respect to the Nassion-Point A (NA) plane, the Sella-Sella-Nassion (SN) plane, the palatal plane, and the Franckfort Horizontal (FH) plane, while C4 presented the highest angulations of the upper incisor with respect to the same planes. (A more detailed description of the supplementary variables that describe each cluster can be found in Supplementary Table S1).

3.5. Gender and Maturation Stage Distribution in Each Proportional Sub-Phenotypic Pattern

Regarding gender and CVMS, their distribution was homogenous in all of the four clusters generated ($p > 0.05$).

4. Discussion

Cluster analysis for the phenotypic classification of skeletal Class III malocclusion is being increasingly used to establish specific sub-phenotypes within the large variations of this malocclusion [23–27,34,40,41]. The establishment of appropriate, specific, distinguishable, and easy-to-use clinical sub-phenotypes would facilitate future studies focused on treatment outcomes, relapse prognosis, or even diagnostic characterization of this particular malocclusion, which may ultimately lead to more appropriate therapeutic protocols for each sub-phenotype.

In this study, 212 lateral cephalometric radiographs of subjects with skeletal Class III malocclusion were analyzed. Twenty-six skeletal proportional variables were used to perform principal component analysis and subsequent cluster analysis. Eight main axes were obtained that represented 85.1% of the total variance, allowing for subsequent cluster analysis which generated two possible configurations of four or six clusters. The six-cluster model was discarded as three of these clusters were highly similar, with no identifiable differences being apparent during graphical recreation. Therefore, the six-cluster model would complicate the clinical diagnosis of this type of malocclusion, contrary to the main objective of this type of analysis. In comparison with other well-designed studies that use skeletal, dental, soft tissue, and some proportional variables for multivariate analysis, in this study, only proportional variables were used to construct the final Class III sub-phenotypes. This method allows us to obtain clinically simplified clusters unaffected by the differences in raw values, which could be affected by gender or other factors. Several studies have demonstrated the differences in anterior facial height and other variables between men and women as well as between ethnic groups [28–32]. Linear measurements in men are higher than in women, with greater mandibular size and facial height. Zacharopoulos et al. [30] conducted a study with the aim of providing an anthropometric facial profile in a Greek population. They observed statistically significant differences in the head and face region between genders, and when compared against published data on North American Caucasians, statistically significant differences were observed. Similarly, Celebi et al. [31] analyzed the sexual dimorphism of facial features in Italian and Egyptian populations and observed that some features, including total facial height, upper facial height, lower facial height, and mandibular measurements were significantly greater in both Italian and Egyptian men than in women. In addition, they also found significant differences in facial morphology between the two sample populations. Due to these existing differences, some generated clusters have been composed mainly or entirely of males or females. Moreover, in a previous study [33] we concluded that in 66.6% of the clusters generated, a gender effect was involved. Specifically, two clusters from the previous study were composed mainly of males (85.7% and 79.4%), while two others were composed mainly or entirely of women (73.4% and 100%). Few studies indicate the total number of each gender in the different subgroups identified. Nevertheless, differences in gender within clusters can be observed in other studies; for instance, in Li et al. [34], two of the four characterized clusters were disproportionately made up of females (67.4% and 75%).

In the present study, the most severe sub-phenotype of skeletal Class III malocclusion was observed in C1, which accounted for the smallest proportion of the sample population (18.4%) among all subgroups, similar to the case in previous studies [26,33,34,41]. However, in this case, gender distribution was proportional. C1 showed a Class III malocclusion of mixed maxillary–mandibular origin [42], with the largest maxillary–mandibular difference, the smallest maxillary size, and a relatively high mandibular size of all four clusters. The highest anterior facial height was also observed in C1, but the mandibular plane was normal. The low frequency of severe Class III malocclusion observed here and in several previous studies may be due to the selection process: the selection of an ANB <1 or 0 [26,33,34,41] and a Wits appraisal <0 or −2 mm [26,33,34] may allow for the inclusion of less severe skeletal Class III malocclusion subjects.

The third type of skeletal Class III phenotype (C3) contained the highest percentage of the sample population (38.68%) and represented a skeletal Class III malocclusion with a proportionally increased mandibular ramus, a proportionally decreased mandibular body, and a greater total mandibular size. The C3 cluster represented a skeletal Class III malocclusion of mixed origin and a mesofacial pattern with a decreased mandibular size compared to the rest of the clusters. Despite possessing the greatest maxillary length of all subgroups, C3 still possesses a mesofacial pattern and a slight maxillary retrusion. These characteristics are similar to what was observed in clusters that represented a large portion of the sample in previous studies [26,34,41] that confirm skeletal Class III of mixed origin as the most frequent type of skeletal Class III malocclusion [42].

The second most representative cluster in this study, C4 (22.17%), was characterized by less severe skeletal malocclusion of mandibular origin, with the smallest maxillo-mandibular difference and a diminished anterior facial height and mandibular plane. Similar characteristics were described in sub-phenotypes found in previous studies that showed a mild skeletal Class III malocclusion of mixed maxillary–mandibular origin, with a flat mandibular plane [26,33].

Finally, C2 represented 20.75% of the total sample population and was characterized by a malocclusion of maxillary origin, a proportionally smaller mandibular ramus, a posterior facial height proportionally lower than the anterior facial height, and a more retracted maxillary–mandibular position. When compared with the supplementary skeletal measurements, C2 demonstrated the lowest SNA and SNB angles of all subgroups. This type of Class III has been described in previous studies, also representing the second most frequent type of Class III malocclusion (19.5%) [42]. Similar characteristics were found in other studies, where the clusters representing a skeletal Class III malocclusion of maxillary origin were the second most representative clusters [33] or even the most representative [26,41]. Despite the observation of a skeletal Class III malocclusion of maxillary origin in previous studies, the sub-phenotype found in the present study (C2) has not been previously characterized [34]. This could be due to the different ethnic origin of the populations [28]; a skeletal malocclusion of maxillary origin is described in Caucasian samples [26,33] or in samples with a greater Caucasian component [41] but not in Asian samples [7].

This configuration of four clusters is comparable to that found in previous studies. However, this type of analysis has led to models with 3 [24,27,40], 4 [34], 5 [26,41], 6 [33], 7 [23], and 14 [25] clusters. The variations in the number of clusters identified may be due to differences in the type of cluster analysis employed, whether hierarchical [24] or diffuse [27,40], in comparison with the mixed principal component analyses used in our study. The reduction to four clusters found may also be a result of the use of proportional variables for multivariate analyses instead of linear, angular, and proportional skeletal variables; using proportional variables enabled us to avoid gender-dependent effects on clustering, thus reducing the number of clinical clusters. The large number of subgroups found in other studies [23,25] could be due, among other reasons, to the lack of principal component analysis prior to cluster analysis or to the inclusion of dental Class III malocclusion subjects, thus including subgroups with Class III dental characteristics in addition to Class III skeletal features [25].

The supplementary variables obtained in this study complement the proportional variables described above. The soft tissue variables correlated to the corresponding skeletal patterns, for example, the cluster that had the proportionally greatest lower facial height (C1) also possessed the greatest soft tissue proportions, as was true for the cluster that presented with the lowest facial height (C4). On the other hand, the position of the lower lip with respect to the S Line and E-Plane was more related to the inclination and position of the lower incisor with respect to the A-Pg plane. We observed that the lowest retrusion of the lower lip in C1 coincided with the highest inclination and protrusion of the lower incisor with respect to the A-Pg plane, while the highest retrusion of the lower lip in C4 coincided with the lowest inclination and protrusion of the lower incisor (see Supplementary Table S1). These results are consistent with multiple studies that have established that the labial position depends fundamentally on the position and inclination of the lower incisors [43,44], while the soft tissues closest to their respective skeletal parts follow a pattern closer to them [45].

The use of principal component analysis established a total of eight principal axes, which were used in subsequent cluster analysis. The eight principal components obtained in this study accounted for 85.1% of the total variance, higher than that observed in other studies, where the total variance ranged from 67% [41] to 81.2% [26] with a number of principal components ranging from five [41] to six [26,34]. The higher percentage of total variance accounted for by the current model may be due to the use of a set of variables focused on the proportional skeleton. Despite the use of a smaller group of variables for cluster analysis, the first three principal components accounted for 51.4% of the total variance, results that are in agreement with previous studies [26,34,41]. The use of proportional variables to obtain the principal components makes it difficult to compare with other studies. In spite of this, similarities with other studies can be observed in the first principal components, since they described sagittal and vertical variables [26,34,41]. In our study, PC1 describe mandibular proportions, i.e., it represents the relationship of the mandible with respect to the cranial and maxillary base among others (SN/GoMe; ANS – PNS/Me – Go; ASN – PNS/Go – Pg); this representation is similar to PC1 of previous articles describing sagittal parameters [26,41]. PC2 and PC3 describe proportions related to anterior facial height (UFH; LFH/TFH; Face Ht Ratio) and proportions related to posterior–anterior height (S – Go/N – Me; PFH:AFH, Ar – Go/ANS – Me), respectively, and their results are comparable with those of previous articles where vertical parameters are described in PC2 [33,34] or vertical and sagittal parameters in PC3 [33,41]. In previous studies that used skeletal, dental, and soft tissue variables to obtain principal components, parameters indicating the position of the lower incisor were part of principal components, (PC2 [41], PC3 [26,34]) and explained a high percentage of variance (14.66% [41], 13.25% [26], 12.16% [34]). The differences between our study and these previous works are primarily due to the use of skeletal proportional variables instead of skeletal, dental, and soft tissue variables. This type of analysis may aid future genetic studies, since an increasing number of studies are performing first principal component analysis to relate principal components to genetics [6,46]. Genes involved in vertical craniofacial discrepancies and others involved in horizontal discrepancies have been identified, as well as those involved in the mandibular prognathism observed in different ethnicities [6,7,47].

The differences found between ethnicities both in the phenotypic sub-classification of skeletal Class III malocclusions [28], as well as in the genes involved in mandibular prognathism [6,7,47], show the need for an appropriate classification of this malocclusion in different ethnicities to facilitate future studies on prognosis and treatment outcomes. The present diagnostic tool might modify, or at least classify, current treatment plan strategies based on skeletal pattern. This method might be useful to analyze how these sub-phenotypes respond to different orthopedic and orthodontic Class III treatment strategies based on the results of future randomized clinical trials aimed at analyzing the effects of any Class III therapy. To achieve this, precise but feasible skeletal Class III classifications may help configure Class III subtypes that provide a clear and simple diagnostic tool without being affected by gender- or ethnicity-dependent effects.

5. Conclusions

The classification of skeletal Class III malocclusion by cluster analysis after a principal component analysis based on proportional variables, provides a clear, concise sub-phenotypic classification and avoids potential gender-dependent effects that can occur when raw values are used. This classification is more clinically useful and may facilitate diagnoses, as well as improving future studies on treatment outcomes, prognoses, or even diagnoses of this malocclusion.

Supplementary Materials: The following are available online at http://www.mdpi.com/2077-0383/9/9/3048/s1, Table S1: Mean values of proportional skeletal variables and supplementary variables, Table S2: Explanation of cephalometric measurements and abbreviations.

Author Contributions: The study was designed by A.I.-L., who wrote the manuscript and reviewed the figures and tables. L.d.F.-V. collected the data, interpreted the data under the supervision of A.I.-L., and wrote the manuscript. C.M., J.A.A., R.O., and J.C.P.-F. assisted in collecting the study sample and reviewed the manuscript, tables, and figures. All authors have read and agreed to the published version of the manuscript.

Funding: This research was funded by G/6400100/3000 (Complutense University, Madrid, Spain).

Acknowledgments: We thank our Statistics services and the Departamento de Especialidades Clínicas Odontológicas (DECO) Department) for their contribution to this research. G/6400100/3000 (Complutense University, Madrid, Spain).

Conflicts of Interest: The authors declare no conflict of interest.

References

1. Lin, Y.; Guo, R.; Hou, L.; Fu, Z.; Li, W. Stability of maxillary protraction therapy in children with Class III malocclusion: A systematic review and meta-analysis. *Clin. Oral Investig.* **2018**, *22*, 2639–2652. [CrossRef] [PubMed]
2. Wendl, B.; Kamenica, A.; Droschl, H.; Jakse, N.; Weiland, F.; Wendl, T.; Wendl, M. Retrospective 25-year follow-up of treatment outcomes in Angle Class III patients: Success versus failure. *J. Orofac. Orthop.* **2017**, *78*, 129–136. [CrossRef] [PubMed]
3. Chen, C.M.; Ko, E.C.; Cheng, J.H.; Tseng, Y.C. Correlation between changes in the gonial area and postoperative stability in the treatment of mandibular prognathism. *J. Stomatol. Oral Maxillofac. Surg.* **2019**, *120*, 414–418. [CrossRef] [PubMed]
4. Saito, F.; Kajii, T.S.; Oka, A.; Ikuno, K.; Iida, J. Genome-wide association study for mandibular prognathism using microsatellite and pooled DNA method. *Am. J. Orthod. Dentofac. Orthop.* **2017**, *152*, 382–388. [CrossRef]
5. Doraczynska-Kowalik, A.; Nelke, K.H.; Pawlak, W.; Sasiadek, M.M.; Gerber, H. Genetic Factors Involved in Mandibular Prognathism. *J. Craniofac. Surg.* **2017**, *28*, 422–431. [CrossRef]
6. Cruz, C.V.; Mattos, C.T.; Maia, J.C.; Granjeiro, J.M.; Reis, M.F.; Mucha, J.N.; Vilella, B.; Ruellas, A.C.; Luiz, R.R.; Costa, M.C.; et al. Genetic polymorphisms underlying the skeletal Class III phenotype. *Am. J. Orthod. Dentofac. Orthop.* **2017**, *151*, 700–707. [CrossRef]
7. Liu, H.; Wu, C.; Lin, J.; Shao, J.; Chen, Q.; Luo, E. Genetic Etiology in Nonsyndromic Mandibular Prognathism. *J. Craniofac. Surg.* **2017**, *28*, 161–169. [CrossRef]
8. Genno, P.G.; Nemer, G.M.; Zein Eddine, S.B.; Macari, A.T.; Ghafari, J.G. Three novel genes tied to mandibular prognathism in eastern Mediterranean families. *Am. J. Orthod. Dentofac. Orthop.* **2019**, *156*, 104–112. [CrossRef]
9. Jiang, Q.; Mei, L.; Zou, Y.; Ding, Q.; Cannon, R.D.; Chen, H.; Li, H. Genetic Polymorphisms in FGFR2 Underlie Skeletal Malocclusion. *J. Dent. Res.* **2019**, *98*, 1340–1347. [CrossRef]
10. Lin, M.; Xie, C.; Yang, H.; Wu, C.; Ren, A. Prevalence of malocclusion in Chinese schoolchildren from 1991 to 2018: A systematic review and meta-analysis. *Int. J. Paediatr. Dent.* **2020**, *30*, 144–155. [CrossRef]
11. Piao, Y.; Kim, S.J.; Yu, H.S.; Cha, J.Y.; Baik, H.S. Five-year investigation of a large orthodontic patient population at a dental hospital in South Korea. *Korean J. Orthod.* **2016**, *46*, 137–145. [CrossRef] [PubMed]
12. Steinmassl, O.; Steinmassl, P.A.; Schwarz, A.; Crismani, A. Orthodontic Treatment Need of Austrian Schoolchildren in the Mixed Dentition Stage. *Swiss Dent. J.* **2017**, *127*, 122–128. [PubMed]
13. Perillo, L.; Masucci, C.; Ferro, F.; Apicella, D.; Baccetti, T. Prevalence of orthodontic treatment need in southern Italian schoolchildren. *Eur. J. Orthod.* **2010**, *32*, 49–53. [CrossRef] [PubMed]
14. Thilander, B.; Pena, L.; Infante, C.; Parada, S.S.; de Mayorga, C. Prevalence of malocclusion and orthodontic treatment need in children and adolescents in Bogota, Colombia. An epidemiological study related to different stages of dental development. *Eur. J. Orthod.* **2001**, *23*, 153–167. [CrossRef] [PubMed]
15. Narayanan, R.K.; Jeseem, M.T.; Kumar, T.A. Prevalence of Malocclusion among 10–12-year-old Schoolchildren in Kozhikode District, Kerala: An Epidemiological Study. *Int. J. Clin. Pediatr. Dent.* **2016**, *9*, 50–55. [PubMed]
16. Borzabadi-Farahani, A.; Borzabadi-Farahani, A.; Eslamipour, F. Malocclusion and occlusal traits in an urban Iranian population. An epidemiological study of 11- to 14-year-old children. *Eur. J. Orthod.* **2009**, *31*, 477–484. [CrossRef]
17. Bilgic, F.; Gelgor, I.E.; Celebi, A.A. Malocclusion prevalence and orthodontic treatment need in central Anatolian adolescents compared to European and other nations' adolescents. *Dental Press J. Orthod.* **2015**, *20*, 75–81. [CrossRef] [PubMed]
18. Borzabadi-Farahani, A.; Eslamipour, F.; Shahmoradi, M. Functional needs of subjects with dentofacial deformities: A study using the index of orthognathic functional treatment need (IOFTN). *J. Plast. Reconstr. Aesthet. Surg.* **2016**, *69*, 796–801. [CrossRef]
19. Eslamian, L.; Borzabadi-Farahani, A.; Badiee, M.R.; Le, B.T. An Objective Assessment of Orthognathic Surgery Patients. *J. Craniofac. Surg.* **2019**, *30*, 2479–2482. [CrossRef]
20. Olkun, H.K.; Borzabadi-Farahani, A.; Uckan, S. Orthognathic Surgery Treatment Need in a Turkish Adult Population: A Retrospective Study. *Int. J. Environ. Res. Public Health* **2019**, *16*, 1881. [CrossRef]
21. Bailey, L.J.; Haltiwanger, L.H.; Blakey, G.H.; Proffit, W.R. Who seeks surgical-orthodontic treatment: A current review. *Int. J. Adult Orthodon. Orthognath. Surg.* **2001**, *16*, 280–292. [PubMed]

22. Ireland, A.J.; Atack, N.E.; Cunningham, S.J.; House, K.; Cobourne, M.T.; Hunt, N.P.; Sherriff, M.; Sandy, J.R. National British Orthodontic Society (BOS) Orthognathic Audit 2017–2018. *J. Orthod.* **2019**, *46*, 287–296. [CrossRef] [PubMed]
23. Hong, S.X.; Yi, C.K. A classification and characterization of skeletal class III malocclusion on etio-pathogenic basis. *Int. J. Oral Maxillofac. Surg.* **2001**, *30*, 264–271. [CrossRef] [PubMed]
24. Abu Alhaija, E.S.; Richardson, A. Growth prediction in Class III patients using cluster and discriminant function analysis. *Eur. J. Orthod.* **2003**, *25*, 599–608. [CrossRef] [PubMed]
25. Li, S.; Xu, T.M.; Lin, J.X. Analysis of treatment templates of Angle's Class III malocclusion patients. *Hua Xi Kou Qiang Yi Xue Za Zhi* **2009**, *27*, 637–641. [PubMed]
26. Moreno Uribe, L.M.; Vela, K.C.; Kummet, C.; Dawson, D.V.; Southard, T.E. Phenotypic diversity in white adults with moderate to severe Class III malocclusion. *Am. J. Orthod. Dentofac. Orthop.* **2013**, *144*, 32–42. [CrossRef]
27. Auconi, P.; Scazzocchio, M.; Cozza, P.; McNamara, J.A., Jr.; Franchi, L. Prediction of Class III treatment outcomes through orthodontic data mining. *Eur. J. Orthod.* **2015**, *37*, 257–267. [CrossRef]
28. de Frutos-Valle, L.; Martin, C.; Alarcon, J.A.; Palma-Fernandez, J.C.; Iglesias-Linares, A. Subclustering in Skeletal Class III Phenotypes of Different Ethnic Origins: A Systematic Review. *J. Evid. Based Dent. Pract.* **2019**, *19*, 34–52. [CrossRef]
29. Amini, F.; Mashayekhi, Z.; Rahimi, H.; Morad, G. Craniofacial morphologic parameters in a Persian population: An anthropometric study. *J. Craniofac. Surg.* **2014**, *25*, 1874–1881. [CrossRef]
30. Zacharopoulos, G.V.; Manios, A.; Kau, C.H.; Velagrakis, G.; Tzanakakis, G.N.; de Bree, E. Anthropometric Analysis of the Face. *J. Craniofac. Surg.* **2016**, *27*, 71–75. [CrossRef]
31. Celebi, A.A.; Kau, C.H.; Femiano, F.; Bucci, L.; Perillo, L. A Three-Dimensional Anthropometric Evaluation of Facial Morphology. *J. Craniofac. Surg.* **2018**, *29*, 304–308. [CrossRef] [PubMed]
32. Lipiec, K.; Ryniewicz, W.I.; Groch, M.; Wieczorek, A.; Loster, J.E. The Evaluation of Anthropometric Measurements of Young Polish Women's Faces. *J. Craniofac. Surg.* **2019**, *30*, 709–712. [CrossRef] [PubMed]
33. de Frutos-Valle, L.; Martin, C.; Alarcon, J.A.; Palma-Fernandez, J.C.; Ortega, R.; Iglesias-Linares, A. Sub-clustering in skeletal Class III malocclusion phenotypes via principal component analysis in a Southern European population. *Sci. Rep.* **2020**. submitted.
34. Li, C.; Cai, Y.; Chen, S.; Chen, F. Classification and characterization of class III malocclusion in Chinese individuals. *Head Face Med.* **2016**, *12*, 31. [CrossRef] [PubMed]
35. Baccetti, T.; Franchi, L.; McNamara, J.A., Jr. An improved version of the cervical vertebral maturation (CVM) method for the assessment of mandibular growth. *Angle Orthod.* **2002**, *72*, 316–323.
36. World Medical Association Declaration of Helsinki: Ethical principles for medical research involving human subjects. *JAMA* **2013**, *310*, 2191–2194. [CrossRef] [PubMed]
37. Doka, G. The 'Excel 3D Scatter Plot' v2.1—The Manual. 2006–2013. Available online: https://www.doka.ch/Excel3Dscatterplot.htm (accessed on 19 January 2020).
38. Shrout, P.E.; Fleiss, J.L. Intraclass correlations: Uses in assessing rater reliability. *Psychol. Bull.* **1979**, *86*, 420–428. [CrossRef]
39. Galvão, M.C.d.S.; Sato, J.R.; Coelho, E.C. Dahlberg formula: A novel approach for its evaluation. *Dental Press J. Orthod.* **2012**, *17*, 115–124. [CrossRef]
40. Auconi, P.; Scazzocchio, M.; Defraia, E.; McNamara, J.A.; Franchi, L. Forecasting craniofacial growth in individuals with class III malocclusion by computational modelling. *Eur. J. Orthod.* **2014**, *36*, 207–216. [CrossRef]
41. Bui, C.; King, T.; Proffit, W.; Frazier-Bowers, S. Phenotypic characterization of Class III patients. *Angle Orthod.* **2006**, *76*, 564–569.
42. Ellis, E., III; McNamara, J.A., Jr. Components of adult Class III malocclusion. *J. Oral Maxillofac. Surg.* **1984**, *42*, 295–305. [CrossRef]
43. Alkadhi, R.M.; Finkelman, M.D.; Trotman, C.A.; Kanavakis, G. The role of lip thickness in upper lip response to sagittal change of incisor position. *Orthod. Craniofac. Res.* **2019**, *22*, 53–57. [CrossRef] [PubMed]
44. Ali, B.; Shaikh, A.; Fida, M. Factors affecting treatment decisions for Class I malocclusions. *Am. J. Orthod. Dentofacial Orthop.* **2018**, *154*, 234–237. [CrossRef] [PubMed]

45. Zednikova Mala, P.; Krajicek, V.; Veleminska, J. How tight is the relationship between the skeletal and soft-tissue facial profile: A geometric morphometric analysis of the facial outline. *Forensic Sci. Int.* **2018**, *292*, 212–223. [CrossRef]
46. da Fontoura, C.S.; Miller, S.F.; Wehby, G.L.; Amendt, B.A.; Holton, N.E.; Southard, T.E.; Allareddy, V.; Moreno Uribe, L.M. Candidate Gene Analyses of Skeletal Variation in Malocclusion. *J. Dent. Res.* **2015**, *94*, 913–920. [CrossRef]
47. Ko, J.M.; Suh, Y.J.; Hong, J.; Paeng, J.Y.; Baek, S.H.; Kim, Y.H. Segregation analysis of mandibular prognathism in Korean orthognathic surgery patients and their families. *Angle Orthod.* **2013**, *83*, 1027–1035. [CrossRef]

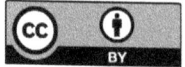

© 2020 by the authors. Licensee MDPI, Basel, Switzerland. This article is an open access article distributed under the terms and conditions of the Creative Commons Attribution (CC BY) license (http://creativecommons.org/licenses/by/4.0/).

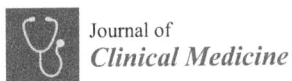

Article

Evaluation of the Reliability, Reproducibility and Validity of Digital Orthodontic Measurements Based on Various Digital Models among Young Patients

Seo-Hyun Park [1,2,†], Soo-Hwan Byun [2,3,4,†], So-Hee Oh [1,2,3], Hye-Lim Lee [1], Ju-Won Kim [2,3,4], Byoung-Eun Yang [2,3,4,*] and In-Young Park [2,3,5,*]

[1] Division of Pediatric Dentistry, Hallym University Sacred Heart Hospital, Anyang 14066, Korea; park070676@gmail.com (S.-H.P.); colfman@hanmail.net (S.-H.O.); onlylove0210@naver.com (H.-L.L.)
[2] Graduate School of Clinical Dentistry, Hallym University, Chuncheon 24252, Korea; purheit@hallym.or.kr (S.-H.B.); kjw9199@hallym.or.kr (J.-W.K.)
[3] Institute of Clinical Dentistry, Hallym University, Chuncheon 24252, Korea
[4] Division of Oral and Maxillofacial Surgery, Hallym University Sacred Heart Hospital, Anyang 14066, Korea
[5] Division of Orthodontics, Hallym University Sacred Heart Hospital, Anyang 14066, Korea
* Correspondence: face@hallym.ac.kr (B.-E.Y.); park.iy2875@gmail.com (I.-Y.P.); Tel.: +82-31-380-3870 (B.-E.Y. & I.-Y.P.)
† These authors contributed equally to this work.

Received: 8 July 2020; Accepted: 20 August 2020; Published: 24 August 2020

Abstract: The advantages of intraoral model scanning have yielded recent developments. However, few studies have explored the orthodontic clinical use of this technique particularly among young patients. This study aimed to evaluate the reliability, reproducibility and validity of the orthodontic measurements: tooth width, arch length and arch length discrepancy in each digital model obtained by model scanner and intraoral scanner, relative to a plaster model. Arch length measured using two methods: curved arch length (CAL) measured automatically by digital program and sum of sectional liner arch length (SLAL) measured sum of anterior and posterior liner arch lengths. Arch length discrepancy calculated each arch length measurement methods: curved arch length discrepancy (CALD) and sum of sectional liner arch length discrepancy (SLALD). Forty young patients were eligible for the study. A plaster model (P), model-scanned digital model (MSD) and intraoral scanned digital model (ISD) were acquired from each patient. The reliability of the measurements was evaluated using Pearson's correlation coefficient, while the reproducibility was evaluated using the intraclass correlation coefficient. The validity was assessed by a paired t-test. All measurements measured in P, MSD and ISD exhibited good reliability and reproducibility. Most orthodontic measurements despite of CAL in MSD exhibited high validity. Only the SLAL and SLALD in ISD group differed significantly, despite of the good validity of the tooth width, CAL and CALD. The measurements based on the digital program appeared high reliability, reproducibility and accurate than conventional measurement. However, SLAL and SLALD in ISD group appeared shorter because of distortion during intraoral scanning. However, this could be compensated by using digital programed curved arch. Although the validity of SLAL and SLALD in the ISD group differed statistically, the difference is not considered clinically significant. Although MSD and ISD are acceptable for a clinical space analysis, clinicians should be aware of digital model-induced errors.

Keywords: digital model; intraoral scanner; intraoral scanned digital model; digital orthodontic measurement; tooth width; arch length; arch length discrepancy

1. Introduction

Accurate measurements and a study model analysis are crucial components of a successful orthodontic treatment. Although treatment planning requires an analysis of crowding and spacing in the patient's mouth, measurements of the tooth width (TW) and arch length (AL) are highly recommended as determinants of the arch length discrepancy (ALD) [1]. A plaster model is typically used for standard studies. However, this type of model has some disadvantages related to volumetric deformation, which can lead to errors, and is more likely to be damaged during storage and transportation [2,3]. Comparatively, a digital model has some advantages such as the ease of production and storage, good mobility and long-term economic benefits. In addition, a digital model provides immediate access to 3D data [4].

Three main methods are used to obtain the digital models: scanning of a plaster model with a 3D model scanner, direct scanning of the oral cavity with an intraoral scanner and obtaining a model via cone-beam computed tomography (CBCT). Previous studies demonstrated that a model-scanned digital model (MSD) produced using a 3D model scanner shows high accuracy with the conventional plaster model [4–7]. Additionally, the clinical compatibility and validity of MSD were approved for orthodontic measurements such as the size of the teeth, length and the width of the arch, Bolton ratio and occlusion [5,6,8–10]. Some researchers reported that the MSD provided a better accurate depiction than a plaster model [11]. MSDs have several advantages, but also share some disadvantages with plaster models, including undercutting and distortion of the impression around the bracket, as well as induction of the gagging reflex. However, intraoral scanners can resolve these disadvantages to some extent, which has led to rapid development in the field of intraoral scanned digital models (ISD). Specifically due to these advantages, many dental college hospitals are increasingly using various types of intraoral scanners for a variety of patients and are providing education and research to numerous dentists and medical personnel.

Some previous studies reported that ISD provides a higher level of accuracy with the MSD or plaster model at shorter scan lengths. However, the accuracy of the whole arch model was relatively poor when compared to plaster models and it remains uncertain whether such models could be used in clinical prosthodontics applications [12–14]. In addition, in the field of oral and maxillofacial surgery, research is being conducted on the use of models acquired with intraoral scanners in various orthognathic and implant surgery [15,16]. Further, earlier studies observed that the clinical use of the full arch should be approached carefully because of the risk of distortion when scanning more than half of the arch length [14,17–21].

Although existing orthodontics studies have explored the clinical validity of ISDs, only a few studies have comprehensively evaluated the reliability and reproducibility with validity of these models [22–25]. No studies have yet analyzed and compared orthodontic measurement aspects, such as arch length discrepancy, through the full arch by MSD and ISD among younger patients. This study aimed to evaluate the reliability, reproducibility and validity of the TW, AL and ALD as measured using different two methods, the sum of anterior and posterior sectional liner arch and automatically designed curved arch, on an MSD and ISD relative to a plaster model to determine the clinical application for a space analysis.

2. Materials and Methods

2.1. Patients Inclusion Criteria and Group Classification

The study population comprised 40 patients who visited the Hallym Sacred Heart Hospital Dental Clinic for an orthodontic diagnosis during January 2018–January 2019. The collection of the patients' data was approved by the Institutional Review Board (IRB) of Hallym University Medical Center (IRB number: 2019-08-006-001). The number of specimens required for this study was estimated using a significance level of $\alpha = 0.05$, 95% power and an effect size of 0.80 at G power (version 3.010, Franx Faul. Universitat Kiel, Germany). The sample included 20 male and 20 female patients aged 12–18 years; the mean ages of males and females were 13.6 and 12.7 years, respectively. The inclusion criteria were full eruption to the first permanent molar, no history of restoration or orthodontic treatment with no maxillofacial deformity and no missing or malformed teeth. Figure 1 depicts the process of model development for each patient.

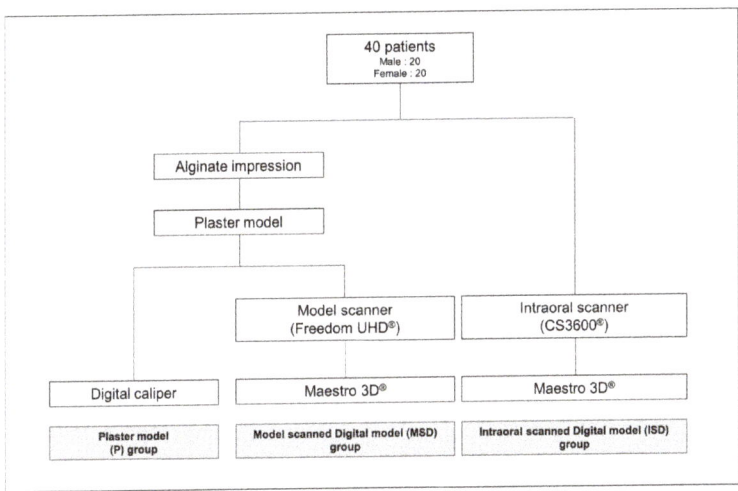

Figure 1. Illustration of the flow chart of model production according to model type.

First, a plaster model was obtained from each patient using an impression taken with alginate (Cavex Impressional; Cavex Holland BV, Haarlem, The Netherlands) and was immediately produced by white stone (Ryoka Dental; Mie-Ken, Japan) in proportions according to the manufacturer's instructions (Figure 2A). Examiner A, who had sufficient education and experience in scanning, produced a MSD using a Freedom UHD® 3D scanner (Dof Inc., Seongdong-gu, Seoul, Korea) according to the manufacturer's protocol same condition on every model. An experienced dentist with sufficient scanning experience then scanned the patient's ISD and obtained measurements using a CS3600® intraoral scanner and software (Carestream Dental, Atlanta, GA, USA). As indicated by the manufacturer, scanning was initiated at the anterior labial surface to the lingual surface area and followed the buccal and occlusal surfaces of the posterior teeth to the left and right lingual surfaces. All digital models were saved as stereolithography language (STL) files, which are approved by the indicated software (Figure 2B,C).

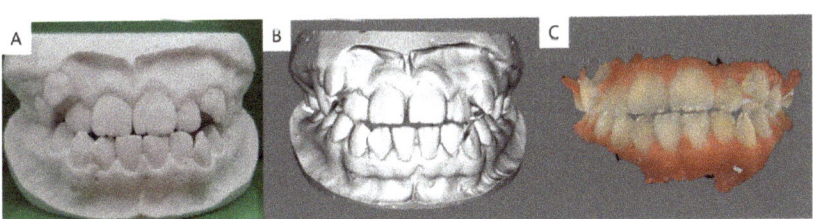

Figure 2. A representative plaster model and images scanned using a model scanner and intraoral scanner. (**A**) Plaster model. (**B**) Stereolithography language (STL) file format image scanned using the Freedom UHD® 3D scanner(Dof Inc., Seongdong-gu, Seoul, Korea) (**C**) Object code (OBJ) file format image scanned using CS3600®(Carestream Dental, Atlanta, GA, USA). The latter was converted to a STL file for measurements.

2.2. Orthodontic Measurements

Measurements were performed by 4 specialists of orthodontics of Hallym Sacred Heart Hospital dental clinic who were sufficiently trained in the indicated methods. Examiner A performed 2 sets of measurements at an interval of 2 weeks. Vernier calipers (CD-20PSX, Mitutoyo Corp, Kawasaki, Japan) with a self-tolerance error of <0.02 mm were used to measure the plaster model. Maestro 3D dental studio® (AGE Solutions, Pisa, Italy) software was used for digital model measurements. All measurements were made in 0.01 mm increments.

The following model analysis criteria were applied. The AL and ALD were analyzed for each arch. For all teeth, the TW was measured as the longest mesial-distal width parallel to the occlusal plane (Figure 3A). In the digital model, the measurement point was set at the height of the contour, and recalibration was practiced using a coronal 2-dimensional sectional view. The AL was measured in 2 ways. First, the sectional liner arch length (SLAL) was defined as the sum of the anterior arch length (AAL), left arch length (LAL) and right arch length (RAL) and was measured parallel to the occlusal plane. The AAL was defined as the linear distance between the midpoint of the mesial height of the contour of both central incisors to the mesial height of the contour of each canine, and the LAL and RAL were defined as the linear distances between the mesial height of the contour of the canine to the mesial height of the contour of the first permanent molar on the indicated side (Figure 3B). Second, the digital curved arch length (CAL) was defined as the total length of the arch formed from the left mesial surface of the first permanent molar to the corresponding point on the other side of the automatically constructed arch curve (Figure 3C). This was determined using the mesial surface of each first permanent molar and canine and the center point of the central incisor and the digital arch length measuring mode in the Maestro 3D dental studio® (AGE Solutions, Pisa, Italy) program.

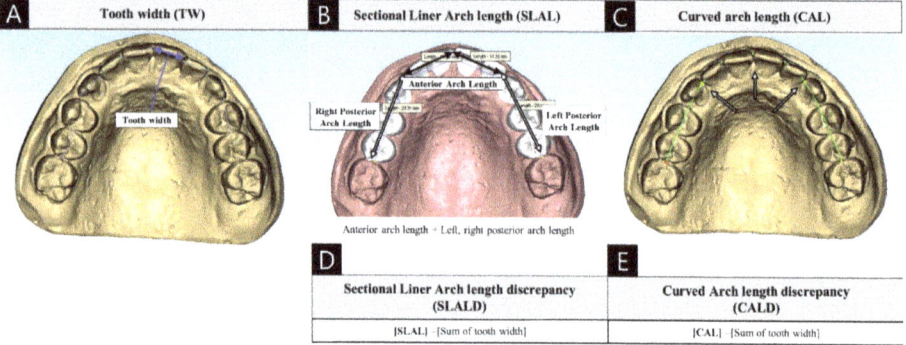

Figure 3. (**A**) Measurement of the mesial-distal width of the tooth and the arch length. (**B**) Sectional liner arch length (SLAL) measured using Maestro 3D®. (**C**) Automatically designed curved arch length (CAL) using Maestro 3D®. (**D**) Definition of sectional full arch length discrepancy (SLALD). (**E**) Definition of digital full arch length discrepancy (CALD).

The ALD was defined as the difference between the available space (AS) and required space (RS). The AS was defined as the AL of each arch, and the RS was defined as the sum of the tooth mesial-distal width from the left second premolar to the right second molar for each arch. Each SLAL and CAL were calculated together with the sectional full arch length discrepancy (SLALD) and digital full arch length discrepancy (CALD) (Figure 3D,E).

2.3. Statistical Methods

The collected data were subjected to statistical processing using the IBM SPSS Statistics software program (Version 24.0, IBM SPSS Inc., Chicago, IL, USA). The reliability was analyzed using Pearson's correlation coefficients of the measured TW, AAL, LAL, RAL and CAL. The significance level of

Pearson's correlation coefficients was verified as $p < 0.0001$. Subsequently, the reproducibility was evaluated using the intraclass correlation coefficients (ICC) between the data collected by Examiners A, B, C and D. An ICC ≥ 0.9 was considered to indicate excellent reproducibility, while values of 0.75 to <0.9, 0.5 to <0.75 and <0.5 were considered good, moderate and poor, respectively. Finally, the validity of the space analysis, including the SLAL, CAL and CALD, was evaluated using a paired t-test to explore the differences between the Group P and Groups MSD and ISD. The first value measured by examiner A was reported as the representative value if the reliability and reproducibility were good.

3. Results

3.1. Reliability

Nearly all data collected by examiner A were highly reliable (Table 1, $p < 0.0001$). Very high reliability was also observed for the AAL, LAL and RAL in all 3 groups as measured by examiner A ($p < 0.0001$). For the mandible AAL, the highest reliability was observed in Group MSD. For the CAL, good reliability was achieved in all 3 groups (Table S1).

3.2. Reproducibility

All data from Examiner A, B, C and D exhibited significant reproducibility (Table S2). For the TW, the values measured by examiner A, B, C and D exhibited excellent or good reproducibility in all 3 groups. Although the ICCs in all groups indicate adequate reproducibility, Groups MSD and ISD yielded higher levels of reproducibility than Group P. The AAL, LAL, RAL and CAL measured by examiners A, B, C and D also exhibited significant reproducibility in all 3 groups. For AAL, LAL and RAL, the ICCs at the anterior and posterior teeth were excellent or good in Group P, good in Group MSD and moderate or good in Group ISD. For the CAL, however, the ICCs determined for Groups MSD and ISD were excellent.

3.3. Validity

In Group MSD, every measured TW was longer than the corresponding value in Group P, except for the lower left canine and first premolar. The greatest error was measured in the upper right first premolar (Table 1). The average error ranged from −0.123 to 0.001 mm, and the standard variation ranged 0.196 from 0.278. Both upper central incisors, the upper right lateral incisor and canine, both lower lateral incisors, the lower left canine and the first premolar seemed to be measured similarly.

Table 1. Validity of tooth widths and arch lengths measured using each digital model.

Verification	p-MSD			P-ISD			Verification	P-MSD			P-ISD		
	Mean	SD	p Value	Mean	SD	p Value		Mean	SD	p Value	Mean	SD	p Value
#15	0.088	0.223	0.000 ***	−0.096	0.297	0.001 **	#35	−0.061	0.251	0.009 **	−0.017	0.312	0.542
#14	−0.123	0.250	0.000 ***	0.105	0.296	0.000 ***	#34	0.001	0.218	0.917	0.020	0.264	0.418
#13	−0.075	0.222	0.000 ***	0.078	0.293	0.004 **	#33	0.001	0.265	0.959	0.035	0.319	0.227
#12	−0.042	0.216	0.037 *	−0.007	0.231	0.747	#32	−0.034	0.196	0.056	−0.033	0.197	0.070
#11	−0.023	0.197	0.207	0.028	0.317	0.340	#31	−0.061	0.200	0.001 ***	−0.008	0.268	0.731
#21	−0.033	0.226	0.116	−0.011	0.254	0.358	#41	−0.063	0.202	0.001 ***	−0.026	0.222	0.201
#22	−0.034	0.258	0.150	0.002	0.282	0.954	#42	−0.039	0.242	0.082	−0.008	0.264	0.751
#23	−0.040	0.239	0.068	−0.056	0.270	0.024 *	#43	−0.070	0.278	0.007 **	−0.032	0.342	0.310
#24	−0.107	0.226	0.000 ***	−0.106	0.251	0.000 ***	#44	−0.062	0.225	0.003 **	−0.056	0.280	0.032 *
#25	−0.086	0.255	0.000 ***	0.060	0.271	0.008 **	#45	−0.070	0.260	0.004 **	−0.029	0.275	0.259
Maxilla							Mandible						
AAL	0.013	1.244	0.908	0.389	1.497	0.005 **	AAL	0.060	1.055	0.535	0.270	1.046	0.006 **
LAL	−0.204	0.882	0.013 *	0.076	1.094	0.451	LAL	−0.136	0.832	0.015 *	0.133	1.178	0.219
RAL	−0.209	1.119	0.043 *	0.045	1.085	0.146	RAL	−0.160	0.730	0.018 *	0.120	0.844	0.121

Paired t-test (*: $p < 0.05$, **: $p < 0.01$, ***: $p < 0.001$, unit = mm). P = plaster, MSD = model scanned digital model, ISD = intraoral scanned digital model, AAL = anterior arch length, LAL = left arch length, RAL = right arch length, CAL = curved arch length, SD = standard deviation.

In Group ISD, every measured TW was longer than the corresponding value in Group P, except the upper right central incisor and canine, upper left lateral incisor, lower left canine and first premolar. The average of error ranged from −0.106 to 0.078 mm, and the standard variation ranged from 0.196 to 0.278. Both upper central incisors and lateral incisors, the lower central incisor, lateral incisor, canine and first premolar and lower left first premolar seemed to be measured similarly. The tooth with the greatest error was upper left first premolar.

Regarding the SLAL between Groups P and MSD, the average error values were similar with a maxilla SLAL of 0.013 mm and a mandible SLAL of 0.060 mm. Neither difference was significant. However, the data from the maxilla and mandible LAL and RAL yielded significantly greater average error values ranging from −0.209 to −0.136 (Table 1, $p < 0.05$). However, the SLAL values of −0.399 mm in the maxilla and −0.236 mm in the mandible were not significant (Table 2).

Regarding the SLAL between Groups P and ISD, the average error values were significantly higher in the latter relative to the former, with a maxilla SLAL of 0.389 mm and mandible SLAL of 0.270 mm. However, the maxilla and mandible LAL and RAL measurements were similar between the groups, with no significant differences (average error: −0.136 to 0.133 mm; Table 1). The SLAL error values of 0.519 mm in the maxilla and 0.523 mm in the mandible indicated that this value was significantly lower in Group ISD than in Group P (Table 2, $p < 0.05$).

Table 2. Validity of arch length and arch length discrepancy measured by two methods.

	P-MSD			P-ISD				P-MSD			P-ISD		
	Mean	SD	p Value	Mean	SD	p Value		Mean	SD	p Value	Mean	SD	p Value
Maxilla							Mandible						
SLAL	−0.399	2.328	0.063	0.519	2.695	0.000 *	SLAL	−0.236	1.641	0.118	0.523	2.070	0.007 *
CAL	−0.755	2.113	0.000 *	0.022	1.695	0.059	CAL	−0.649	2.013	0.000 *	−0.173	1.887	0.067
RS	−0.649	1.120	0.000 *	−0.233	1.234	0.197	RS	−0.456	1.191	0.000 *	−0.153	1.351	0.216
SLALD	0.250	2.410	0.257	0.752	3.084	0.009 *	SLALD	0.221	1.789	0.179	0.676	2.390	0.002 *
CALD	−0.106	2.998	0.321	0.255	2.929	0.117	CALD	0.193	2.410	0.257	−0.040	1.084	0.718

Paired t-test (*: $p < 0.05$, unit = mm), RS = required space, SLAL = sectional liner arch length, CAL = curved arch length, SLALD = sectional liner arch length discrepancy, CALD = curved arch length discrepancy.

3.4. Validity of the Space Analysis

When the SLALD was measured, the average error values between Groups P group and MSD were 0.250 mm in the maxilla and 0.221 mm in the mandible, and these differences were not significant (Table 2). However, the CAL was significantly higher in Group MSD because of the differences resulting from curved and straight measurements. The average error value between Groups P and ISD were 0.752 mm in the maxilla and 0.676 mm in the mandible, and both SLALD values were significantly smaller in the ISD group than in the P group (Table 2, $p < 0.05$).

When the CALD was measured, the average error values between Groups P and MSD were 0.106 mm in the maxilla and 0.193 mm in the mandible, and these differences were not significant (Table 2). The average error values between Groups P and ISD were 0.255 mm in the maxilla and 0.040 mm in the mandible, and neither difference was significant (Table 2, $p < 0.05$).

4. Discussion

This study evaluated the reliability, reproducibility, and validity of the TW and AL measured using the MSD and ISD and the analyzed ALD in 40 young patients with permanent dentition. Notably, the TW, AAL, LAL and RAL measured in Groups P, MSD and ISD were very highly reliable and adequately reproducible. In the validity evaluation, most TW, AL and ALD values in Group MSD group and the TW values in Group ISD were highly valid. In comparison, the AL and ALD in Group ISD had relatively low validity, and the average total AL values in the maxilla and mandible were significantly smaller than those in Group P by 0.519 and 0.523 mm, respectively. Similarly, the average

ALD values in the maxilla and mandible in Group ISD were significantly smaller than those in Group P by 0.752 and 0.676 mm, respectively.

An intraoral scanner can more efficiently evaluate oral conditions in patients with an undercut, orthodontic appliance, gag reflex or thicker soft tissue, which can increase the difficulty and reduce the accuracy of impression modeling [7,20,26]. Particularly, conventional impression modeling induces anxiety and the gagging reflex in pediatric patients, who find oral scanner-based modeling to be relatively more comfortable [17,20,27,28]. The proportion of pediatric orthodontic patients who begin orthodontic treatment at an early age has increased recently in response to the emerging aesthetic emphasis on an ideal appearance and dentition, and the use of an intraoral scanner, rather than an impression, could reduce discomfort and improve the process of orthodontic diagnosis and treatment [26,28]. An ISD is digitalized and saved immediately, which could also reduce the time required for the digital setup of a clear aligner and other orthodontic appliances and decrease the error associated with the impression step [23,29]. In the future, it would be preferable for additional research to confirm the reproducibility of the intra-premises scan model performed by individuals of various occupations (i.e., dental hygienists, nurses, students), rather than dentist-guaranteed.

Measurements of lengths in a diagnostic model are influenced by factors such as the contact between adjacent teeth, the undercut of the teeth, intraoral orthodontic appliances or soft tissue. Regarding contact methods, Vernier caliper measurements of plaster models provide better accuracy. However, a non-contact measurement method is recommended when the measurement range is wide or the measurement location is easily deformed because the accuracy of a contact method decreases when the measurement area is complex or difficult to reach. The digital model measurement is a non-contact method and can accurately reach areas that are difficult to access using a Vernier caliper or that are affected by severe crowding or orthodontic appliances. Digital models also enable a visual determination of the 3D tooth inclination or axis [30]. The height of the arch height, difference in height between marginal ridges, angles between teeth, overjet and overbite tend to be measured inaccurately by Vernier calipers. In such cases, 3D methods can provide more accurate measurements. Although digital measurement methods may require significant learning curves and adjustment periods, these methods have the advantage of saving considerable time for both patients and clinicians [17,20]. In addition, the point where the measurement was performed can be recorded, which may be helpful for future re-measurements.

In this study, the use of the Maestro 3D dental studio® (AGE Solutions, Pisa, Italy) provided higher levels of reliability and reproducibility in terms of the TW measurements when compared to the Vernier caliper-based measurements. Specifically, the digital method was highly reproducible. Potentially, the coronal sectional view with a 3D tooth axis, which can be automatically visualized during measurement via a digital measurement program, could enable a set measurement point and help the clinician to measure this point more reproducibly, compared to a plaster model. Further, future research should confirm digital measurement while analyzing various digital programs. The superimposition of a digital model obtained from CBCT on this digital model, could further enable the more accurate measurement of the position of the tooth and the angle of the root in the alveolar bone.

The digital scanners used currently in clinical settings form the measurements using laser reflections. However, the laser may be reflected diffusely in areas such as adjacent surfaces, which can increase the possibility of error and reduce the reproducibility [31,32]. When the model scanner was used, the plaster model was constantly irradiated with lasers in various directions, and additional areas were scanned to increase the accuracy. However, a plaster model can easily cause physical errors due to air bubbles or stone surface defects, and impressions may be deformed or distorted at the undercut due to structural dental issues such as orthodontic appliances and interdental areas.

The digital model cannot be set as an accurate measurement point if it cannot directly reach the surface. Therefore, the ability to measure areas without data (e.g., inside bubbles) is limited. In this study, we observed significant differences in the LAL and RAL in Group MSD. These values were presumed to have been affected by the validity of the measurement points on adjacent surfaces, which were due to the error in the impression of the adjacent surfaces. In Group MSD, the SLAL tended to be measured overall, but again, the values did not differ significantly from those in Group P. Presumably, the error between the measurement points resulting from those measured in parts was reduced, which eliminated any significant differences.

In comparison, the ISD can provide digital images without defects from brackets or adjacent surfaces, which often cause surface defects or bubbles in stone models. Here, the TW measurements in Group ISD were most valid, indicating that the accurate measurement of a short span (e.g., TW) affected the impression without damaging the proximal and tooth surfaces. However, the SLAL value was significantly smaller in Group ISD than in Group P. Particularly, a significant error occurred in the AAL in Group ISD, and this may be due to the scanning method recommended by the CS3600® (Carestream Dental, Atlanta, GA, USA) manufacturer. Further, when digitalizing the anterior dental arch during the intraoral scanning process, the shape and size of the straight head of the intraoral scanner prevents a smooth transition from the labial surface to the lingual surface. Another cause of errors in intraoral scans is distortion that occurs during the process of superimposition of the scanned images. As a result, it is a known issue that errors appear larger in a long span scan image [12,18,22,33,34]. Although the tooth shape can be obtained relatively accurately, the errors are thought to arise in the form or length of the arch due to distortions in the labial width, alveolar bone shape and occlusal plane of the arch form. We expect that this distortion was caused by the intraoral scan rather than by a digital measurement issue (e.g., an error in the approach to the measuring point) (Figure 4). However, we attributed the similarity to the ability to measure the length of the curved form, which was difficult to measure in the stone model. In other words, the error of the straight-line distance measured by the intraoral scanner can be compensated by measuring the curved distance.

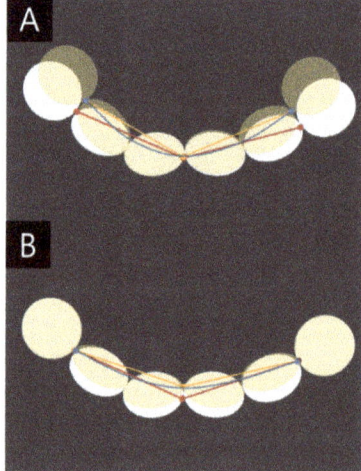

Figure 4. Illustration of differences in the sectional anterior arch length measurement caused by a distortion of intraoral scanning (**A**) and arch shape distortion. (**B**). Tooth labial-lingual width distortion. Red line: actual, yellow line: difference by distortion, blue line: curved arch.

In addition to the scanning method, errors may be caused by saliva, surrounding soft tissues, patient coordination and movement, the scanner head size, acquisition time, acquisition skill and acquisition range. Accordingly, further studies of the clinical validity of the ISD are warranted. Our study evaluated the validity of the measured values corresponding to the full arch span.

In last years, some studies evaluated clinical reliability and validity of the 3D measurements of features such as the palatal volume, occlusal relation, arch height, overjet and overbite, which are difficult to measure accurately using a Vernier caliper and stone models in MSD or CBCT digital model [35]. A study of the validity of 3D measurements in ISD would also be helpful.

Although we observed significant errors in the SLAL and SLALD in Group ISD, the relatively small error values in the maxilla and mandible would not significantly affect a diagnostic and treatment plan. However, the CAL and CALD produced using the digital program were deemed highly valid for clinical use. Therefore, dental analytic measurements based on an ISD may be clinically acceptable. The MSD is recommended for an orthodontic diagnosis that requires a measurement over a long span (e.g., full arch or alveolar ridge width) and a digital model for storage. The ISD is recommended when the predicted error of a stone model would be large due to the difficulty of impression taking, the interdental area or the presence of an orthodontic appliance. Moreover, if a space analysis such as the ALD is required in ISD, a digital program could be used to analyze the CAL and CALD while reducing the error. The resulting data would be highly valid for an orthodontic diagnosis.

5. Conclusions

In summary, the TW values obtained in Group ISD were more valid than those obtained in Group MSD. However, the former group yielded less valid SLAL and SLALD values. The CAL and CALD values in both groups exhibited high validity when compared with the corresponding values in Group P. Therefore, clinicians should be aware of the errors that may occur when using an MSD or ISD for a spatial analysis during the course of diagnosis and treatment. The appropriate impression method should be determined according to the individual situation.

Supplementary Materials: The following are available online at http://www.mdpi.com/2077-0383/9/9/2728/s1, Table S1: Reliability of tooth widths and arch lengths in each group; Table S2: Reproducibility of the tooth widths and arch lengths in each group.

Author Contributions: Conceptualization, S.-H.P., B.-E.Y. and I.-Y.P.; data collection and analysis, S.-H.P. and I.-Y.P.; investigation, B.-E.Y., H.-L.L., S.-H.O., J.-W.K., and S.-H.B.; writing—original draft preparation, S.-H.P.; writing—review and editing, S.-H.B. and I.-Y.P.; supervision, B.-E.Y. and I.-Y.P. All authors have read and agreed to the published version of the manuscript.

Funding: This research was supported by Hallym University Research Fund 2019 (HURF-2019-33). This work was supported by the Medical Device Technology Development Program (20006006, development of artificial intelligence-based augmented reality surgery system for oral and maxillofacial surgery) funded by the Ministry of Trade, Industry, and Energy.

Conflicts of Interest: The authors declare no potential conflicts of interest with respect to the authorship and/or publication of this article.

References

1. Richter, A.E.; Arruda, A.O.; Peters, M.C.; Sohn, W. Incidence of caries lesions among patients treated with comprehensive orthodontics. *Am. J. Orthod. Dentofac. Orthop.* **2011**, *139*, 657–664. [CrossRef] [PubMed]
2. Crosby, D.R.; Alexander, C.G. The occurrence of tooth size discrepancies among different malocclusion groups. *Am. J. Orthod. Dentofac. Orthop.* **1989**, *95*, 457–461. [CrossRef]
3. Schirmer, U.R.; Wiltshire, W.A. Manual and computer-aided space analysis: A comparative study. *Am. J. Orthod. Dentofac. Orthop.* **1997**, *112*, 676–680. [CrossRef]
4. Motohashi, N.; Kuroda, T. A 3D computer-aided design system applied to diagnosis and treatment planning in orthodontics and orthognathic surgery. *Eur. J. Orthod.* **1999**, *21*, 263–274. [CrossRef] [PubMed]
5. Zilberman, O.; Huggare, J.A.; Parikakis, K.A. Evaluation of the validity of tooth size and arch width measurements using conventional and three-dimensional virtual orthodontic models. *Angle Orthod.* **2003**, *73*, 301–306. [CrossRef] [PubMed]
6. Fleming, P.S.; Marinho, V.; Johal, A. Orthodontic measurements on digital study models compared with plaster models: A systematic review. *Orthod. Craniofac. Res.* **2011**, *14*, 1–16. [CrossRef]
7. Rossini, G.; Parrini, S.; Castroflorio, T.; Deregibus, A.; Debernardi, C.L. Diagnostic accuracy and measurement sensitivity of digital models for orthodontic purposes: A systematic review. *Am. J. Orthod. Dentofac. Orthop.* **2016**, *149*, 161–170. [CrossRef]

8. Santoro, M.; Galkin, S.; Teredesai, M.; Nicolay, O.F.; Cangialosi, T.J. Comparison of measurements made on digital and plaster models. *Am. J. Orthod. Dentofac. Orthop.* **2003**, *124*, 101–105. [CrossRef]
9. Stevens, D.R.; Flores-Mir, C.; Nebbe, B.; Raboud, D.W.; Heo, G.; Major, P.W. Validity, reliability, and reproducibility of plaster vs digital study models: Comparison of peer assessment rating and Bolton analysis and their constituent measurements. *Am. J. Orthod. Dentofac. Orthop.* **2006**, *129*, 794–803. [CrossRef]
10. Tomassetti, J.J.; Taloumis, L.J.; Denny, J.M.; Fischer, J.R., Jr. A comparison of 3 computerized Bolton tooth-size analyses with a commonly used method. *Angle Orthod.* **2001**, *71*, 351–357. [CrossRef]
11. Mullen, S.R.; Martin, C.A.; Ngan, P.; Gladwin, M. Accuracy of space analysis with emodels and plaster models. *Am. J. Orthod. Dentofac. Orthop.* **2007**, *132*, 346–352. [CrossRef] [PubMed]
12. Jeong, I.D.; Lee, J.J.; Jeon, J.H.; Kim, J.H.; Kim, H.Y.; Kim, W.C. Accuracy of complete-arch model using an intraoral video scanner: An in vitro study. *J. Prosthet. Dent.* **2016**, *115*, 755–759. [CrossRef] [PubMed]
13. Malik, J.; Rodriguez, J.; Weisbloom, M.; Petridis, H. Comparison of Accuracy between a Conventional and Two Digital Intraoral Impression Techniques. *Int. J. Prosthodont.* **2018**, *31*, 107–113. [CrossRef] [PubMed]
14. Kihara, H.; Hatakeyama, W.; Komine, F.; Takafuji, K.; Takahashi, T.; Yokota, J.; Oriso, K.; Kondo, H. Accuracy and practicality of intraoral scanner in dentistry: A literature review. *J. Prosthodont. Res.* **2019**. [CrossRef] [PubMed]
15. An, X.; Yang, H.W.; Choi, B.H. Digital Workflow for Computer-Guided Implant Surgery in Edentulous Patients with an Intraoral Scanner and Old Complete Denture. *J. Prosthodont.* **2019**, *28*, 715–718. [CrossRef]
16. Resnick, C.M.; Doyle, M.; Calabrese, C.E.; Sanchez, K.; Padwa, B.L. Is It Cost Effective to Add an Intraoral Scanner to an Oral and Maxillofacial Surgery Practice? *J. Oral Maxillofac. Surg.* **2019**, *77*, 1687–1694. [CrossRef]
17. Grunheid, T.; McCarthy, S.D.; Larson, B.E. Clinical use of a direct chairside oral scanner: An assessment of accuracy, time, and patient acceptance. *Am. J. Orthod. Dentofac. Orthop.* **2014**, *146*, 673–682. [CrossRef]
18. Goracci, C.; Franchi, L.; Vichi, A.; Ferrari, M. Accuracy, reliability, and efficiency of intraoral scanners for full-arch impressions: A systematic review of the clinical evidence. *Eur. J. Orthod.* **2016**, *38*, 422–428. [CrossRef]
19. Camardella, L.T.; Breuning, H.; de Vasconcellos Vilella, O. Accuracy and reproducibility of measurements on plaster models and digital models created using an intraoral scanner. *J. Orofac. Orthop.* **2017**, *78*, 211–220. [CrossRef]
20. Sfondrini, M.F.; Gandini, P.; Malfatto, M.; Di Corato, F.; Trovati, F.; Scribante, A. Computerized Casts for Orthodontic Purpose Using Powder-Free Intraoral Scanners: Accuracy, Execution Time, and Patient Feedback. *Biomed. Res. Int.* **2018**, *2018*, 4103232. [CrossRef] [PubMed]
21. Tomita, Y.; Uechi, J.; Konno, M.; Sasamoto, S.; Iijima, M.; Mizoguchi, I. Accuracy of digital models generated by conventional impression/plaster-model methods and intraoral scanning. *Dent. Mater. J.* **2018**, *37*, 628–633. [CrossRef] [PubMed]
22. Ender, A.; Attin, T.; Mehl, A. In vivo precision of conventional and digital methods of obtaining complete-arch dental impressions. *J. Prosthet. Dent.* **2016**, *115*, 313–320. [CrossRef] [PubMed]
23. Zhang, F.; Suh, K.J.; Lee, K.M. Validity of Intraoral Scans Compared with Plaster Models: An In-Vivo Comparison of Dental Measurements and 3D Surface Analysis. *PLoS ONE* **2016**, *11*, e0157713. [CrossRef] [PubMed]
24. Nedelcu, R.; Olsson, P.; Nystrom, I.; Ryden, J.; Thor, A. Accuracy and precision of 3 intraoral scanners and accuracy of conventional impressions: A novel in vivo analysis method. *J. Dent.* **2018**, *69*, 110–118. [CrossRef]
25. Sun, L.; Lee, J.S.; Choo, H.H.; Hwang, H.S.; Lee, K.M. Reproducibility of an intraoral scanner: A comparison between in-vivo and ex-vivo scans. *Am. J. Orthod. Dentofac. Orthop.* **2018**, *154*, 305–310. [CrossRef]
26. Jimenez-Gayosso, S.I.; Lara-Carrillo, E.; Lopez-Gonzalez, S.; Medina-Solis, C.E.; Scougall-Vilchis, R.J.; Hernandez-Martinez, C.T.; Colome-Ruiz, G.E.; Escoffie-Ramirez, M. Difference between manual and digital measurements of dental arches of orthodontic patients. *Medicine* **2018**, *97*, e10887. [CrossRef]
27. Burhardt, L.; Livas, C.; Kerdijk, W.; van der Meer, W.J.; Ren, Y. Treatment comfort, time perception, and preference for conventional and digital impression techniques: A comparative study in young patients. *Am. J. Orthod. Dentofac. Orthop.* **2016**, *150*, 261–267. [CrossRef]
28. Mangano, A.; Beretta, M.; Luongo, G.; Mangano, C.; Mangano, F. Conventional Vs Digital Impressions: Acceptability, Treatment Comfort and Stress Among Young Orthodontic Patients. *Open Dent. J.* **2018**, *12*, 118–124. [CrossRef]

29. Ting-Shu, S.; Jian, S. Intraoral Digital Impression Technique: A Review. *J. Prosthodont.* **2015**, *24*, 313–321. [CrossRef]
30. Kim, E.-J.; Hwang, H.-S. Reproducibility and accuracy of tooth size measurements obtained by the use of computer. *Korean J. Orthod.* **1998**, *29*, 563–573.
31. Flugge, T.V.; Schlager, S.; Nelson, K.; Nahles, S.; Metzger, M.C. Precision of intraoral digital dental impressions with iTero and extraoral digitization with the iTero and a model scanner. *Am. J. Orthod. Dentofac. Orthop.* **2013**, *144*, 471–478. [CrossRef] [PubMed]
32. Gul Amuk, N.; Karsli, E.; Kurt, G. Comparison of dental measurements between conventional plaster models, digital models obtained by impression scanning and plaster model scanning. *Int. Orthod.* **2019**, *17*, 151–158. [CrossRef] [PubMed]
33. Muallah, J.; Wesemann, C.; Nowak, R.; Robben, J.; Mah, J.; Pospiech, P.; Bumann, A. Accuracy of full-arch scans using intraoral and extraoral scanners: An in vitro study using a new method of evaluation. *Int. J. Comput. Dent.* **2017**, *20*, 151–164. [PubMed]
34. Muller, P.; Ender, A.; Joda, T.; Katsoulis, J. Impact of digital intraoral scan strategies on the impression accuracy using the TRIOS Pod scanner. *Quintessence Int.* **2016**, *47*, 343–349. [CrossRef] [PubMed]
35. Shahen, S.; Carrino, G.; Carrino, R.; Abdelsalam, R.; Flores-Mir, C.; Perillo, L. Palatal volume and area assessment on digital casts generated from cone-beam computed tomography scans. *Angle Orthod.* **2018**, *88*, 397–402. [CrossRef]

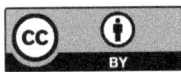

© 2020 by the authors. Licensee MDPI, Basel, Switzerland. This article is an open access article distributed under the terms and conditions of the Creative Commons Attribution (CC BY) license (http://creativecommons.org/licenses/by/4.0/).

Review

Mechanistic Insight into Orthodontic Tooth Movement Based on Animal Studies: A Critical Review

Hyeran Helen Jeon *, Hellen Teixeira and Andrew Tsai

Department of Orthodontics, School of Dental Medicine, University of Pennsylvania, 240 South 40th Street, Philadelphia, PA 19104-6030, USA; hellen@dental.upenn.edu (H.T.); andrewts@dental.upenn.edu (A.T.)
* Correspondence: hjeon@upenn.edu; Tel.: +1-215-898-5792

Abstract: Alveolar bone remodeling in orthodontic tooth movement (OTM) is a highly regulated process that coordinates bone resorption by osteoclasts and new bone formation by osteoblasts. Mechanisms involved in OTM include mechano-sensing, sterile inflammation-mediated osteoclastogenesis on the compression side and tensile force-induced osteogenesis on the tension side. Several intracellular signaling pathways and mechanosensors including the cilia and ion channels transduce mechanical force into biochemical signals that stimulate formation of osteoclasts or osteoblasts. To date, many studies were performed in vitro or using human gingival crevicular fluid samples. Thus, the use of transgenic animals is very helpful in examining a cause and effect relationship. Key cell types that participate in mediating the response to OTM include periodontal ligament fibroblasts, mesenchymal stem cells, osteoblasts, osteocytes, and osteoclasts. Intercellular signals that stimulate cellular processes needed for orthodontic tooth movement include receptor activator of nuclear factor-κB ligand (RANKL), tumor necrosis factor-α (TNF-α), dickkopf Wnt signaling pathway inhibitor 1 (DKK1), sclerostin, *transforming growth factor* beta (*TGF-β*), and bone morphogenetic proteins (BMPs). In this review, we critically summarize the current OTM studies using transgenic animal models in order to provide mechanistic insight into the cellular events and the molecular regulation of OTM.

Keywords: orthodontic tooth movement; animal studies; mechanosensing; osteoclastogenesis; osteogenesis

1. Introduction

Alveolar bone remodeling in orthodontic tooth movement (OTM) requires the coordinated action of different cell types, including periodontal ligament (PDL) fibroblasts, mesenchymal stem cells, inflammatory cells, osteoblasts, osteocytes, and osteoclasts. Generally, OTM is composed of three stages on the compression side; (i) a gradual compression of the PDL, which may last from about 4–7 days, (ii) the hyalinization period, when cell death due to lack of blood supply in the compressed area of the PDL occurs, which may last from 7–14 days or more, and (iii) the secondary period, which is characterized by direct bone resorption so that the tooth will continue to move [1–3]. On the tension side, the PDL is stretched and blood flow is activated, stimulating osteoblastic activity and osteoid deposition and mineralization. On mechanical force loading, cells around the tooth sense either compression or tension and release multiple cytokines and growth factors that stimulate subsequent biological responses. The process by which cells transmit mechanical forces and generate biological responses is essential for bone remodeling in OTM [4].

On the compression side, multinucleated osteoclasts initiate bone resorption to allow tooth movement to occur in the direction of the applied force, which is a rate limiting step in OTM. In addition, a sterile inflammatory response is induced by the generation of proinflammatory cytokines such as tissue necrosis factor (TNF), interleukin-1 (IL-1), prostaglandins, and IL-6, along with matrix metalloproteinases (MMPs) within a short time after the application of pressure [5–10]. The response to mechanical stress induces transitory inflammation that is pathogen-free. In addition, prostaglandins are secreted when cells are mechanically deformed and focal adhesion kinase, the mechanosensor in PDL cells, is known to be related with this process [11]. Therefore, both sterile inflammation and mechano-transduction are important for OTM [12]. Cells experiencing compressive forces induce osteoclastogenesis through up-regulation of receptor activator of nuclear factor kappa-B ligand (RANKL) [13]. Proinflammatory cytokines induce RANKL expression to stimulate osteoclastogenesis, further contributing to bone resorption in OTM [14]. On the tension side, PDL cells are stretched and proliferate with increased PDL width, followed by new bone formation, eventually returning to a normal PDL width [15]. Progenitor cells in the PDL and alveolar bone proliferate and differentiate into osteoblasts to produce new bone. The osteogenic transcription factor Runx2 and bone matrix proteins osteocalcin and osteopontin are significantly up-regulated by tension forces [7]. The mechano-response, osteoclastogenesis and osteogenesis are important components of OTM as they represent simultaneous bone remodeling processes in response to mechanical loading.

Human studies examining changes induced by orthodontic forces have frequently examined gingival crevicular fluid after orthodontic force loading. While important, these studies do not establish the cause and effect relationships. Transgenic mouse models are ideal in delineating the molecular actions of specific genes, as they facilitate lineage-specific gene deletion to well-defined cell types [16]. In addition, inducible transgenic mice models are available, allowing the induction of a transgene or the deletion of an endogenous gene in a time- and tissue-specific manner to address limitations of global constitutive germ-line deletion [17].

In this review, we focus on the roles of various mechanosensory cells, cytokine expression and signaling pathways in OTM that have been identified by animal models and summarize the possible cellular mechanosensors. A better understanding of the cellular processes in OTM may one day benefit our patients by expediting tooth movement, preventing relapse and improving treatment stability through the modification of specific genes which are critical for the orthodontic bone remodeling.

2. Cytokines, Mechanosensory Cells, and Intracellular Signaling Pathways in OTM
2.1. Cytokines in OTM
2.1.1. RANKL

RANKL is a member of the TNF cytokine family and is critical for osteoclastogenesis [18]. During OTM, RANKL is highly expressed in periodontal tissue on the compression and tension side [13,19]. Numerous cell types in OTM have been shown to express RANKL including PDL fibroblasts, mesenchymal stem cells, lymphocytes, osteoblasts, and osteocytes, particularly in response to inflammatory cytokines [9,13,20–22].

Human gingival crevicular fluid (GCF) samples have been used for cytokine analysis during OTM as it is non-invasive and convenient. Human GCF isolated from the tooth 24 h after orthodontic forces application, the early phase of OTM, had shown a significant increase in the levels of RANKL, IL-1β, IL-6, and TNF-α, while the levels of osteoprotegerin (OPG) had remained significantly lower when compared to the control teeth [7,23–25]. Furthermore, Garlet et al. examined the cytokine expression on the PDL of extracted human teeth after OTM [7]. After 7 days of OTM, teeth were extracted and PDL cells on both compression and tension sides were collected for real-time PCR analysis. On the compression side, tumor necrosis factor alpha (TNF-α), RANKL, and matrix metalloproteinases (MMPs) were highly expressed. On the tension side, IL-10, tissue inhibitors of metalloproteinase 1 *(TIMP-1)*, type I collagen, OPG, and osteocalcin were highly expressed. The same author tested chemokine expression on the extracted teeth after OTM and found that the compression side exhibited higher expression of monocyte chemoattractant protein-1 (MCP-1/CCL2), macrophage inflammatory protein-1α (MIP-1α/CCL3) and RANKL, which predominate bone resorption activity, while the tension side presented higher expression of osteocalcin.

Consistent with human studies, animal models demonstrated bone resorption activity with proinflammatory cytokines and osteoclastic markers on the compression side and bone formation activity with the osteogenic markers on the tension side. To further apply the findings to clinical orthodontics, several animal studies have examined the modulation of RANKL to accelerate OTM [26–28]. Injection of RANKL during OTM increases osteoclastogenesis and the rate of tooth movement [26]. Indeed, the rate of OTM is increased by 130% with RANKL injection [28]. Local RANKL gene transfer in animals with OTM increases RANKL protein expression and osteoclastogenesis without any systemic effects, accelerating the amount of tooth movement [27]. The authors proposed that local RANKL gene transfer might be a useful tool to accelerate orthodontic tooth movement, even the ankylosed teeth. Conversely, daily local RANKL antibody injection reduces the rate OTM by 70% [22]. In a comparison of RANKL gene transduction compared to periodontal accelerated osteogenic orthodontics, gene transduction led to more prolonged osteoclastogenesis and a greater rate of tooth movement during OTM [29].

In vitro compressive force causes an increase of RANKL expression and a decrease of OPG expression in human PDL cells, consistent with the human GCF and animal studies results. PDL fibroblasts are distorted under compressive force and express higher amounts of RANKL, TNF-α, MMPs, IL-1β and prostaglandins on the compression side [30]. Experimental compressive forces on the PDL resulted in a 16.7-fold increase in RANKL secretion and a 2.9-fold decrease in OPG secretion when compared to the control [23].

Taken together, studies with RANKL indicate that this cytokine is a central pro-osteoclastogenic factor that is expressed in response to mechanical forces. Interestingly, RANKL is also expressed on the tension side [19]. Thus, early induction of RANKL and osteoclastogenesis in response to tension may initiate a formation of bone remodeling that leads to increased bone formation on the tension side. This concept warrants further investigation.

2.1.2. Sclerostin

Sclerostin, encoded by the SOST gene and is primarily produced by mature osteocytes in response to OTM, promotes bone resorption and inhibits new bone formation [31,32]. Sclerostin stimulates RANKL expression by osteocytes, negatively regulates expression of BMP proteins and prevents canonical Wnt signaling [33,34]. Sclerostin expression is initially induced on the compression side in OTM models and gradually diminishes after 5–7 days, demonstrating their effect in the early phase of OTM [31,35]. During OTM, sclerostin KO mice have a 20% reduction in osteoclasts and reduced RANKL expression on the compression side with a reduced rate of tooth movement [35]. Local injection of sclerostin on the compression side doubles RANKL expression, reduces OPG expression by 30%, increases osteoclastogenesis by 150% and accelerates tooth movement [36]. In addition, in vitro studies showed that rhSCL-supplement enhanced the expression of RANKL and the RANKL/OPG ratio in osteocytes, supporting the in vivo finding. In addition, the intensity of sclerostin expression is closely related with the force magnitude [37]. On the tension side, sclerostin expression is immediately decreased and maintained at low levels during OTM, negating their negative effect on new bone formation [31]. These studies suggest that sclerostin can be a key factor in OTM by regulating both bone resorption and formation.

2.1.3. Bone Morphogenetic Proteins (BMPs)

It is well known that BMPs induce new bone formation and that the expression of BMPs increases on the tension side during OTM, stimulating the differentiation of mesenchymal stem cells to osteoblasts [30,38]. Noggin, an inhibitor of several bone morphogenetic proteins (BMPs), prevents mechanical force-induced osteoblast differentiation. BMP-3 expression is gradually increased on the tension side until 14 days in rodent models of OTM, the mid-stage in OTM [39]. One study examined the effect of BMP2 injection on tension side and found that local injection of BMP-2 on the tension side did not accelerate OTM, indicating that new bone formation per se is not a rate limiting step in OTM [40].

2.1.4. Transforming Growth Factor (TGF)-β

TGF-β signaling is involved in many cellular processes, including cell migration, proliferation, differentiation, and cellular homeostasis [41]. A previous study with extracted human teeth after OTM showed that TGF-β expression was similarly increased in both the compression and tension sides [7]. In OTM, its role on the compression side is complex as TGF-β has both positive and negative effects on osteoclastogenesis [42]. In some studies, TGF-β has been reported to inhibit osteoclastic activity. However, other studies found that TGF-β actually induces bone resorption, depending on the cell types involved, TGF-β concentration, and inducing mechanism [42,43]. Its expression on the tension side is significantly greater than that on the compression side [7,44–46]. TGF- β is generally known for its anabolic activity, regulating osteoblast differentiation from progenitors on the tension side [47]. Pretreatment with a TGF-β receptor inhibitor inhibits mechanical force-induced bone mineralization in vitro, suggesting that TGF-β could play a role in osteogenesis in response to tension forces during OTM.

Combining all, the findings from the animal studies could be the base foundation for the studies to expedite the OTM in humans. For example, RANKL or sclerostin can be given on the compression side to accelerate the osteoclastogenesis or BMPs can be given on the tension side to support the new bone formation. As previously mentioned, the new bone formation itself on the tension side cannot make the tooth movement faster while their effects are more important in the late phase in OTM. Therefore, many studies to speed up the velocity of OTM have been focused on the osteoclastogenic markers on the compression side.

2.2. The Mechanosensory Cells in OTM

PDL cells, osteocytes, and osteoblasts are the principal mechanosensory cells that produce various cytokines to regulate alveolar bone remodeling in OTM, by converting mechanical force into intracellular signals [48–51] (Figure 1). The role of mechanosensors in these cells during OTM will be reviewed later in this paper.

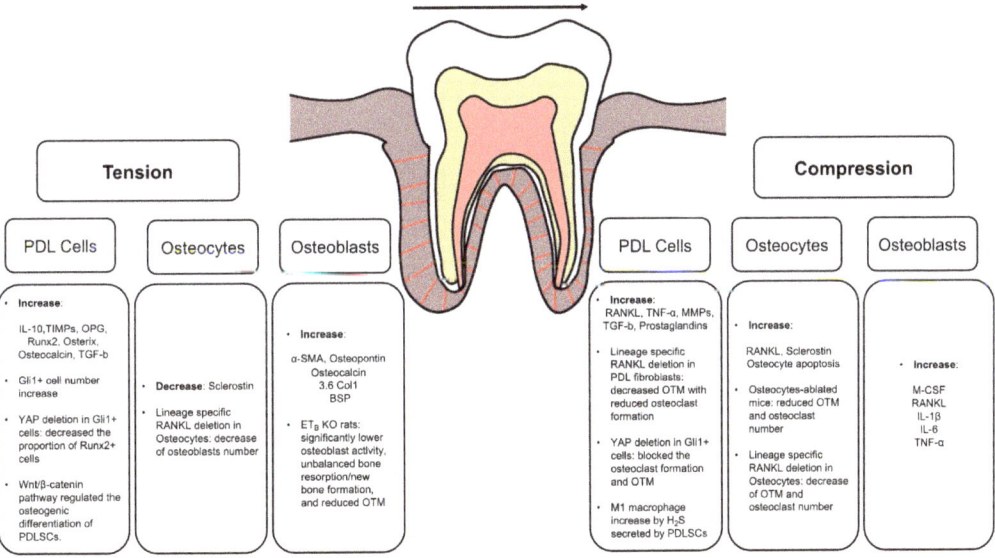

Figure 1. Cytokines and Mechanosensory cells in OTM.

2.2.1. Periodontal Ligament Cells

Periodontal Ligament Fibroblasts

The periodontal ligament (PDL) is a fibrous tissue that connects teeth with alveolar bone and transmits mechanical stimuli [52]. The PDL comprises of heterogenous cell types including fibroblasts, progenitor cells, bone-lining cells, osteoclasts, endothelial cells, nerve cells and others [53]. PDL fibroblasts constitute 50–60% of the total PDL cellularity and contribute to bone resorption in OTM as a main source of RANKL [21]. Interestingly, PDL fibroblasts have some characteristics similar to those of osteoblasts, expressing a 2.3 kb regulatory unit of Col1α1 promoter typical of osteoblasts and osteocytes [54,55] and bone-associated proteins such as alkaline phosphatase [56]. Indeed, PDL fibroblasts are more similar to tendon cells than skin fibroblasts in many respects [30,57].

On the compression side, the experimental mice with RANKL deletion in PDL fibroblasts showed significantly less osteoclast formation with narrower PDL space compared to control mice, leading to severely impaired OTM [21]. In addition, our recent study found that this up-regulation of RANKL depends on NF-κB activation [58]. NF-κB inhibition in PDL fibroblasts blocked the OTM with significantly reduced osteoclastogenesis, narrower PDL width, higher bone volume fraction and reduced RANKL expression compared to wild type mice. Both studies support the critical role of PDL fibroblasts via NF-κB activation in OTM.

Periodontal Ligament Stem Cells

Mesenchymal stem cells reside in the PDL, giving rise to PDL, alveolar bone, and cementum during alveolar bone remodeling. Gli1+ cells have been identified as the multipotent stem cells in adult mouse PDL [59]. Complete removal of Gli1+ cells using the inhibitors or by the genetic ablation significantly reduce OTM by 60% and diminish osteoclast formation by more than 80% [60]. On the tension side, Gli1+ increases its cell number and differentiate into osteoblasts with increased Runx2 expression during OTM [60].

Mesenchymal stem cells reside in the PDL, giving rise to PDL, alveolar bone, and cementum function as mechanosensory cells during OTM [60]. Yes-associated protein (YAP) and the paralogue transcriptional coactivator with PDZ-binding motif (TAZ), the downstream effectors of the Hippo signaling pathway, have been identified as important regulators during mechanotransduction [61]. Recent rodent OTM studies showed that YAP and TAZ expression were up-regulated with nuclear translocation in the PDL cells on both compression and tension side [62,63]. Moreover, YAP and TAZ expression were proportional to the applied orthodontic force. A recent study investigated the role of Gli1+ cells through Yes-associated protein (YAP) activation in mouse OTM models [60].Lineage-specific deletion of the YAP in Gli1+ cells significantly reduced OTM by 50% with decreased osteoclast formation by more than 80% on compression side. On the tension side, the same transgenic mice with the YAP deletion in Gli1+ cells showed a significantly decreased proportion of Runx2+ cells by more than 80%. In vitro cyclic stretch promoted the osteogenic differentiation of human PDL cells [62]. Moreover, the nuclear translocation of YAP was significantly increased with increased expression of connective tissue growth factor (CTGF) and cysteine-rich angiogenic inducer 61 (CYR61) mRNA, the target gene of YAP. Furthermore, knockdown of YAP suppressed the cyclic stretch induced osteogenesis in human PDL cells, while overexpression of YAP enhanced osteogenesis. Both in vivo and in vitro data supportthe role of YAP as the mechanical sensor and important regulator of the osteogenic differentiation in PDL cells under tensile force. In addition, the level of tension is important in the osteogenic differentiation as the magnitude of tension differentially regulates osteogenic and osteoclastic process [64]. Tension with a magnitude of 12% could increase osteogenic differentiation and proliferation of mesenchymal stem cells whereas tension above 12% would up-regulate the function of mesenchymal stem cells to regulate osteoclast differentiation, demonstrating the importance of the light force during OTM especially for the patients with poor bony support such as periodontitis [65,66].

Mechanical force-induced hydrogen sulfide (H_2S), produced by PDL mesenchymal stem cells, supports macrophage polarization toward an inflammatory, M1 phenotype and promotes osteoclast activity in OTM [67,68]. These cells express cystathionine-β-synthase that generates H_2S. Treatment with an inhibitor of H_2S reduces osteoclast formation and OTM by almost half. The generation of M1 macrophages is increased 5.6-fold after orthodontic force loading. An H_2S blocker reduces M1 macrophage formation by 70%, and an H_2S donor enhances it 1.4-fold. This shows that PDL mesenchymal stem cells can increase the expression of M1-macrophages, which are main source of several proinflammatory cytokines such as IL-1β, IL-6, and TNF-α, leading to the RANKL stimulation.

2.2.2. Osteocytes

Osteocytes are terminally differentiated from osteoblasts and embedded in the bone matrix. They are the most abundant cells in the adult skeleton, comprising 90–95% of all bone cells [12,51]. They are the primary mechanosensory cells in bone and regulate both osteoclast and osteoblast formation and function during mechanical force-induced bone remodeling [69,70]. They have dendritic processes that interact with other osteocytes and bone-lining cells. Mechanical loading stimulates dentin matrix protein 1 (DMP1) expression in osteocytes *in vivo*, which is a key molecule in regulating osteocyte formation, maturation, phosphate regulation and regulating mineralization [71,72]. In addition to RANKL, osteocytes produce sclerostin, M-CSF, OPG, and other cytokines during OTM.

As the early findings in OTM, osteocyte apoptosis peaks at 24 h on the compression side in mouse OTM models, as measured by TUNEL and caspase-3 immunofluorescence stain [73]. Osteoclastogenesis was evident after 72 h and continued to increase up to 7 days. Apoptotic osteocytes were preferentially located close to osteoclasts, suggesting that dying osteocytes produce active signaling to recruit osteoclasts [73–75].

Osteocytes can be also an important source of RANKL in OTM mouse models [22,76,77]. Osteocyte-deleted mice have a 60% reduction in osteoclasts and a 50% reduction in tooth movement compared to normal controls [78]. Under basal conditions osteocyte ablation negatively affects bone quality by increasing intracortical porosity, osteoblastic dysfunction, and adipose tissue proliferation in the marrow space [79]. These mice showed a severe osteopetrotic phenotype due to a lack of osteoclasts. The mice with lineage-specific RANKL deletion in osteocytes decreased OTM by 40% and osteoclast number by 60% compared with WT mice [22]. In vitro, osteocytes express a higher amount of RANKL and have a greater capacity to support osteoclastogenesis than osteoblasts and bone marrow stromal cells [77]. Interestingly, the osteoblast number on the tension side was significantly reduced in the same transgenic mice, possibly through a coupling mechanism.

2.2.3. Osteoblasts

Osteoblasts are bone forming cells, accounting for the 4–6% of total bone cells and differentiate from mesenchymal stem cells [80]. Runx2 and osterix are transcription factors that promote osteoblastic differentiation from mesenchymal stem cells. The fate of osteoblasts includes: (1) apoptosis, (2) become bone-lining cells or (3) form osteocytes. Bone-lining cells maintain homeostasis of bone and contain osteoblast progenitors [81]. Osteoblasts are mechanosensory cells and convert the mechanical signals into biological responses, producing various cytokines such as prostaglandin, OPG, RANKL and BMPs [82,83]. In OTM, bone-lining cells and osteoblasts express M-CSF and RANKL and produce other factors that positively influence osteoclastogenesis, including IL- 1β, IL-6 and TNF-α [84–86].

Osteoblast differentiation is an important process on the tension side during OTM. The initial response to OTM on the tension side is a proliferation of osteoblast progenitors that express α-SMA, which peaks at 2 days after initiating OTM while osteoid formation in mice peak at 4 days, the early phase of OTM, represented by osteopontin, osteocalcin, and bone sialoprotein in mouse OTM models [87,88]. Endothelin B receptors (ET$_B$) play an important role in alveolar bone modeling in the late stage of OTM in the rat animal model [89]. To examine the role of osteoblasts in OTM, ET$_B$ knockout rats (ET$_B$-KO) exhibited decreased OTM after 35 days, a late stage in OTM, by 27% compared to the ET$_B$-WT mice. The alveolar bone volume in the ET$_B$-KO appliance group was significantly less due to diminished osteoblast activity, but osteoclast volume was not significantly different compared to the ET$_B$-WT appliance group. In addition, the expression levels of osteocalcin and DMP1, the osteoblast activity markers, were significantly down-regulated by 70% in the ET$_B$-KO appliance group compared to the ET$_B$-WT appliance group. However, the expression of cathepsin K, an osteoclast activity marker, did not show any statistical difference. In summary, ET$_B$ knockout rats (ET$_B$-KO) have significantly lower osteoblast activity, unbalanced bone resorption/new bone formation, and reduced OTM with increased tooth mobility compared with control group, explaining the role of osteoblasts in the late stage of OTM.

Taken together, identifying the roles of each cells during OTM is critical and use of the transgenic mouse with each cell type-specific gene deletion can be a great tool for these studies.

2.3. Intracellular Signaling Pathways Stimulated by Mechanical Force

In OTM, various signaling pathways are activated, which mediate the response of mechanosensory cells that modulate bone resorption and formation. The function of Wnt/β-Catenin signaling, and Yes-associated protein and transcriptional coactivator with PDZ-binding motif (YAP/TAZ) signaling participate in bone remodeling in tooth movement.

Wnt/β-catenin signaling is critical for bone homeostasis [49,50]. β-catenin is a transcription factor that is activated by canonical Wnt signaling and translocates to the nucleus in osteoblasts lineage cells subjected to mechanical stimulation [90]. During OTM, Wnt/β-catenin signaling modulate expression of osteogenesis- and osteoclastogenesis-related factors in response to mechanotransduction [91–93]. Mice with global loss-of-function Lrp5, a Wnt receptor, have low bone mineral density and impaired osteogenic response to mechanical loading [94]. Conversely, mice with gain-of function mutations in the Lrp5 gene have significantly increase bone mineral density and bone mass in response to mechanical forces [95,96]. In OTM, a gain-of-function mutation in Lrp5 decreases orthodontic tooth movement by reducing osteoclast- mediated bone resorption and increasing alveolar bone mass [97]. Consistent with this, constitutive Wnt signaling increases osteogenic gene expression and reduces RANKL expression and osteoclast activity [98]. Conversely, viral transduction of DKK1, a Wnt inhibitor, increases osteoclast activity and reduces osteogenic markers, resulting in increased PDL width [98]. In a rat OTM model, the expression of Wnt3a, Wnt10b, and β-catenin is stronger on the tension side, consistent with Wnt induced bone formation observed under tension. In contrast, Dkk-1 levels are much higher on the compression side, consistent with reduced Wnt signaling and greater bone resorption on the compression side [99].

Yes-associated protein (YAP) and transcriptional coactivator with PDZ-binding motif (TAZ) play a key role in the mechanotransduction process [63,100]. YAP senses extracellular mechanical signals and translocates into nucleus to function as the coactivator of other transcription factors [62]. During OTM, YAP/TAZ signaling is observed in osteoblasts, osteocytes, osteoclasts and PDL fibroblasts and increases proportionally with the degree of orthodontic force [62,63]. Conditional deletion of YAP in PDL mesenchymal stem cells decreases osteoclast formation by 80% on the compression side and reduces tooth movement by half. In vitro cyclic stretch stimulates proliferation of PDL fibroblasts and osteoblast differentiation via YAP activation [62,101]. YAP knockdown suppresses mechanical forced-induced osteogenesis while overexpression of YAP enhances osteogenesis in PDL fibroblasts [62].

3. Possible Mechanosensors

Cells sense their mechanical environment through cell-cell or cell-matrix adhesions during physiologic growth and development and during mechanical loading. Mechanosensing occurs by mechanical force-induced conformational changes in cellular molecules, including force-activated cytoskeleton, integrins, ion channels and cell-cell adhesions, consequently affecting cellular gene expression and its function and regulating orthodontic bone remodeling (Figure 2).

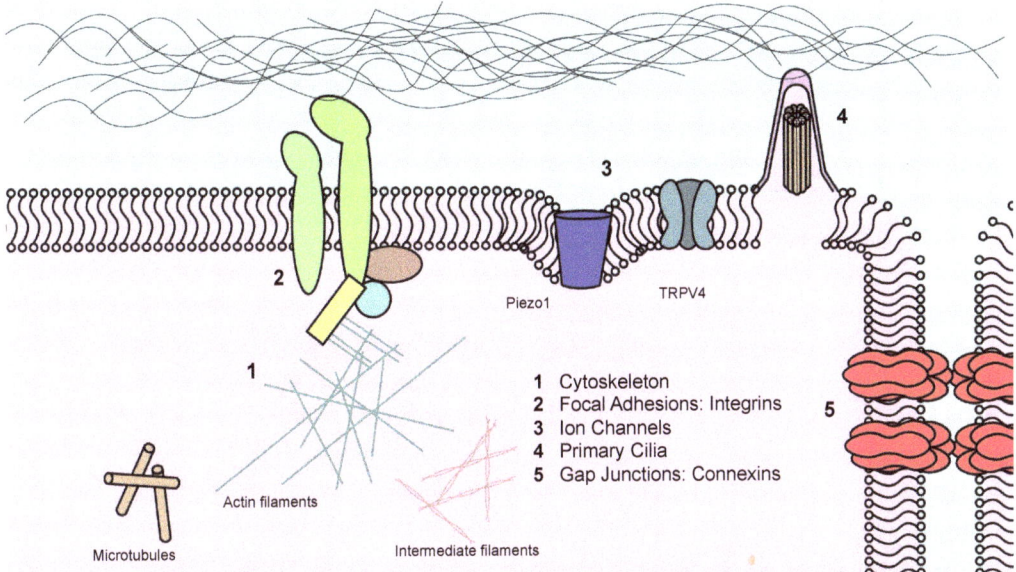

Figure 2. Possible Mechanosensors in Orthodontic Tooth Movement. (1) Cytoskeletons, (2) Focal adhesions: integrins, (3) Ion channels, (4) Primary cilia, and (5) Gap Junctions: connexins. TRPV4: transient receptor potential cation channel subfamily V member 4.

3.1. Cytoskeleton

Cellular cytoskeletons provide structural frameworks for the cell and are largely comprised of microtubules, actin, and intermediate filaments [102]. Cytoskeletons play a role in the response to mechanical force and are responsible for cell motility [103]. For example, cilia and flagella are mainly composed of microtubules and move as a result of microtubules sliding. In OTM, PDL and alveolar bone cells are reconstructed and their cellular cytoskeleton changes stimulate the elaboration of multiple cytokines and growth factors, mediating the cell morphology, differentiation, and proliferation [102,104,105]. On the tension side, cytoskeletal reorganization influences the differentiation of osteoprogenitors to osteoblasts and bone formation, stressing the critical role of cytoskeleton to influence both compression and tension sides during OTM [106].

3.2. Focal Adhesions (FAs)

Focal adhesions are integrin-associated proteins that connect intracellular actin filaments and extracellular matrix proteins [51,107]. Orthodontic force-induced stress on the extracellular matrix can be transmitted to cells through focal adhesions to induce proliferation and differentiation of several cells in the PDL and alveolar bone, leading to the balanced bone remodeling in response to the applied force [104]. Focal adhesions are involved in mechanosensing and downstream signaling through focal adhesion kinase in osteoblasts [108] and osteocytes [109,110]. Gene deletion that results in loss of focal adhesions in osteoblasts reduce mechanical responses to fluid flow [108]. Mechanical forces through focal adhesion kinases stimulate Wnt/β-catenin signaling in osteocytes [109].

3.3. Primary Cilia

Primary cilia are non-motile protruding organelles from the cell membrane and are observed in chondrocytes, mesenchymal stem cells, osteoblasts and osteocytes as mechanosensors [111,112]. Changes in fluid flow stimulate numerous cells via primary cilia [113], which may be important in OTM. Blocking primary cilia formation inhibits the expression of osteopontin, prostaglandins and cyclooxygenase-2 in osteoblasts or osteocytes and reduces their response to fluid flow. Tensile forces promote the osteogenic differentiation and proliferation of PDL mesenchymal stem cells via primary cilia that are needed for osteoblast differentiation and bone formation [114]. Lineage-specific deletion of key ciliary proteins including the IFT80, IFT88, Kif3a, Evc and polycystin in osteoblasts or osteoblast precursors leads to cilia loss, impairs osteoblast differentiation, reduces osteoid formation, and inhibits bone mineralization in response to mechanical loading in vivo [114–116]. On this basis, it may have a role in bone formation on tension side during OTM.

A calcium channel complex composed of the polycystin-1 and polycystin-2 is located at the base of primary cilium and mediates the effect of cilia bending [117]. When the primary cilium is bent by dynamic fluid flow, a Ca^{2+} signal is transduced proportional to the degree of distortion. This bending motion opens Ca^{2+}-permeable ion channels and stimulates formation of inositol (1,3,5)-trisphosphate (IP3) that is transmitted through gap junctions, thereby transmitting the ciliary signal to neighboring cells [4,118–120]. Loss of polycystin-1 function in vivo leads to reduced formation of osteoblasts, a reduced anabolic response to mechanical loading and the development of osteopenia [121]. Conditional deletion of polycystin-1 under the control of a regulatory element of the Wnt1 promoter has been used in OTM studies [122]. Conditional polycystin-1 deletion blocks the tooth movement with reduced osteoclast formation on the compression side. This study demonstrates that the calcium channels in primary cilia play an important role in the transduction of mechanical signals to induce bone resorption.

3.4. Gap Junctions: Connexins

Connexins are gap junction proteins that connect two neighboring cells [123,124]. Connexin 43 (Cx43) is the most abundant connexin in bone and modulates bone resorption and formation activity by regulating osteoprotegerin and sclerostin levels [74,125]. During OTM, Cx43 is strongly expressed in osteoclasts and PDL cells on the compression side and in osteoblasts and osteocytes on the tension side in vivo [124]. In vitro studies with PDL fibroblasts report that mechanical tension increases Cx43, up-regulating the expression of Runx2 and osterix, and down-regulating RANKL expression [126]. Suppression of Cx43 reduces the induction of osteogenic markers but promotes RANKL expression [126,127]. Given its function in regulating the response of osteoblasts and osteocytes to mechanical forces, it is reasonable to speculate that connexins play a role in OTM.

3.5. Ion Channels

Ion channels are pore-forming membrane proteins that facilitate direct ion passage through the cell membrane [51]. Mechanical force-activated ion channels increase membrane permeability and trigger the influx of extracellular calcium, demonstrating their role in mechanotransduction in osteocytes and PDL fibroblasts [51,128,129]. Piezo1 ion channel and transient receptor potential cation channel subfamily V member 4 (TRPV4) are key factors in the mechanotransduction of osteocytes and PDL fibroblasts under mechanical loading. Conditional deletion of Piezo1 in osteoblasts and osteocytes significantly reduced bone mass and strength in mice [130]. Conversely, administration of a Piezo1 agonist to adult mice increased bone mass in a way that mimicked the effects of mechanical loading, demonstrating that Piezo1 is a mechanosensitive ion channel by which osteoblast lineage cells sense and respond to changes in mechanical load. In vitro mechanical stimulation of mature osteocytes activates Piezo1, which rapidly activates Akt and down-regulates sclerostin [131]. Piezo1 and TRPV4 increase their expression 8 h after mechanical loading, followed by the increased expression of M-CSF, RANKL and COX2 [128]. However, pretreatment with the inhibitors of Piezo1 and TRPV4 suppressed the related cytokine expression. Fluid shear stress on osteocytes activates TRPV4 to rapidly increase intracellular Ca^{2+} levels, which activates Ca^{2+}/calmodulin-dependent kinase (CaMK) II and down-regulates sclerostin [132,133]. This is functionally important as shown by in vivo and in vitro studies that conditional deletion of Piezo1 in osteoblasts and osteocytes reduces bone mass and strength [130], while administration of a Piezo1 agonist increases bone mass, mimicking the effects of mechanical loading. It is likely that ion channel proteins are important in OTM.

4. Conclusions

Orthodontic tooth movement is a highly coordinated process in which various cells, cytokines, and complex mechanisms are involved. To date, numbers of OTM studies have been performed, but many are in vitro studies or examined the global deletion of a specific gene or cell type. Transgenic animal studies with the cell type-specific gene deletion can provide the insight into the key cellular and molecular mechanisms in OTM by establishing the cause and effect relationships. Findings from those studies could be applied for our daily orthodontic practice in the future, accelerating osteoclastogenesis and reducing treatment time. Conversely, blocking osteoclastogenesis can be applied to prevent orthodontic relapse. In addition, increasing osteogenesis can greatly help the maxillary expansion procedure, reducing the retention period of 5 to 6 months. The RANKL gene transfer to expedite the OTM is just one example. Furthermore, the findings from the transgenic animal studies can contribute to the development of precision orthodontics in the future so that we can provide patient-specific orthodontic treatment.

One of the limitations of this review is that animal studies that specifically examined mechanosensors are rare and many of them were conducted in vitro. Mechanosensors play a critical role in the mechanotransduction process and further investigation is needed. In addition, several OTM studies used slightly different amount of orthodontic force and time points. The use of standardized OTM methods would greatly help compare the outcomes from multiple animal OTM studies. Lastly, applying the findings from rodent studies to humans does warrant some modification considering the species differences, for example when considering the time periods in OTM.

Author Contributions: Conceptualization, H.H.J.; writing—original draft preparation, H.H.J.; writing—review and editing, H.H.J., H.T. and A.T. All authors have read and agreed to the published version of the manuscript

Funding: This research was supported by the Schoenleber Pilot Grant from the University of Pennsylvania School of Dental Medicine (HHJ) and the Orthodontic Faculty Development Fellowship Award from the American Association of Orthodontists Foundation (HHJ).

Institutional Review Board Statement: Not applicable.

Informed Consent Statement: Not applicable.

Data Availability Statement: Not applicable.

Acknowledgments: We greatly appreciate Dana Graves for his helpful discussion and guidance.

Conflicts of Interest: The authors declare no conflict of interest.

References

1. Reitan, K. Clinical and histologic observations on tooth movement during and after orthodontic treatment. *Am. J. Orthod.* **1967**, *53*, 721–745. [CrossRef]
2. Profit, W.R.; Fields, H.W.; Larson, B.E.; Sarver, D.M. *Contemporary Orthodontics*, 6th ed.; Mosby: Maryland Heights, MO, USA, 2018.
3. von Bohl, M.; Kuijpers-Jagtman, A.M. Hyalinization during orthodontic tooth movement: A systematic review on tissue reactions. *Eur. J. Orthod.* **2009**, *31*, 30–36. [CrossRef]

4. Temiyasathit, S.; Jacobs, C.R. Osteocyte primary cilium and its role in bone mechanotransduction. *Ann. N. Y. Acad. Sci.* **2010**, *1192*, 422–428. [CrossRef]
5. Uematsu, S.; Mogi, M.; Deguchi, T. Interleukin (IL)-1 beta, IL-6, tumor necrosis factor-alpha, epidermal growth factor, and beta 2-microglobulin levels are elevated in gingival crevicular fluid during human orthodontic tooth movement. *J. Dent. Res.* **1996**, *75*, 562–567. [CrossRef] [PubMed]
6. Ren, Y.; Hazemeijer, H.; de Haan, B.; Qu, N.; de Vos, P. Cytokine profiles in crevicular fluid during orthodontic tooth movement of short and long durations. *J. Periodontol.* **2007**, *78*, 453–458. [CrossRef]
7. Garlet, T.P.; Coelho, U.; Silva, J.S.; Garlet, G.P. Cytokine expression pattern in compression and tension sides of the periodontal ligament during orthodontic tooth movement in humans. *Eur. J. Oral Sci.* **2007**, *115*, 355–362. [CrossRef]
8. Rubartelli, A.; Lotze, M.T.; Latz, E.; Manfredi, A. Mechanisms of sterile inflammation. *Front. Immunol.* **2013**, *4*, 398. [CrossRef]
9. Klein, Y.; Fleissig, O.; Polak, D.; Barenholz, Y.; Mandelboim, O.; Chaushu, S. Immunorthodontics: In vivo gene expression of orthodontic tooth movement. *Sci. Rep.* **2020**, *10*, 8172. [CrossRef]
10. Meikle, M.C. The tissue, cellular, and molecular regulation of orthodontic tooth movement: 100 years after Carl Sandstedt. *Eur. J. Orthod.* **2006**, *28*, 221–240. [CrossRef]
11. Kang, Y.G.; Nam, J.H.; Kim, K.H.; Lee, K.S. FAK pathway regulates PGE(2) production in compressed periodontal ligament cells. *J. Dent. Res.* **2010**, *89*, 1444–1449. [CrossRef] [PubMed]
12. Krishnan, V.; Davidovitch, Z. On a path to unfolding the biological mechanisms of orthodontic tooth movement. *J. Dent. Res.* **2009**, *88*, 597–608. [CrossRef]
13. Yamaguchi, M. RANK/RANKL/OPG during orthodontic tooth movement. *Orthod. Craniofac. Res.* **2009**, *12*, 113–119. [CrossRef] [PubMed]
14. Glantschnig, H.; Fisher, J.E.; Wesolowski, G.; Rodan, G.A.; Reszka, A.A. M-CSF, TNFalpha and RANK ligand promote osteoclast survival by signaling through mTOR/S6 kinase. *Cell Death Differ.* **2003**, *10*, 1165–1177. [CrossRef] [PubMed]
15. Garlet, T.P.; Coelho, U.; Repeke, C.E.; Silva, J.S.; Cunha Fde, Q.; Garlet, G.P. Differential expression of osteoblast and osteoclast chemmoatractants in compression and tension sides during orthodontic movement. *Cytokine* **2008**, *42*, 330–335. [CrossRef] [PubMed]
16. Cho, A.; Haruyama, N.; Kulkarni, A.B. Generation of transgenic mice. *Curr. Protoc. Cell Biol.* **2009**, *19*, 11. [CrossRef]
17. Elefteriou, F.; Yang, X. Genetic mouse models for bone studies-strengths and limitations. *Bone* **2011**, *49*, 1242–1254. [CrossRef]
18. Kim, T.; Handa, A.; Iida, J.; Yoshida, S. RANKL expression in rat periodontal ligament subjected to a continuous orthodontic force. *Arch. Oral Biol.* **2007**, *52*, 244–250. [CrossRef] [PubMed]
19. Otero, L.; Garcia, D.A.; Wilches-Buitrago, L. Expression and Presence of OPG and RANKL mRNA and Protein in Human Periodontal Ligament with Orthodontic Force. *Gene Regul. Syst. Biol.* **2016**, *10*, 15–20. [CrossRef] [PubMed]
20. Yan, Y.; Liu, F.; Kou, X.; Liu, D.; Yang, R.; Wang, X.; Song, Y.; He, D.; Gan, Y.; Zhou, Y. T Cells Are Required for Orthodontic Tooth Movement. *J. Dent. Res.* **2015**, *94*, 1463–1470. [CrossRef]
21. Yang, C.Y.; Jeon, H.H.; Alshabab, A.; Lee, Y.J.; Chung, C.H.; Graves, D.T. RANKL deletion in periodontal ligament and bone lining cells blocks orthodontic tooth movement. *Int. J. Oral Sci.* **2018**, *10*, 3. [CrossRef]
22. Shoji-Matsunaga, A.; Ono, T.; Hayashi, M.; Takayanagi, H.; Moriyama, K.; Nakashima, T. Osteocyte regulation of orthodontic force-mediated tooth movement via RANKL expression. *Sci. Rep.* **2017**, *7*, 8753. [CrossRef]
23. Nishijima, Y.; Yamaguchi, M.; Kojima, T.; Aihara, N.; Nakajima, R.; Kasai, K. Levels of RANKL and OPG in gingival crevicular fluid during orthodontic tooth movement and effect of compression force on releases from periodontal ligament cells in vitro. *Orthod. Craniofac. Res.* **2006**, *9*, 63–70. [CrossRef]
24. Ren, Y.; Vissink, A. Cytokines in crevicular fluid and orthodontic tooth movement. *Eur. J. Oral Sci.* **2008**, *116*, 89–97. [CrossRef]
25. Meeran, N.A. Biological response at the cellular level within the periodontal ligament on application of orthodontic force—An update. *J. Orthod. Sci.* **2012**, *1*, 2–10. [CrossRef]
26. Li, C.; Chung, C.J.; Hwang, C.J.; Lee, K.J. Local injection of RANKL facilitates tooth movement and alveolar bone remodelling. *Oral Dis.* **2019**, *25*, 550–560. [CrossRef] [PubMed]
27. Kanzaki, H.; Chiba, M.; Arai, K.; Takahashi, I.; Haruyama, N.; Nishimura, M.; Mitani, H. Local RANKL gene transfer to the periodontal tissue accelerates orthodontic tooth movement. *Gene Ther.* **2006**, *13*, 678–685. [CrossRef] [PubMed]
28. Chang, J.H.; Chen, P.J.; Arul, M.R.; Dutra, E.H.; Nanda, R.; Kumbar, S.G.; Yadav, S. Injectable RANKL sustained release formulations to accelerate orthodontic tooth movement. *Eur. J. Orthod.* **2020**, *42*, 317–325. [CrossRef]
29. Iglesias-Linares, A.; Moreno-Fernandez, A.M.; Yanez-Vico, R.; Mendoza-Mendoza, A.; Gonzalez-Moles, M.; Solano-Reina, E. The use of gene therapy vs. corticotomy surgery in accelerating orthodontic tooth movement. *Orthod. Craniofac. Res.* **2011**, *14*, 138–148. [CrossRef]
30. Li, Y.; Jacox, L.A.; Little, S.H.; Ko, C.C. Orthodontic tooth movement: The biology and clinical implications. *Kaohsiung J. Med. Sci.* **2018**, *34*, 207–214. [CrossRef] [PubMed]
31. Odagaki, N.; Ishihara, Y.; Wang, Z.; Ei Hsu Hlaing, E.; Nakamura, M.; Hoshijima, M.; Hayano, S.; Kawanabe, N.; Kamioka, H. Role of Osteocyte-PDL Crosstalk in Tooth Movement via SOST/Sclerostin. *J. Dent. Res.* **2018**, *97*, 1374–1382. [CrossRef] [PubMed]
32. Morse, A.; McDonald, M.M.; Kelly, N.H.; Melville, K.M.; Schindeler, A.; Kramer, I.; Kneissel, M.; van der Meulen, M.C.; Little, D.G. Mechanical load increases in bone formation via a sclerostin-independent pathway. *J. Bone Miner. Res.* **2014**, *29*, 2456–2467. [CrossRef]

33. Wijenayaka, A.R.; Kogawa, M.; Lim, H.P.; Bonewald, L.F.; Findlay, D.M.; Atkins, G.J. Sclerostin stimulates osteocyte support of osteoclast activity by a RANKL-dependent pathway. *PLoS ONE* **2011**, *6*, e25900. [CrossRef] [PubMed]
34. Galea, G.L.; Lanyon, L.E.; Price, J.S. Sclerostin's role in bone's adaptive response to mechanical loading. *Bone* **2017**, *96*, 38–44. [CrossRef]
35. Shu, R.; Bai, D.; Sheu, T.; He, Y.; Yang, X.; Xue, C.; He, Y.; Zhao, M.; Han, X. Sclerostin Promotes Bone Remodeling in the Process of Tooth Movement. *PLoS ONE* **2017**, *12*, e0167312. [CrossRef]
36. Lu, W.; Zhang, X.; Firth, F.; Mei, L.; Yi, J.; Gong, C.; Li, H.; Zheng, W.; Li, Y. Sclerostin injection enhances orthodontic tooth movement in rats. *Arch. Oral Biol.* **2019**, *99*, 43–50. [CrossRef] [PubMed]
37. Robling, A.G.; Niziolek, P.J.; Baldridge, L.A.; Condon, K.W.; Allen, M.R.; Alam, I.; Mantila, S.M.; Gluhak-Heinrich, J.; Bellido, T.M.; Harris, S.E.; et al. Mechanical stimulation of bone in vivo reduces osteocyte expression of Sost/sclerostin. *J. Biol. Chem.* **2008**, *283*, 5866–5875. [CrossRef] [PubMed]
38. Kamiya, N.; Mishina, Y. New insights on the roles of BMP signaling in bone-A review of recent mouse genetic studies. *Biofactors* **2011**, *37*, 75–82. [CrossRef]
39. Gao, Y.; Zhang, M.; Tian, X.; Wang, M.; Zhang, F. Experimental animal study on BMP-3 expression in periodontal tissues in the process of orthodontic tooth movement. *Exp. Ther. Med.* **2019**, *17*, 193–198. [CrossRef]
40. Iglesias-Linares, A.; Yanez-Vico, R.M.; Moreno-Fernandez, A.M.; Mendoza-Mendoza, A.; Solano-Reina, E. Corticotomy-assisted orthodontic enhancement by bone morphogenetic protein-2 administration. *J. Oral Maxillofac. Surg.* **2012**, *70*, e124–e132. [CrossRef] [PubMed]
41. Manokawinchoke, J.; Pavasant, P.; Sawangmake, C.; Limjeerajarus, N.; Limjeerajarus, C.N.; Egusa, H.; Osathanon, T. Intermittent compressive force promotes osteogenic differentiation in human periodontal ligament cells by regulating the transforming growth factor-beta pathway. *Cell Death Dis.* **2019**, *10*, 761. [CrossRef]
42. Quinn, J.M.; Itoh, K.; Udagawa, N.; Hausler, K.; Yasuda, H.; Shima, N.; Mizuno, A.; Higashio, K.; Takahashi, N.; Suda, T.; et al. Transforming growth factor beta affects osteoclast differentiation via direct and indirect actions. *J. Bone Miner. Res.* **2001**, *16*, 1787–1794. [CrossRef]
43. Itonaga, I.; Sabokbar, A.; Sun, S.G.; Kudo, O.; Danks, L.; Ferguson, D.; Fujikawa, Y.; Athanasou, N.A. Transforming growth factor-beta induces osteoclast formation in the absence of RANKL. *Bone* **2004**, *34*, 57–64. [CrossRef]
44. Wang, L.L.; Zhu, H.; Liang, T. Changes of transforming growth factor beta 1 in rat periodontal tissue during orthodontic tooth movement. *Chin. J. Dent. Res.* **2000**, *3*, 19–22.
45. Uematsu, S.; Mogi, M.; Deguchi, T. Increase of transforming growth factor-beta 1 in gingival crevicular fluid during human orthodontic tooth movement. *Arch. Oral Biol.* **1996**, *41*, 1091–1095. [CrossRef]
46. Nagai, M.; Yoshida, A.; Sato, N.; Wong, D.T. Messenger RNA level and protein localization of transforming growth factor-beta1 in experimental tooth movement in rats. *Eur. J. Oral Sci.* **1999**, *107*, 475–481. [CrossRef] [PubMed]
47. Van Schepdael, A.; Vander Sloten, J.; Geris, L. A mechanobiological model of orthodontic tooth movement. *Biomech. Model. Mechanobiol.* **2013**, *12*, 249–265. [CrossRef] [PubMed]
48. Masella, R.S.; Meister, M. Current concepts in the biology of orthodontic tooth movement. *Am. J. Orthod. Dentofac. Orthop.* **2006**, *129*, 458–468. [CrossRef]
49. Qin, L.; Liu, W.; Cao, H.; Xiao, G. Molecular mechanosensors in osteocytes. *Bone Res.* **2020**, *8*, 23. [CrossRef]
50. Huang, H.; Yang, R.; Zhou, Y.H. Mechanobiology of Periodontal Ligament Stem Cells in Orthodontic Tooth Movement. *Stem Cells Int.* **2018**, *2018*, 6531216. [CrossRef]
51. Klein-Nulend, J.; Bakker, A.D.; Bacabac, R.G.; Vatsa, A.; Weinbaum, S. Mechanosensation and transduction in osteocytes. *Bone* **2013**, *54*, 182–190. [CrossRef]
52. Mabuchi, R.; Matsuzaka, K.; Shimono, M. Cell proliferation and cell death in periodontal ligaments during orthodontic tooth movement. *J. Periodontal Res.* **2002**, *37*, 118–124. [CrossRef] [PubMed]
53. Seo, B.M.; Miura, M.; Gronthos, S.; Bartold, P.M.; Batouli, S.; Brahim, J.; Young, M.; Robey, P.G.; Wang, C.Y.; Shi, S. Investigation of multipotent postnatal stem cells from human periodontal ligament. *Lancet* **2004**, *364*, 149–155. [CrossRef]
54. Zheng, J.; Chen, S., Albiero, M.L.; Vieira, G.H.A.; Wang, J.; Feng, J.Q.; Graves, D.T. Diabetes Activates Periodontal Ligament Fibroblasts via NF-kappaB In Vivo. *J. Dent. Res.* **2018**, *97*, 580–588. [CrossRef]
55. Dacquin, R.; Starbuck, M.; Schinke, T.; Karsenty, G. Mouse alpha1(I)-collagen promoter is the best known promoter to drive efficient Cre recombinase expression in osteoblast. *Dev. Dyn.* **2002**, *224*, 245–251. [CrossRef]
56. Giannopoulou, C.; Cimasoni, G. Functional characteristics of gingival and periodontal ligament fibroblasts. *J. Dent. Res.* **1996**, *75*, 895–902. [CrossRef]
57. Basdra, E.K.; Komposch, G. Osteoblast-like properties of human periodontal ligament cells: An in vitro analysis. *Eur. J. Orthod.* **1997**, *19*, 615–621. [CrossRef]
58. Hyeran Helen Jeon, C.-Y.Y.; Shin, M.K.; Wang, J.; Patel, J.H.; Chung, C.; Graves, D.T. Osteoblast lineage cells and periodontal ligament fibroblasts regulate orthodontic tooth movement that is dependent on Nuclear Factor-kappa B (NF-kB) activation. *Angle Orthod.* **2021**, in press.
59. Men, Y.; Wang, Y.; Yi, Y.; Jing, D.; Luo, W.; Shen, B.; Stenberg, W.; Chai, Y.; Ge, W.P.; Feng, J.Q.; et al. Gli1+ Periodontium Stem Cells Are Regulated by Osteocytes and Occlusal Force. *Dev. Cell* **2020**, *54*, 639–654 e636. [CrossRef] [PubMed]

60. Liu, A.Q.; Zhang, L.S.; Chen, J.; Sui, B.D.; Liu, J.; Zhai, Q.M.; Li, Y.J.; Bai, M.; Chen, K.; Jin, Y.; et al. Mechanosensing by Gli1(+) cells contributes to the orthodontic force-induced bone remodelling. *Cell Prolif.* **2020**, *53*, e12810. [CrossRef]
61. Dupont, S.; Morsut, L.; Aragona, M.; Enzo, E.; Giulitti, S.; Cordenonsi, M.; Zanconato, F.; Le Digabel, J.; Forcato, M.; Bicciato, S.; et al. Role of YAP/TAZ in mechanotransduction. *Nature* **2011**, *474*, 179–183. [CrossRef] [PubMed]
62. Yang, Y.; Wang, B.K.; Chang, M.L.; Wan, Z.Q.; Han, G.L. Cyclic Stretch Enhances Osteogenic Differentiation of Human Periodontal Ligament Cells via YAP Activation. *Biomed. Res. Int.* **2018**, *2018*, 2174824. [CrossRef]
63. Sun, B.; Wen, Y.; Wu, X.; Zhang, Y.; Qiao, X.; Xu, X. Expression pattern of YAP and TAZ during orthodontic tooth movement in rats. *J. Mol. Histol.* **2018**, *49*, 123–131. [CrossRef] [PubMed]
64. Zhang, L.; Liu, W.; Zhao, J.; Ma, X.; Shen, L.; Zhang, Y.; Jin, F.; Jin, Y. Mechanical stress regulates osteogenic differentiation and RANKL/OPG ratio in periodontal ligament stem cells by the Wnt/beta-catenin pathway. *Biochim. Biophys. Acta* **2016**, *1860*, 2211–2219. [CrossRef]
65. Pelaez, D.; Acosta Torres, Z.; Ng, T.K.; Choy, K.W.; Pang, C.P.; Cheung, H.S. Cardiomyogenesis of periodontal ligament-derived stem cells by dynamic tensile strain. *Cell Tissue Res.* **2017**, *367*, 229–241. [CrossRef]
66. Chen, J.; Zhang, W.; Backman, L.J.; Kelk, P.; Danielson, P. Mechanical stress potentiates the differentiation of periodontal ligament stem cells into keratocytes. *Br. J. Ophthalmol.* **2018**, *102*, 562–569. [CrossRef]
67. Liu, F.; Wen, F.; He, D.; Liu, D.; Yang, R.; Wang, X.; Yan, Y.; Liu, Y.; Kou, X.; Zhou, Y. Force-Induced H2S by PDLSCs Modifies Osteoclastic Activity during Tooth Movement. *J. Dent. Res.* **2017**, *96*, 694–702. [CrossRef] [PubMed]
68. He, D.; Liu, F.; Cui, S.; Jiang, N.; Yu, H.; Zhou, Y.; Liu, Y.; Kou, X. Mechanical load-induced H2S production by periodontal ligament stem cells activates M1 macrophages to promote bone remodeling and tooth movement via STAT1. *Stem Cell Res. Ther.* **2020**, *11*, 112. [CrossRef] [PubMed]
69. Huang, H.; Williams, R.C.; Kyrkanides, S. Accelerated orthodontic tooth movement: Molecular mechanisms. *Am. J. Orthod. Dentofac. Orthop.* **2014**, *146*, 620–632. [CrossRef] [PubMed]
70. Florencio-Silva, R.; Sasso, G.R.; Sasso-Cerri, E.; Simoes, M.J.; Cerri, P.S. Biology of Bone Tissue: Structure, Function, and Factors That Influence Bone Cells. *Biomed. Res. Int.* **2015**, *2015*, 421746. [CrossRef]
71. Dallas, S.L.; Prideaux, M.; Bonewald, L.F. The osteocyte: An endocrine cell . . . and more. *Endocr. Rev.* **2013**, *34*, 658–690. [CrossRef]
72. Gluhak-Heinrich, J.; Ye, L.; Bonewald, L.F.; Feng, J.Q.; MacDougall, M.; Harris, S.E.; Pavlin, D. Mechanical loading stimulates dentin matrix protein 1 (DMP1) expression in osteocytes in vivo. *J. Bone Miner. Res.* **2003**, *18*, 807–817. [CrossRef]
73. Moin, S.; Kalajzic, Z.; Utreja, A.; Nihara, J.; Wadhwa, S.; Uribe, F.; Nanda, R. Osteocyte death during orthodontic tooth movement in mice. *Angle Orthod.* **2014**, *84*, 1086–1092. [CrossRef]
74. Bivi, N.; Condon, K.W.; Allen, M.R.; Farlow, N.; Passeri, G.; Brun, L.R.; Rhee, Y.; Bellido, T.; Plotkin, L.I. Cell autonomous requirement of connexin 43 for osteocyte survival: Consequences for endocortical resorption and periosteal bone formation. *J. Bone Miner. Res.* **2012**, *27*, 374–389. [CrossRef]
75. Kogianni, G.; Mann, V.; Noble, B.S. Apoptotic bodies convey activity capable of initiating osteoclastogenesis and localized bone destruction. *J. Bone Miner. Res.* **2008**, *23*, 915–927. [CrossRef]
76. Xiong, J.; Onal, M.; Jilka, R.L.; Weinstein, R.S.; Manolagas, S.C.; O'Brien, C.A. Matrix-embedded cells control osteoclast formation. *Nat. Med.* **2011**, *17*, 1235–1241. [CrossRef]
77. Nakashima, T.; Hayashi, M.; Fukunaga, T.; Kurata, K.; Oh-Hora, M.; Feng, J.Q.; Bonewald, L.F.; Kodama, T.; Wutz, A.; Wagner, E.F.; et al. Evidence for osteocyte regulation of bone homeostasis through RANKL expression. *Nat. Med.* **2011**, *17*, 1231–1234. [CrossRef]
78. Matsumoto, T.; Iimura, T.; Ogura, K.; Moriyama, Y.; Yamaguchi, A. The role of osteocytes in bone resorption during orthodontic tooth movement. *J. Dent. Res.* **2013**, *92*, 340–345. [CrossRef]
79. Tatsumi, S.; Ishii, K.; Amizuka, N.; Li, M.; Kobayashi, T.; Kohno, K.; Ito, M.; Takeshita, S.; Ikeda, K. Targeted ablation of osteocytes induces osteoporosis with defective mechanotransduction. *Cell Metab.* **2007**, *5*, 464–475. [CrossRef]
80. Kassem, M.; Abdallah, B.M.; Saeed, H. Osteoblastic cells: Differentiation and trans-differentiation. *Arch. Biochem. Biophys.* **2008**, *473*, 183–187. [CrossRef]
81. Matic, I.; Matthews, B.G.; Wang, X.; Dyment, N.A.; Worthley, D.L.; Rowe, D.W.; Grcevic, D.; Kalajzic, I. Quiescent Bone Lining Cells Are a Major Source of Osteoblasts During Adulthood. *Stem Cells* **2016**, *34*, 2930–2942. [CrossRef]
82. Kohli, S.S.; Kohli, V.S. Role of RANKL-RANK/osteoprotegerin molecular complex in bone remodeling and its immunopathologic implications. *Indian J. Endocrinol. Metab.* **2011**, *15*, 175–181. [CrossRef] [PubMed]
83. Wang, L.; Li, J.Y.; Zhang, X.Z.; Liu, L.; Wan, Z.M.; Li, R.X.; Guo, Y. Involvement of p38MAPK/NF-kappaB signaling pathways in osteoblasts differentiation in response to mechanical stretch. *Ann. Biomed. Eng.* **2012**, *40*, 1884–1894. [CrossRef]
84. Matsuo, K.; Irie, N. Osteoclast-osteoblast communication. *Arch. Biochem. Biophys.* **2008**, *473*, 201–209. [CrossRef]
85. Zhang, S.; Wang, X.; Li, G.; Chong, Y.; Zhang, J.; Guo, X.; Li, B.; Bi, Z. Osteoclast regulation of osteoblasts via RANKRANKL reverse signal transduction in vitro. *Mol. Med. Rep.* **2017**, *16*, 3994–4000. [CrossRef] [PubMed]
86. Boyce, B.F.; Xing, L. The RANKL/RANK/OPG pathway. *Curr. Osteoporos. Rep.* **2007**, *5*, 98–104. [CrossRef]
87. Holland, R.; Bain, C.; Utreja, A. Osteoblast differentiation during orthodontic tooth movement. *Orthod. Craniofac. Res.* **2019**, *22*, 177–182. [CrossRef]

88. Uribe, F.; Kalajzic, Z.; Bibko, J.; Nanda, R.; Olson, C.; Rowe, D.; Wadhwa, S. Early effects of orthodontic forces on osteoblast differentiation in a novel mouse organ culture model. *Angle Orthod.* **2011**, *81*, 284–291. [CrossRef] [PubMed]
89. Ibrahimi Disha, S.; Furlani, B.; Drevensek, G.; Plut, A.; Yanagisawa, M.; Hudoklin, S.; Prodan Zitnik, I.; Marc, J.; Drevensek, M. The role of endothelin B receptor in bone modelling during orthodontic tooth movement: A study on ETB knockout rats. *Sci. Rep.* **2020**, *10*, 14226. [CrossRef] [PubMed]
90. Premaraj, S.; Souza, I.; Premaraj, T. Mechanical loading activates beta-catenin signaling in periodontal ligament cells. *Angle Orthod.* **2011**, *81*, 592–599. [CrossRef] [PubMed]
91. Kramer, I.; Halleux, C.; Keller, H.; Pegurri, M.; Gooi, J.H.; Weber, P.B.; Feng, J.Q.; Bonewald, L.F.; Kneissel, M. Osteocyte Wnt/beta-catenin signaling is required for normal bone homeostasis. *Mol. Cell. Biol.* **2010**, *30*, 3071–3085. [CrossRef]
92. Chen, B.; Li, X.D.; Liu, D.X.; Wang, H.; Xie, P.; Liu, Z.Y.; Hou, G.Q.; Chang, B.; Du, S.X. Canonical Wnt signaling is required for Panax notoginseng saponin-mediated attenuation of the RANKL/OPG ratio in bone marrow stromal cells during osteogenic differentiation. *Phytomedicine* **2012**, *19*, 1029–1034. [CrossRef]
93. Fu, H.D.; Wang, B.K.; Wan, Z.Q.; Lin, H.; Chang, M.L.; Han, G.L. Wnt5a mediated canonical Wnt signaling pathway activation in orthodontic tooth movement: Possible role in the tension force-induced bone formation. *J. Mol. Histol.* **2016**, *47*, 455–466. [CrossRef] [PubMed]
94. Sawakami, K.; Robling, A.G.; Ai, M.; Pitner, N.D.; Liu, D.; Warden, S.J.; Li, J.; Maye, P.; Rowe, D.W.; Duncan, R.L.; et al. The Wnt co-receptor LRP5 is essential for skeletal mechanotransduction but not for the anabolic bone response to parathyroid hormone treatment. *J. Biol. Chem.* **2006**, *281*, 23698–23711. [CrossRef] [PubMed]
95. Cui, Y.; Niziolek, P.J.; MacDonald, B.T.; Zylstra, C.R.; Alenina, N.; Robinson, D.R.; Zhong, Z.; Matthes, S.; Jacobsen, C.M.; Conlon, R.A.; et al. Lrp5 functions in bone to regulate bone mass. *Nat. Med.* **2011**, *17*, 684–691. [CrossRef]
96. Niziolek, P.J.; Warman, M.L.; Robling, A.G. Mechanotransduction in bone tissue: The A214V and G171V mutations in Lrp5 enhance load-induced osteogenesis in a surface-selective manner. *Bone* **2012**, *51*, 459–465. [CrossRef] [PubMed]
97. Holland, R.; Bain, C.; Alrasheed, R.S.; Robling, A.G.; Utreja, A. The effect of overexpression of Lrp5 on orthodontic tooth movement. *Orthod. Craniofac. Res.* **2020**. [CrossRef] [PubMed]
98. Lim, W.H.; Liu, B.; Mah, S.J.; Yin, X.; Helms, J.A. Alveolar bone turnover and periodontal ligament width are controlled by Wnt. *J. Periodontol.* **2015**, *86*, 319–326. [CrossRef] [PubMed]
99. Lu, J.; Duan, Y.; Zhang, M.; Wu, M.; Wang, Y. Expression of Wnt3a, Wnt10b, beta-catenin and DKK1 in periodontium during orthodontic tooth movement in rats. *Acta Odontol. Scand.* **2016**, *74*, 217–223. [CrossRef] [PubMed]
100. Pocaterra, A.; Romani, P.; Dupont, S. YAP/TAZ functions and their regulation at a glance. *J. Cell Sci.* **2020**, *133*, jcs230425. [CrossRef]
101. Huelter-Hassler, D.; Tomakidi, P.; Steinberg, T.; Jung, B.A. Orthodontic strain affects the Hippo-pathway effector YAP concomitant with proliferation in human periodontal ligament fibroblasts. *Eur. J. Orthod.* **2017**, *39*, 251–257. [CrossRef]
102. Klein-Nulend, J.; Bacabac, R.G.; Bakker, A.D. Mechanical loading and how it affects bone cells: The role of the osteocyte cytoskeleton in maintaining our skeleton. *Eur. Cells Mater.* **2012**, *24*, 278–291. [CrossRef]
103. Feller, L.; Khammissa, R.A.; Schechter, I.; Thomadakis, G.; Fourie, J.; Lemmer, J. Biological Events in Periodontal Ligament and Alveolar Bone Associated with Application of Orthodontic Forces. *Sci. World J.* **2015**, *2015*, 876509. [CrossRef]
104. Feller, L.; Khammissa, R.A.; Schechter, I.; Moodley, A.; Thomadakis, G.; Lemmer, J. Periodontal Biological Events Associated with Orthodontic Tooth Movement: The Biomechanics of the Cytoskeleton and the Extracellular Matrix. *Sci. World J.* **2015**, *2015*, 894123. [CrossRef]
105. McBeath, R.; Pirone, D.M.; Nelson, C.M.; Bhadriraju, K.; Chen, C.S. Cell shape, cytoskeletal tension, and RhoA regulate stem cell lineage commitment. *Dev. Cell* **2004**, *6*, 483–495. [CrossRef]
106. Pan, J.; Wang, T.; Wang, L.; Chen, W.; Song, M. Cyclic strain-induced cytoskeletal rearrangement of human periodontal ligament cells via the Rho signaling pathway. *PLoS ONE* **2014**, *9*, e91580. [CrossRef] [PubMed]
107. Geiger, B.; Bershadsky, A.; Pankov, R.; Yamada, K.M. Transmembrane crosstalk between the extracellular matrix–cytoskeleton crosstalk. *Nat. Rev. Mol. Cell Biol.* **2001**, *2*, 793–805. [CrossRef]
108. Young, S.R.; Gerard-O'Riley, R.; Kim, J.B.; Pavalko, F.M. Focal adhesion kinase is important for fluid shear stress-induced mechanotransduction in osteoblasts. *J. Bone Miner. Res.* **2009**, *24*, 411–424. [CrossRef] [PubMed]
109. Santos, A.; Bakker, A.D.; Zandieh-Doulabi, B.; de Blieck-Hogervorst, J.M.; Klein-Nulend, J. Early activation of the beta-catenin pathway in osteocytes is mediated by nitric oxide, phosphatidyl inositol-3 kinase/Akt, and focal adhesion kinase. *Biochem. Biophys. Res. Commun.* **2010**, *391*, 364–369. [CrossRef]
110. Chen, C.S.; Tan, J.; Tien, J. Mechanotransduction at cell-matrix and cell-cell contacts. *Annu. Rev. Biomed. Eng.* **2004**, *6*, 275–302. [CrossRef] [PubMed]
111. Yuan, X.; Yang, S. Cilia/Ift protein and motor -related bone diseases and mouse models. *Front. Biosci.* **2015**, *20*, 515–555. [CrossRef]
112. Song, J.; Wang, L.; Fan, F.; Wei, J.; Zhang, J.; Lu, Y.; Fu, Y.; Wang, S.; Juncos, L.A.; Liu, R. Role of the Primary Cilia on the Macula Densa and Thick Ascending Limbs in Regulation of Sodium Excretion and Hemodynamics. *Hypertension* **2017**, *70*, 324–333. [CrossRef] [PubMed]
113. Whitfield, J.F. Primary cilium–is it an osteocyte's strain-sensing flowmeter? *J. Cell Biochem.* **2003**, *89*, 233–237. [CrossRef]
114. Yuan, X.; Yang, S. Primary Cilia and Intraflagellar Transport Proteins in Bone and Cartilage. *J. Dent. Res.* **2016**, *95*, 1341–1349. [CrossRef] [PubMed]

115. Yang, S.; Wang, C. The intraflagellar transport protein IFT80 is required for cilia formation and osteogenesis. *Bone* **2012**, *51*, 407–417. [CrossRef]
116. Qiu, N.; Xiao, Z.; Cao, L.; Buechel, M.M.; David, V.; Roan, E.; Quarles, L.D. Disruption of Kif3a in osteoblasts results in defective bone formation and osteopenia. *J. Cell Sci.* **2012**, *125*, 1945–1957. [CrossRef] [PubMed]
117. Nauli, S.M.; Alenghat, F.J.; Luo, Y.; Williams, E.; Vassilev, P.; Li, X.; Elia, A.E.; Lu, W.; Brown, E.M.; Quinn, S.J.; et al. Polycystins 1 and 2 mediate mechanosensation in the primary cilium of kidney cells. *Nat. Genet.* **2003**, *33*, 129–137. [CrossRef]
118. Wang, P.; Tang, C.; Wu, J.; Yang, Y.; Yan, Z.; Liu, X.; Shao, X.; Zhai, M.; Gao, J.; Liang, S.; et al. Pulsed electromagnetic fields regulate osteocyte apoptosis, RANKL/OPG expression, and its control of osteoclastogenesis depending on the presence of primary cilia. *J. Cell Physiol.* **2019**, *234*, 10588–10601. [CrossRef] [PubMed]
119. Delaine-Smith, R.M.; Sittichokechaiwut, A.; Reilly, G.C. Primary cilia respond to fluid shear stress and mediate flow-induced calcium deposition in osteoblasts. *FASEB J.* **2014**, *28*, 430–439. [CrossRef]
120. Malone, A.M.; Anderson, C.T.; Tummala, P.; Kwon, R.Y.; Johnston, T.R.; Stearns, T.; Jacobs, C.R. Primary cilia mediate mechanosensing in bone cells by a calcium-independent mechanism. *Proc. Natl. Acad. Sci. USA* **2007**, *104*, 13325–13330. [CrossRef]
121. Xiao, Z.; Zhang, S.; Mahlios, J.; Zhou, G.; Magenheimer, B.S.; Guo, D.; Dallas, S.L.; Maser, R.; Calvet, J.P.; Bonewald, L.; et al. Cilia-like structures and polycystin-1 in osteoblasts/osteocytes and associated abnormalities in skeletogenesis and Runx2 expression. *J. Biol. Chem.* **2006**, *281*, 30884–30895. [CrossRef]
122. Shalish, M.; Will, L.A.; Fukai, N.; Hou, B.; Olsen, B.R. Role of polycystin-1 in bone remodeling: Orthodontic tooth movement study in mutant mice. *Angle Orthod.* **2014**, *84*, 885–890. [CrossRef] [PubMed]
123. Riquelme, M.A.; Cardenas, E.R.; Xu, H.; Jiang, J.X. The Role of Connexin Channels in the Response of Mechanical Loading and Unloading of Bone. *Int. J. Mol. Sci.* **2020**, *21*, 1146. [CrossRef]
124. Su, M.; Borke, J.L.; Donahue, H.J.; Li, Z.; Warshawsky, N.M.; Russell, C.M.; Lewis, J.E. Expression of connexin 43 in rat mandibular bone and periodontal ligament (PDL) cells during experimental tooth movement. *J. Dent. Res.* **1997**, *76*, 1357–1366. [CrossRef] [PubMed]
125. Plotkin, L.I.; Stains, J.P. Connexins and pannexins in the skeleton: Gap junctions, hemichannels and more. *Cell. Mol. Life Sci.* **2015**, *72*, 2853–2867. [CrossRef]
126. Li, S.; Zhang, H.; Li, S.; Yang, Y.; Huo, B.; Zhang, D. Connexin 43 and ERK regulate tension-induced signal transduction in human periodontal ligament fibroblasts. *J. Orthop. Res.* **2015**, *33*, 1008–1014. [CrossRef]
127. Xu, C.; Fan, Z.; Shan, W.; Hao, Y.; Ma, J.; Huang, Q.; Zhang, F. Cyclic stretch influenced expression of membrane connexin 43 in human periodontal ligament cell. *Arch. Oral Biol.* **2012**, *57*, 1602–1608. [CrossRef]
128. Shen, Y.; Pan, Y.; Guo, S.; Sun, L.; Zhang, C.; Wang, L. The roles of mechanosensitive ion channels and associated downstream MAPK signaling pathways in PDLC mechanotransduction. *Mol. Med. Rep.* **2020**, *21*, 2113–2122. [CrossRef] [PubMed]
129. Jin, Y.; Li, J.; Wang, Y.; Ye, R.; Feng, X.; Jing, Z.; Zhao, Z. Functional role of mechanosensitive ion channel Piezo1 in human periodontal ligament cells. *Angle Orthod.* **2015**, *85*, 87–94. [CrossRef] [PubMed]
130. Li, X.; Han, L.; Nookaew, I.; Mannen, E.; Silva, M.J.; Almeida, M.; Xiong, J. Stimulation of Piezo1 by mechanical signals promotes bone anabolism. *Elife* **2019**, *8*. [CrossRef]
131. Sasaki, F.; Hayashi, M.; Mouri, Y.; Nakamura, S.; Adachi, T.; Nakashima, T. Mechanotransduction via the Piezo1-Akt pathway underlies Sost suppression in osteocytes. *Biochem. Biophys. Res. Commun.* **2020**, *521*, 806–813. [CrossRef]
132. Pei, F.; Liu, J.; Zhang, L.; Pan, X.; Huang, W.; Cen, X.; Huang, S.; Jin, Y.; Zhao, Z. The functions of mechanosensitive ion channels in tooth and bone tissues. *Cell. Signal.* **2021**, *78*, 109877. [CrossRef] [PubMed]
133. Lyons, J.S.; Joca, H.C.; Law, R.A.; Williams, K.M.; Kerr, J.P.; Shi, G.; Khairallah, R.J.; Martin, S.S.; Konstantopoulos, K.; Ward, C.W.; et al. Microtubules tune mechanotransduction through NOX2 and TRPV4 to decrease sclerostin abundance in osteocytes. *Sci. Signal.* **2017**, *10*, eaan5748. [CrossRef] [PubMed]

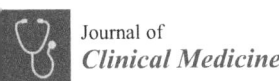

Journal of Clinical Medicine

Review

Application of Vibrational Spectroscopies in the Qualitative Analysis of Gingival Crevicular Fluid and Periodontal Ligament during Orthodontic Tooth Movement

Fabrizia d'Apuzzo [1,*], Ludovica Nucci [1], Ines Delfino [2], Marianna Portaccio [3], Giuseppe Minervini [1], Gaetano Isola [4], Ismene Serino [3], Carlo Camerlingo [5] and Maria Lepore [3]

[1] Multidisciplinary Department of Medical-Surgical and Dental Specialties, University of Campania Luigi Vanvitelli, 80138 Napoli, Italy; ludortho@gmail.com (L.N.); giuseppe.minervini@unicampania.it (G.M.)
[2] Department of Ecological and Biological Sciences, University of Tuscia, 01100 Viterbo, Italy; delfino@unitus.it
[3] Department of Experimental Medicine, University of Campania Luigi Vanvitelli, 80138 Napoli, Italy; mariannabiancaemanuela.portaccio@unicampania.it (M.P.); ismene.serino@unicampania.it (I.S.); maria.lepore@unicampania.it (M.L.)
[4] Department of General Surgery and Medical-Surgical Specialties, University of Catania, 95124 Catania, Italy; gaetanoisola@gmail.com
[5] CNR-SPIN, SuPerconductivity and Other INnovative Materials and Devices Institute, 80078 Pozzuoli, Italy; carlo.camerlingo@spin.cnr.it
* Correspondence: fabrizia.dapuzzo@unicampania.it; Tel.: +39-3384820462

Citation: d'Apuzzo, F.; Nucci, L.; Delfino, I.; Portaccio, M.; Minervini, G.; Isola, G.; Serino, I.; Camerlingo, C.; Lepore, M. Application of Vibrational Spectroscopies in the Qualitative Analysis of Gingival Crevicular Fluid and Periodontal Ligament during Orthodontic Tooth Movement. *J. Clin. Med.* **2021**, *10*, 1405. https://doi.org/10.3390/jcm10071405

Academic Editor: Francisco Mesa

Received: 14 February 2021
Accepted: 24 March 2021
Published: 1 April 2021

Publisher's Note: MDPI stays neutral with regard to jurisdictional claims in published maps and institutional affiliations.

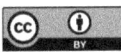

Copyright: © 2021 by the authors. Licensee MDPI, Basel, Switzerland. This article is an open access article distributed under the terms and conditions of the Creative Commons Attribution (CC BY) license (https:// creativecommons.org/licenses/by/ 4.0/).

Abstract: Optical vibrational techniques show a high potentiality in many biomedical fields for their characteristics of high sensitivity in revealing detailed information on composition, structure, and molecular interaction with reduced analysis time. In the last years, we have used these techniques for investigating gingival crevicular fluid (GCF) and periodontal ligament (PDL) during orthodontic tooth treatment. The analysis with Raman and infrared signals of GCF and PDL samples highlighted that different days of orthodontic force application causes modifications in the molecular secondary structure at specific wavenumbers related to the Amide I, Amide III, CH deformation, and CH_3/CH_2. In the present review, we report the most relevant results and a brief description of the experimental techniques and data analysis procedure in order to evidence that the vibrational spectroscopies could be a potential useful tool for an immediate monitoring of the individual patient's response to the orthodontic tooth movement, aiming to more personalized treatment reducing any side effects.

Keywords: vibrational spectroscopies; Raman spectroscopies; infrared spectroscopies; orthodontic tooth movement; gingival crevicular fluid; periodontal ligament

1. Introduction

Orthodontic tooth movement (OTM) is related to remodeling of alveolar bone and periodontal ligament (PDL) with several macroscopic and microscopic biological changes. These events lead to structural modifications of the periodontal ligament (PDL), as well as an increased flow and composition changes of the gingival crevicular fluid (GCF) in the periodontal sulcus. The PDL is a complex, neurovascular, cellular, and connective tissue interposed between the tooth root and the alveolar bone, mainly composed of collagen fibers, whereas the GCF derives from the epithelium lining of the gingival sulcus, thus its characteristics depend on the specific site from which it is collected. Orthodontic force application generates a regular process that is basically characterized by bone deposition at sites of tension and bone resorption on the pressure site upsetting the homeostatic environment of periodontal tissues and locally altering the blood flow and electrochemical conditions. These modifications lead to the generation and propagation of signaling chemical cascades and associated tissue remodeling by delineating biochemical and cellular reactions occurring in tissues and fluids around the teeth [1–3]. In the literature, several in vivo and in vitro studies, both in animal and human samples, investigated the structure and molecular patterns of the PDL and GCF during orthodontic treatment through different analytical methodologies (i.e., immunohistochemistry, immunocytochemistry, confocal laser microscopy, gene arrays real-time PCR (Polymerase Chain Reaction), transmission electron-microscopy, microcomputed tomography) [4–10]. However, these methods are time-consuming and labor-intensive, requiring complex procedures to prepare the samples. In the last years, some optical vibrational techniques as micro-Raman Spectroscopy (µ-RS), Surface-Enhanced Raman Spectroscopy (SERS), and Fourier Transform-Infrared (FT-IR) [11–14] were used for this purpose. Vibrational spectroscopy is the collective term used to describe analytical techniques that measure vibrational energy levels associated with the chemical bonds. The spectra obtained from these analyses are considered like a fingerprint containing signals from the functional groups in the sample. In particular, Raman techniques measure the characteristics Raman emission induced from molecules under monochromatic laser irradiation while IR measures the light absorption by specific molecules using a broadband light source [15]. Raman Spectroscopies (RS) and FT-IR are complementary techniques because the related bands are due to nonpolar and polar functional groups, respectively, thus they are both needed to detect complete biochemical information of the samples. For these reasons, the vibrational spectroscopies have been utilized in an enormous number of fundamental and applied research fields. In the biomedical fields, these techniques show high sensitivity in revealing detailed information on molecular composition, structure, and interactions with non-destructive sampling and reduced analysis time in comparison to other conventional methodologies. In particular, biofluids are ideal samples for routinely clinical assessment with vibrational spectroscopies being easily accessible through minimally invasive collection methods and repeatedly available for monitoring disease progression or therapeutic response [14–22]. Vibrational spectroscopies are thus convenient and reliable techniques in order to obtain an overall biochemical characterization of the main tissue and biofluids involved in the orthodontic tooth movement to properly monitor their microscopic changes during treatment. A comprehensive evaluation of the novel use of these techniques in Orthodontics may provide a wider vision of recent outcomes and future research both for diagnosis and monitoring strategies in this field. In the last years, we devoted great attention to the use of vibrational spectroscopies for monitoring OTM in young and adult patients and this review aims to revise the studies which used these vibrational spectroscopies for the qualitative analysis of PDL and GCF samples collected during the initial phase of OTM in young and adult patients.

2. Materials and Methods

2.1. Study Selection

To retrieve lists of potential articles to be included in the review, the search strategy included the following databases to December 2020: PubMed, PubMed Central, National Library of Medicine's Medline, Embase, Cochrane Central Register of Controlled Clinical Trials, Web of Knowledge, Scopus, Google Scholar, Latin American and Caribbean Health Sciences Literature (LILACs). Abstracts, and presentations from international orthodontic meetings were evaluated. To identify relevant records, the search encompassed an effective combination of Medical Subject Headings (MeSH) terms and free-text terms including 'vibrational spectroscopies', 'Raman spectroscopy', micro-Raman spectroscopy', 'infrared spectroscopy', 'Fourier-Transform infrared spectroscopy', AND 'tooth movement', 'orthodontics', 'orthodontic force application', 'orthodontic treatment', AND 'gingival crevicular fluid', 'periodontal ligament'.

Title and abstract screening were performed to select articles for full-text retrieval by two reviewers. An initial screening of titles and abstracts against the inclusion criteria was performed to identify potentially relevant papers followed by a screening of the full possibly relevant papers. Duplicate articles were removed, and the studies were selected for inclusion independently by both authors. The concordance percentage between the two reviewers was less than 3% and any doubts or disagreements were resolved after discussion.

A total of seven relevant publications including analysis of human GCF and PDL subjected to orthodontic forces with vibrational spectroscopies were selected. The results reported in these publications (see Table 1) are revised in the present paper. In Table 1 information about first authors and year of publication, analytical vibrational techniques, type of sample collected, duration of orthodontic tooth movement and characteristics of subjects are indicated [23–29].

Table 1. Characteristics of the selected studies.

Author, Year [Ref. n°]	Vibrational Spectroscopy	Sample Type	OTM Time (Days)	Subject Number	Age (yrs)
Camerlingo et al., 2014 [23]	µ-RS	PDL	0, 2, 7, 14	3	range 13–21
Jung et al., 2014 [24]	µ-RS	GCF	0, 1, 7, 28	10	range 18–23 mean 20.8 ± 2.5
Camerlingo et al., 2015 [25]	µ-RS	GCF	0/28	3	range 13–26
D'Apuzzo et al., 2017 [26]	µ-RS/SERS	GCF	0, 2, 7, 14	18	range 13–22
Portaccio et al., 2019 [27]	FT-IR	GCF	0, 2, 7, 14	18	range 12–22
Perillo et al., 2020 [28]	µ-RS	PDL	0, 2, 7, 14	11	range 11–24 mean 19.9 ± 4.7
Camerlingo et al., 2020 [29]	µ-RS/FT-IR	PDL	0	3	range 13–22

2.2. Sample Selection

In the studies here considered, the patients were selected according to the following criteria: (1) young subjects, between 11 and 18 years, and adults over 18 years of age with dental malocclusion needing orthodontic treatment; (2) patients treated with any type of orthodontic force application through fixed appliances; (3) patients without treatment were assumed as controls. GCF and PDL samples were collected from these patients at different time intervals of OTM (Figure 1). The GCF was collected from each patient before bracket bonding (T0), and after 1 or 2 (T1), 7 (T2), and 14 or 28 (T3) days of treatment [24–27]. As showed in Figure 1, paper points were inserted into the gingival crevice for about 30 s, then placed into Eppendorf PCR Tubes and stored in a $-80\ °C$ refrigerator before analysis. Specifically, for µ-RS measurements, the paper points were directly examined without any other treatment [25,26], whereas for SERS and FT-IR measurements, 10 µL of distilled water was added in the tubes that were vortexed and then centrifuged [26,27].

The PDL was scarified from the root of extracted premolars using a one-way lancet after surgery, immediately fixed in 4% paraformaldehyde and stored in ethanol solutions until analysis (Figure 1) [23,27].

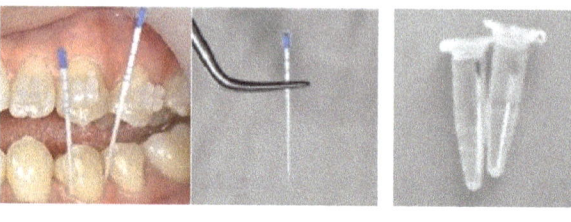
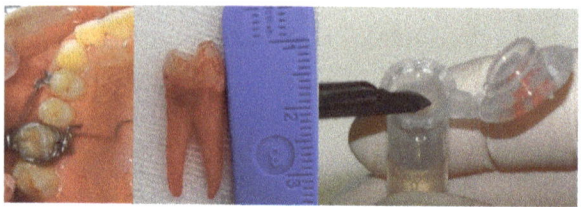

Figure 1. Collection of GCF (line above) and PDL (line below) samples. (Photographs taken at the Orthodontic Program of the University of Campania *Luigi Vanvitelli*).

2.3. Experimental Techniques

2.3.1. Raman Spectroscopy

Raman spectroscopy is considered an effective tool to determine the structure and the chemical composition of materials considering the vibrations of molecules. This technique enables acquiring vibrational spectra of samples by analyzing scattered light due to monochromatic laser excitation [12]. When the laser light beam hits the tissue, it is partly absorbed and partly transmitted or reflected by the sample at the same wavelength of the incident light. Besides, there is a little component that has a wavelength slightly differing from the incident one of a quantity reflecting the typical vibrational modes of the analyzed substance. In biological tissues, the molecular contribution to Raman scattering is mainly related to vibrational transitions which force a molecule to make a transition from a state of vibrational energy E1 to another state E2 (see Reference [30] and References [2–5] therein). Absorption by atoms or molecules occurs only if the difference in energy ΔE is less than or equal to the quantum photon energy $h\upsilon$: $\Delta E = E2 - E1 \leq h\upsilon$, where υ is the light frequency and h the Planck constant.

As shown in Figure 2, an incident photon collides with a molecule that can be either in the fundamental state or in an excited vibrational state. If the impact is of an elastic type, the diffused photon has exactly the same energy and wavelength of that incident (scattering Rayleigh) not altering the energy state of the molecule. On the other hand, if the impact is inelastic (Raman scattering), the diffused photon may have less energy (and consequently less frequency and longer wavelength) or greater energy (higher frequency and shorter wavelength) than the incident photon. The scattered photon has a frequency different from the one of the incident photon due to the lost or gain in energy from a particular vibrational mode of the molecule.

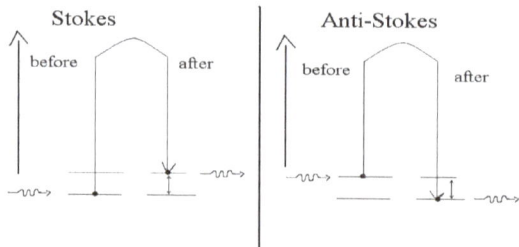

Figure 2. Stokes and Anti-Stokes mechanisms of the Raman scattering.

In the Raman spectrum, lower frequency photons give rise to Stokes lines, whereas higher frequency photons are known as Anti-Stokes lines (Figure 2). Usually, the Anti-Stokes lines have small or negligible intensity compared to the Stokes ones, because the population of the excited states is smaller than the one of the fundamental states.

Raman spectroscopy can offer information on the spatial distributions of organic and inorganic compounds in a sample with a spatial resolution of about 1 μm. Furthermore, Raman spectra exhibit little interference with water, making this technique highly convenient for studying many biological specimens, in vivo too. In Figure 3, a schematic representation of a μ-RS experimental setup is reported. This set up has been used for investigating PDL and CGF samples in References [23,25,26,28,29], and it is equipped with a Helium-Neon laser as a light source, coupled to a 50× optical objective. The Raman signal is dispersed by a grating of 1800 grooves/mm and collected by a liquid N_2 cooled couple charge detector (CCD), then the data are acquired using a dedicated software.

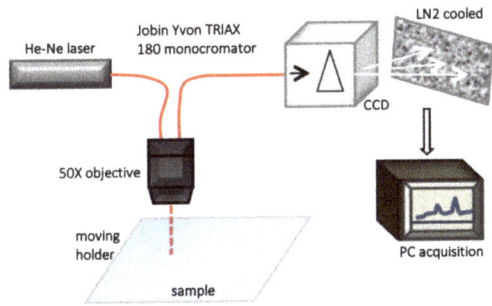

Figure 3. Schematic representation of a micro-Raman spectroscopy experimental setup.

2.3.2. Surface-Enhanced Raman Scattering (SERS)

To enlarge the applicability of Raman techniques on biological tissues and fluids, it is possible to amplify the signal coming from the samples thanks to the Surface Enhanced Raman Spectroscopy (SERS, also named as Surface-Enhanced Raman Scattering). SERS is a vibrational spectroscopy technique that exploits the intensity amplification of Raman signal by metallic nanostructures or metal nanoparticles. At the beginning SERS was adopted to the study of dilute aqueous solutions of a rather simple system such as small molecules or molecular ions, recent nanotechnology, and photonics developments stimulated the application of SERS to more complex bio-systems such as macromolecules, cells, tissues, and bio-fluids. Qualitative and quantitative detection of one or more analytes with SERS can be achieved in a direct or indirect way [31]: in the direct approach (label-free SERS) the spectroscopic signal is due to all those analytes which adsorb on the SERS substrate, whereas in the indirect approach the signal results form a specific SERS label that binds to a target analyte of the sample (see Figure 4). SERS enhancement factor is a very significant parameter in SERS, and it is used for quantifying the overall signal enhancement. To experimentally evaluate SERS enhancement factor measurements of the SERS intensity for the adsorbed molecule on the metal surface, relative to the normal Raman intensity of the "free" molecule in solution are required. The enhancement factor can assume values from 10^{10} to 10^{11}, which allows detecting single molecules.

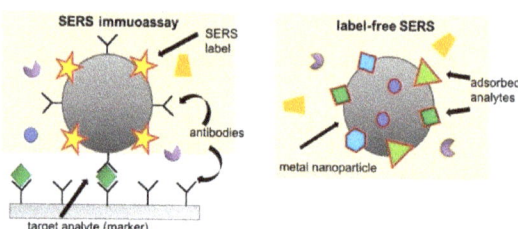

Figure 4. Graphic representation of the two approaches for SERS: the indirect approach (SERS immunoassay) on the left and the direct approach (label-free SERS) on the right.

2.3.3. Infrared Spectroscopy

Fourier Transform Infra-Red (FT-IR) spectroscopy is a technique based on the analysis of the spectral IR radiation absorbed by a sample. The energy of IR radiation absorbed corresponds to the energy necessary to the transition between vibrational states of the functional groups. Thus, the spectral intensity of the radiation absorbed by different biochemical bonds within a sample gives rise to the spectrum of IR absorption characteristic, which comprised several peaks or bands, each referred to a particular mode of vibration characteristic of functional groups in the sample [32].

The main component of FT-IR set-up is an interferometer (Michelson's interferometer) which replaces the monochromator of the traditional IR spectrometer model. It is a modern and powerful optical method for collecting absorption spectra in the infrared field by obtaining qualitative information on the structure of the compounds analyzed, as well as, by means of modern software algorithms, also quantitative data. A FT-IR system separates and recombines a light beam leading the recombined light beam to produces an interference pattern dependent on wavelength or interferogram. In particular, the interferometer (Figure 5) consists of a fixed mirror, a moving mirror forming an angle of 90° with the first one, and a beam splitter mirror which is placed at an angle of 45° with respect to the incident beam. The energy of the beam coming from the source is incident on the splitter and comes from this collimated and divided into two perpendicular rays of equal intensity: one reflecting along a path directed to the fixed mirror, and the other passing the splitter and transmitted to the moving mirror. The first ray is reflected by the fixed mirror again on the splitter, from where it is partially returned to the source and partially transmitted and focused on the detector. On the other hand, the moving mirror slides forward parallel to itself along the other branch of the optical path, continuously modifying the distance between it and the splitter, it reflects the other ray on the splitter from different distances and so also this ray is partially returned to the source and partly reflected towards the detector. The energy reaching the detector is therefore the algebraic sum of the two rays, which is switched from the same detector into an electrical signal, which is amplified and represented by an interferogram. The sample to be investigated is placed between the two arms of the interferometer, the frequencies that correspond to the excitation of vibrational states of functional groups of the molecules of the sample are attenuated and the obtained interferogram is converted into the traditional absorption spectrum through the Fourier Transform.

Some practical advantages offered by the use of FT-IR spectroscopy include a minor dispersion of energy, thus, greater energy reaching the detector; time-saving ability to collect spectra in a very short time, since with the FT-IR all frequencies and wavelengths are simultaneously analyzed and recorded by the detector; high precision and accuracy in the discrimination of wavenumbers with the possibility to superimpose the monochrome radiation of a laser source of known frequency as internal standard; finally, the possibility to obtain spectra from a very wide range of samples at any temperature (the source is sufficiently far from the sample and therefore there is no heating effect of the sample) and pressure with appropriate devices and accessories. Moreover, FT-IR spectroscopy can be equipped with a microscope to allow the microscopic analysis of samples or parts of samples up to one micron in size.

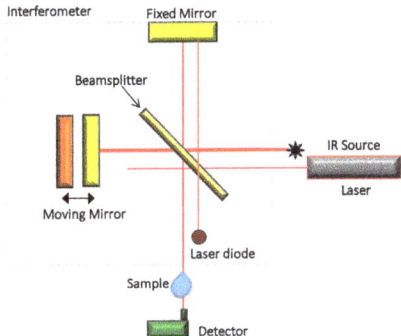

Figure 5. Schematic image of a Fourier-Transform Infrared spectrometer.

2.3.4. Complementarity of Raman and Infrared Spectroscopies

Raman and infrared spectroscopies are chemical analytical methods that provide spectra that contain signals from the functional groups in the sample. Both these techniques are usually coupled to a microscopic approach for biological sample analysis, they are non-destructive, non-invasive, and not time-consuming. These techniques usually require simple or no special preparation procedures for the sample in comparison with the conventional biological methods of analysis. IR measures the light absorption by specific molecules using a broadband light source, the Raman technique measures the characteristics of Raman emission induced from molecules under monochromatic laser irradiation. It is important to underline that FT-IR and Raman spectroscopy are complementary techniques because the bands in FT-IR spectra are due to polar functional groups while the bands in Raman spectra are due to non-polar functional groups. Thus, the use of both the described vibrational spectroscopies is suggested to detect all the qualitative and quantitative information of the samples included in the study.

2.4. Data Analysis

The signal intensity of the spectroscopy response of biomaterials is usually relatively weak, especially in the case of Raman spectroscopy. Moreover, fluorescence mechanisms can often occur affecting the insight of spectral data. Numerical data treatments are generally used for subtracting background spurious signal and decrease the uncorrelated noise component [33–35]. Numerical data processing for removing background signals from the Raman spectra are exhaustively reviewed in Reference [36]. A numerical filtering process based on wavelet algorithms has been also developed for both remove the background signal and improve the signal/noise level [23,24,26,37]. By using special scaled functions, named "wavelets", the method allows a decomposition of the experimental spectrum in components with increasing spectral detail, the provides the basis of a filter bank algorithm able to attenuate both high-frequency signal components (noise) and low-frequency components (smooth background signal). The detail of the method implementation is reported in Camerlingo et al. 2006 [37].

A normalization of the data, with respect to the signal intensity, is also demanding to compare different spectra. Different criteria can be used for this purpose, choosing as normalization reference the intensity of a fixed mode [24] or the total area of the spectral signal or the square standard deviation of data, with respect to the mean intensity value [23,26,28].

Similarities between spectra acquired from analogous samples in equivalent experimental conditions, and differences between spectra from samples collected in different stages of orthodontic treatment can be evidenced by a univariate analysis. A comparison between the intensity of one value of a spectrum and the corresponding value of another spectrum collected from another sample was performed by using a linear regression or univariate analysis of data. This analysis offers a numerical coefficient that spans from 0 for uncorrelated data, to 1 for perfect linear dependence [27].

The deconvolution of the spectrum in elemental components allows to individuate the main modes occurring. Typically, Lorentzian functions were used for modeling Raman spectra, while Gaussian and mixed Gaussian-Lorentzian functions are more indicated in the case of FT-IR spectra and for broad Raman mode components. Their spectral positions, intensities, and widths were evaluated by a fitting procedure. In some case, mainly for FT-IR data, the second derivative of the spectrum is also performed to preliminarily evaluate the local minima which correspond to the vibrational modes [38].

For classification of Raman spectra from PDL sample a multivariate analysis was also adopted. Principal component analysis (PCA) is particularly adequate for analyzing Raman spectra of complex biological samples. The spectral data are decomposed by using a mathematical procedure that decreases the data dimensions to a smaller number of scores and principal components (PC) that give the most important information of the spectra. PCA can be performed not on all the investigated spectral region but only on properly selected intervals, in this case interval-PCA (i-PCA) is executed [26].

3. Results and Discussion

In five of the selected studies, samples were collected before and after 2, 7, and 14 days of OTM [23,26–28], in one after 1, 7, and 28 days [24] and in another only after 28 days [25]. The main Raman modes were identified by the centers of the Lorentzian components evaluated by fitting the spectroscopy data [39] and are reported in Table 2 for PDL and in Table 3 for GCF samples, together with their assignments.

Table 2. μ-RS and FT-IR main peak assignments for PDL samples References [23,28,29,39].

Assignment Mode	Peak Position Raman (cm^{-1})				Peak Position FT-IR (cm^{-1})			
	0	2	7	14	0	2	7	14
PO_2^- asymmetric stretching C-O-P stretching					1239			
Amide III (β-sheet)	1243	1245	1247	1252				
Amide III (random coil)	1258	1265	1266	1273				
Amide III (α-helix)	1309	1307	1310	1307				
CH_2	1450				1455			
Amide II					1544			
Amide I (3_{10}-helix; β-sheet)	1617	1619	1618	1621	1631			
Amide I (α-helix)	1642	1643	1641	1642	1650			
Amide I (β-turn)	1668	1662	1661	1666	1661			
Amide I (β-sheet)	1695	1687	1690	1695	1673			
CH_2 asymmetric stretching	2875				2926			
CH_3 symmetric stretching	2930				2873			
CH_3 asymmetric stretching	2970				2960			

Table 3. μ-RS, SERS, and FT-IR spectroscopy peak position and assignments for GCF samples References [24–27,39].

Assignment Mode	Peak Position SERS (cm^{-1})				Peak Position Raman (cm^{-1})				Peak Position FT-IR (cm^{-1})			
	0	2	7	14	0	2	7	14	0	2	7	14
S–S bond stretching	465											
Phenylalanine	621											
Tyrosine	825											
Deoxyribose bending CO$_2$H of tyrosine	895								897			
PO$_4^{3-}$	946											
PO$_4^{3-}$ ν1 symmetric stretching, apatite					984	985	986	986				
C–H bending phenylalanine	1007				1002							
C–O stretching of carbohydrates									1039	1038	1035	1039
symmetric PO$_2^-$ stretching of nucleic acids									1087	1087	1067	1092
Nucleic acid base PO$_2^-$					1100	1100						
C–O asymmetric stretching and COH bending of lipids									1160	1158	1158	1158
Cytochrome					1167	1167	1167					
Nucleic acid C–N	1176				1176							
Amide III	1242	1242	1242									
PO$_2^-$ asymmetric stretching of nucleic acids									1253	1255	1254	1253
Amide III, CH$_2$ deformation	1276				1280							
CH$_2$/CH$_3$ twisted									1311	1314	1313	1308
Adenine/guanine of nucleic acids	1348	1348	1348		1345	1345	1345					
symmetric bending of CH$_3$ of nucleic acids									1376	1361	1388	1384
Cytochrome			1390									
COO– stretching of aminoacids									1424	1419	1415	1423
CH$_3$ symmetric stretching CH$_2$ lipids/proteins scissoring										1462	1459	
CH$_2$	1470											
Carotene					1540	1540						
Amide II (N–H bending of proteins)									1547	1539	1545	1548
Amide II/cytochrome	1577				1575	1577	1577	1577				
C=C stretching of amino acids									1598	1594	1598	1596

Table 3. *Cont.*

Assignment Mode	Peak Position SERS (cm^{-1})				Peak Position Raman (cm^{-1})				Peak Position FT-IR (cm^{-1})			
	0	2	7	14	0	2	7	14	0	2	7	14
Amide I (β-sheet)					1625	1625	1611					
Amide I (α-helix)	1641				1640	1640						
C=O stretching of proteins (Amide I band)									1656	1650	1655	1655
CH$_3$ symmetric stretching of lipids									2873	2880	2877	2881
CH$_2$ asymmetric stretching of lipids									2927	2930	2929	2916
CH$_3$ asymmetric stretching of lipids									2974	2981	2984	2937
NH stretching of Amide A OH stretching									3356	3357	3359	3365

3.1. Periodontal Ligament Analysis

3.1.1. μ-RS Results

Camerlingo et al. 2014 [23] and Perillo et al. 2020 [28] assessed the changes of PDL from premolars that were extracted from patients under OTM by using the difference observed in Raman spectra collected after 2, 7, and 14 days of orthodontic treatment. In Figure 6, a representative Raman spectrum (a) obtained by averaging all the spectra from the control PDL samples is reported together with the average spectra of the PDL samples after 2 (b), 7 (c), and 14 days (d) of in vivo ~0.5 N force application. In these spectra, the regions related to Amide I and CH$_3$/CH$_2$ bands were prevalent. The contributions at 1600–1700 cm^{-1} (Amide I mode) and 1200–1300 cm^{-1} (Amide III mode) were attributed to protein vibrations and the broadband at 2930 cm^{-1} was due to the CH$_2$/CH$_3$ bond vibrations. A further Raman mode, at about 1450 cm^{-1} is characteristic of CH$_2$ scissoring Raman mode and protein components.

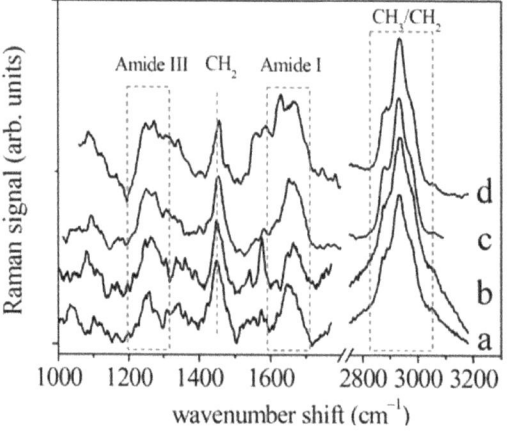

Figure 6. Raman spectra of PDL samples from premolars extracted (**a**) before, (**b**) after 2 days, (**c**) 7, and (**d**) 14 days of orthodontic treatment. Protein and CH$_2$/CH$_3$ contributions were indicated. (Reprinted with permission from Perillo et al., 2020 under Open Access conditions).

The Amide I spectral region of a PDL control sample (Figure 7) presented different components that are usually correlated to the secondary structure of the protein. More in detail, the mode at 1645–1650 cm^{-1} was assigned to the α-helix component dominated the band. The further peaks at about 1620, 1668, and 1680 cm^{-1} were related to β-sheet or collagen 3$_{10}$-helix, β-turn, and β-sheet secondary structure conformations, respectively (see Table 2).

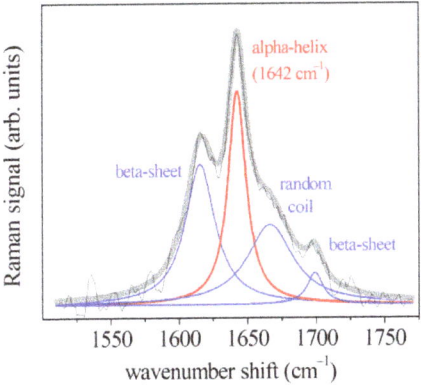

Figure 7. Deconvolution of the average Raman spectrum of PDL in the region of Amide I. This spectrum was evaluated by averaging the Raman spectra of samples collected before OTM. Red and blue lines indicate the α-helix component and the other main components of the Raman band, respectively. (Reprinted with permission from Perillo et al., 2020 under Open Access conditions).

By comparing the Amide I regions of spectra from samples collected at different times, it was possible to notice many changes in the peak centers (in cm^{-1}) of the modes above mentioned (see Table 2). In particular, the intensity of the α-helix Raman mode and the whole Amide I band lowered with respect to the same contributions in control PDL Raman spectra [23,28]. The other components of Amide I band enlarged and increased their intensity in comparison with the α-helix mode. To note, the α-helix mode can be considered as a hierarchical structure in which are present H–bonds at the higher molecular level originated from individual hydrogen (H) bonds. The α-helix is characterized a single-stranded conformation with a spring-like protein structure with 3-4 H–bonds per turn. In the case of collagen, a particular triple helix configuration is considered for α-helix. This structural arrangement is the most effective bond arrangement for ensuring the thermodynamic and mechanical stability together with high elasticity and large deformation capacity. A partially unfolded α-helix structure with a combination of broken and intact H–bonds along the filament axis can be associated to the β-sheet structure. The most relevant changes were observed in Raman spectra after 48 h of tooth movement while they were quite recovered on day 7 of PDL collection. When a strain is applied to the tissue, a stress necessary for the beginning of a modification of the α-helix structure or transformation from the α-helix to the β-sheet conformation, is caused by the above-discussed unfolding-refolding processes, that induces a hydrogen relocation, and an increase in disorder [28].

The Raman spectra of the CH_3/CH_2 modes for PDL samples collected before (a), and after 2 (b), 7 (c), and 14 days (d) of the orthodontic force application are reported in Figure 8.

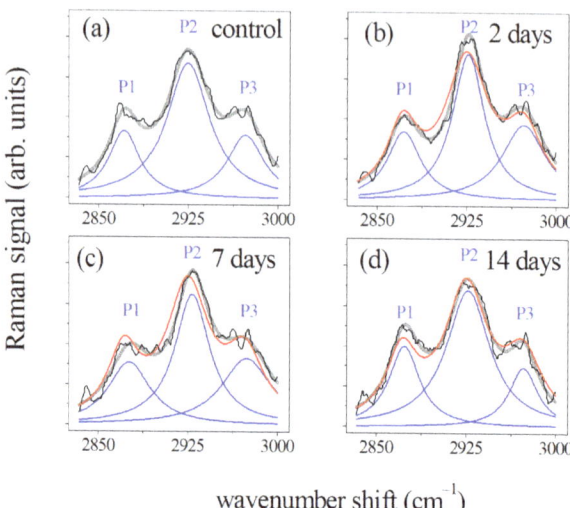

Figure 8. Deconvolution of the average Raman spectra of PDL samples collected before (**a**) and after (**b**) 2, (**c**) 7, and (**d**) 14 days of OTM in the 2800–3000 cm^{-1} spectral region. Black lines indicated the measured spectra and blue lines are related to the main P1, P2, and P3 Lorentzian components of the Raman band. Fit of the experimental data resulting from the deconvolution process are indicated by gray lines. All the band areas were normalized to 1. In the (**b**–**d**) panels the spectra were compared with the Raman response (red line) of the control of (**a**) panel. (Reprinted with permission from Perillo et al., 2020 under Open Access conditions).

These average spectra were normalized according to the procedure previously described and presented a large and predominant peak at 2930 cm^{-1}. This feature is typically attributed to CH$_3$ symmetric stretching vibration. The other two peaks located at 2875 cm^{-1} (P1) and 2970 cm^{-1} (P3), were also assigned to C–H bond modes, in particular, to CH$_2$ asymmetric and CH$_3$ asymmetric stretching modes, respectively [28,38]. The quantitative analysis of these data (see Reference [28]) shown that the intensity of P1 and P2 peaks initially increased after 2 days of force application, then decreased after 7 days of treatment and after manifested an increase after two weeks of force application. A different behavior was noticed for the P3 peak after 14 days of OTM.

3.1.2. FT-IR Results

In Figure 9, an average infrared spectrum acquired from PDL samples collected before OTM is reported. In this Figure also the results of the deconvolution procedure performed by using Lorentzian–Gaussian curves is shown.

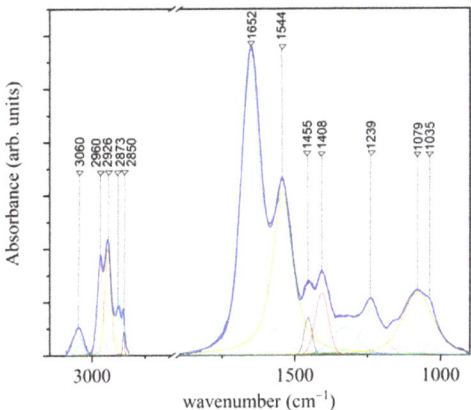

Figure 9. Representative FT-IR spectrum of PDL in the 3100–1000 cm^{-1} with the deconvolution analysis of peaks with Lorentzian–Gaussian curves (blue line: experimental curve). (Reprinted with permission from Camerlingo et al., 2020).

The main features of the spectrum and the related assignments are reported in Table 2. The region associated to C–H bonds in the region 3100–2800 cm^{-1} is mainly related to collagen contribution that has been also evidenced by SEM micrographs [29] and to a lesser extent to lipid content. In the 1750 to 1000 cm^{-1} spectral range, the band at 1656 cm^{-1} is related to the C=O stretching of Amide I (Table 2). By evaluating the subcomponents of the Amide I band, a characterization of the secondary structure of protein component can be obtained. As shown in Figure 10, the deconvolution of this region (1750–1580 cm^{-1}) evidences the presence of different subcomponents. The contribution at 1673 cm^{-1} is attributed to β-turn subcomponent, the ones at 1661 and 1650 cm^{-1} are assigned to the α-helix subcomponent, and the features at 1639 and 1631 cm^{-1} are due to β-sheets contributions.

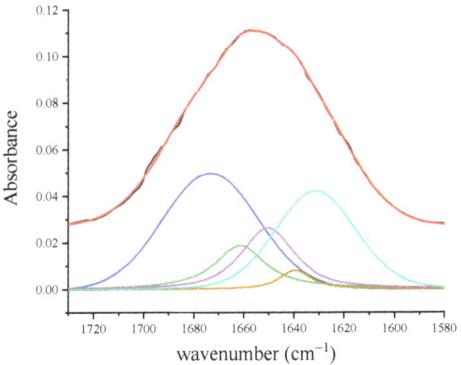

Figure 10. Spectrum of PDL in the Amide I region (1710–1580 cm^{-1}) (black line). Colored lines indicate the different contributions obtained by the deconvolution analysis of peaks using Lorentzian–Gaussian curves. Fit of the experimental data resulting from the deconvolution process is indicated by the red line. (Reprinted with permission from Portaccio et al., 2019).

3.2. Gingival Crevicular Fluid Analysis

3.2.1. SERS Results

Typical SERS spectra with the principal vibrational modes, obtained from GCF samples in the 1000 to 1800 cm^{-1} range before (T0) and after (T1, T2 and T3) the application of an orthodontic force, are reported in Figure 11. The attention was focused on 1000 to

1700 cm^{-1} wavenumber range and on the five main modes at about 1176, 1276, 1348, 1577, and 1641 cm^{-1}. The mode at 1176 cm^{-1} can be attributed to the nucleic acid base C–N. The peaks at 1242 and 1276 cm^{-1} can be due to different components of Amide III (α-helix or β-sheet) and the 1276 cm^{-1} peak may also indicate a contribution from CH$_2$ deformation mode. The structure present at 1348 cm^{-1} can be attributed to adenine and guanine of nucleic acids. The small peak at 1470 cm^{-1} is due to CH$_2$, the one at 1577 cm^{-1} which can be related to Amide II and cytochrome, and the large structure at 1641 cm^{-1} is typical of protein spectra and is related to Amide I (see Table 3). As done for PDL, GCF samples from untreated case (T0) and after 2 (T1), 7 (T2) and 14 (T3) days of OTM have been considered. From T0 to T1 of OTM, the intensity of Raman mode at 1276 cm^{-1} decreases, whereas the Amide I band intensity increases in T1 and decreases in the subsequent T2 and T3 stages (see Figure 11). This behavior can be ascribed to changes in protein concentration.

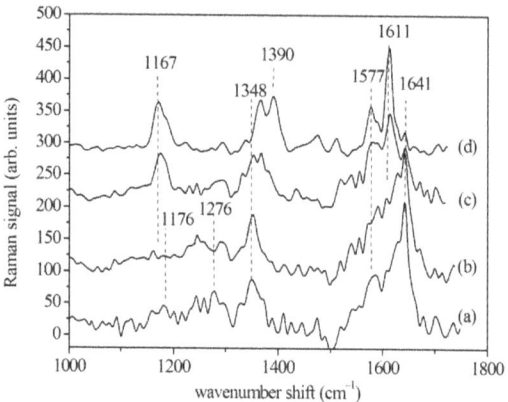

Figure 11. SERS spectra of GCF samples collected before (T0), after 2 (T1), after 7 (T2), and 14 days (T3) the beginning of the OTM. For facilitating the visual inspection, the spectra are arbitrarily shifted along the vertical axis. (Reprinted with permission from d'Apuzzo et al., 2017).

More detailed information can be obtained also in this case from the Amide I band deconvolution (Figure 12). During the OTM, the center of the Amide I band moves toward shorter wavenumber shifts, specifically for T2 and T3 spectra. These changes are related to the decrease in the α-helix subcomponent (located around 1640 cm^{-1}) and the increase in the β-sheet subcomponent (located in the range between 1610 and 1625 cm^{-1}). The percentage of α-helix subcomponent to the Amide I band was evaluated by estimating the ratio of areas of the α-helix peak and the whole Amide I band, and it is shown in Figure 12b for the different stages of the OTM. The present results of the

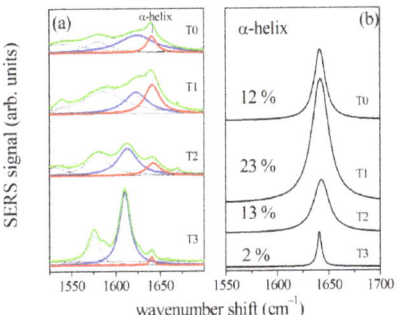

Figure 12. (a) Amide I region of SERS spectra of GCF samples collected from an 18-year-old patient before (T0) the beginning of the OTM, (T1), (T2), and (T3) refer to samples collected after 2, 7, and 14 days after, respectively. Black lines indicate the experimental data that are fitted by a convolution of Lorentzian peaks indicated by green lines. The main components are also plotted using colored lines. Red and blue lines indicate the α-helix and the β-sheet components, respectively. (b) The α-helix component at T0, T1, T2, and T3 stages. Percentage value of the α-helix area normalized to the whole amide I band area is reported for each plot. (Reprinted with permission from d'Apuzzo et al., 2017).

Amide I contributions at the different stages are not in complete agreement with the results reported by Jung et al. [24]. This could be ascribed to different modalities in GCF sampling and to the different days of collection.

3.2.2. μ-RS Results

The μ-Raman analysis was performed on the GCF paper points without any sample manipulation in order to develop an effective approach for monitoring the processes occurring during OTMs. The Raman spectra of the GCF collected using paper cones showed similar features observed in the SERS spectrum above (see Table 3). Much information was obtained by analyzing the 1500 to 1750 cm^{-1} region where the Amide I band is located. In agreement with the SERS results, also μ-RS results show that the center of the band moved toward shorter wavenumber shifts in the days after the beginning of the treatment. As said before these results are not in complete agreement with the outcomes reported by Jung et al. [24] (see Figure 13). This discrepancy cold be due to different modalities in experimental procedure.

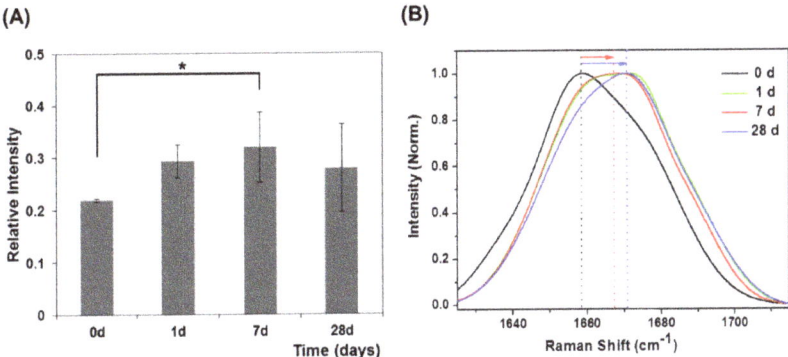

Figure 13. (**A**) Relative intensities in 1667 cm^{-1} Raman peaks during OTM. * Significantly different from day 0 ($p < 0.05$, one-way ANOVA with Turkey's Honest Significance Difference (HSD) post-hoc procedure). (**B**) Normalized average GCF Raman spectra in the 1625–1715 cm^{-1} range during OTM. (Reprinted from Jung et al. 2014 under Open Access conditions).

Jung et al. [24] reported also the results of a ratiometric analysis of Raman spectra collected at different times after starting OTM. As an example, in Figure 14 the intensity ratio between the hydroxyapatite to primarily collagen-dominated matrix band is reported. The values of this ratio indicate significant changes in the amount of mineralization. In particular, hydroxyapatite and collagen ratios decreased at day 7 ($p < 0.05$), indicating a decrease in the mineralization due to a reduction in hydroxyapatite content during the alveolar bone remodeling process. Other intensity ratios able to give interesting information are the ones related to carbonate/Amide I and carbonate apatite/hydroxyapatite bands, also reported in Reference [24].

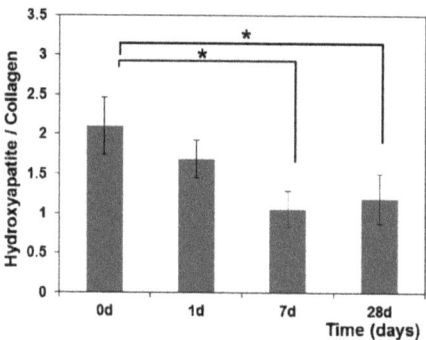

Figure 14. Hydroxyapatite to collagen ratio in GCF during OTM. * Significantly different from day 0 ($p < 0.05$, one-way ANOVA with Turkey's HSD post-hoc procedure). (Reprinted from Jung et al., 2014 under Open Access conditions).

To calculate the percentage of success in matching peak assignments in Raman spectra with the OTM time points, a multivariate analysis (i-PCA) showed that the OTM stage was exactly recovered in 98% of Raman spectra with 100% of correct assignment for T0 and T2 spectra and 92% of T1 spectra. Some T1 spectra were incorrectly assigned as T0 [26]. Thus, the use of Raman spectroscopy and multivariate analysis of GCF spectra can enable to recognize the exact time point of the OTM. This innovative approach might be useful for the clinician for choosing the type of treatment for each patient and speed up and make progress in the orthodontic therapy.

3.2.3. FT-IR Results

FT-IR spectra were preliminarily analyzed using the univariate analysis briefly described in Section 2.3. Such univariate analysis was used to evaluate any correspondences in spectra from samples in the similar experimental conditions and any differences between spectra from GCF samples at different OTM timepoints [27]. The average spectra between 3800 and 800 cm^{-1} for GCF samples before (T0) and after 2 (T1), 7 (T2), and 14 (T3) days of orthodontic treatment are reported in Figures 15 and 16, respectively.

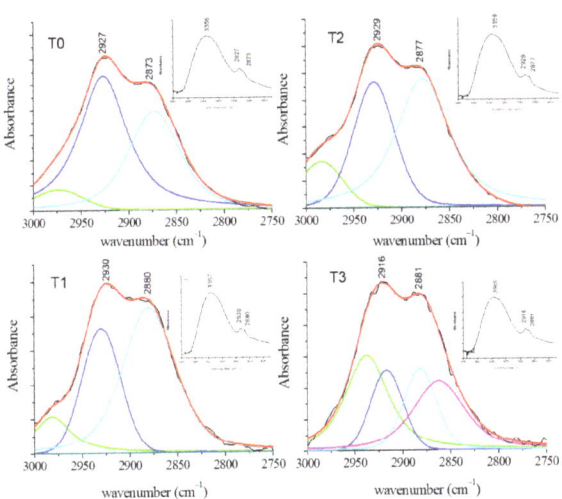

Figure 15. Average FT-IR spectra of GCF samples obtained from patients before (T0) and during OTM in the 3000–2750 cm^{-1} spectral region (black lines). The deconvolution analysis of peaks with Gaussian–Lorentzian curves is shown by colored lines. Red lines indicated the fitted spectra. (Reprinted with permission from Portaccio et al., 2019).

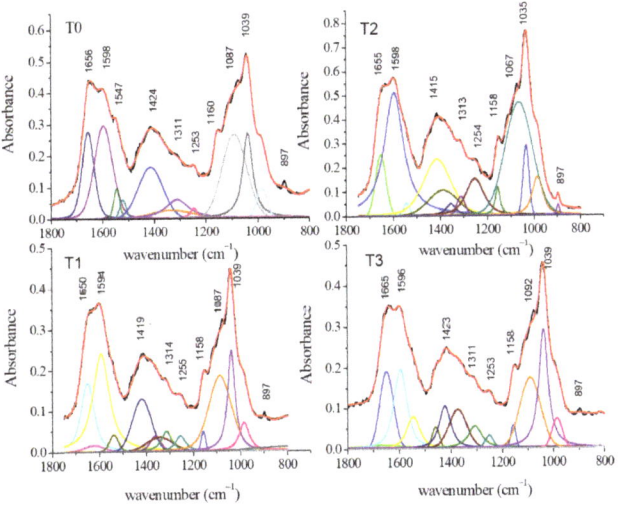

Figure 16. Average FT-IR spectra of GCF samples obtained from patients before (T0) and during OTM in the 1800–800 cm^{-1} spectral region (black lines). The deconvolution analysis of peaks with Gaussian-Lorentzian curves is shown by colored lines. Red lines indicated the fitted spectra. (Reprinted with permission from Portaccio et al., 2019).

The 3000–2800 cm^{-1} region is particularly relevant due to the presence of different features related to lipid contents. GCF samples at T1, T2, and T3 showed several modifications due to shifts of the different contributions over time (Figure 15). In particular, the peaks at 2927 and 2870 cm^{-1} can be assigned to CH_2 antisymmetric and CH_3 symmetric stretching, respectively (see Table 3). Thanks to the deconvolution procedure it is possible to evidence a third small component centered at 2974 cm^{-1} that can be due to antisymmetric CH_3 stretching mode of lipids. The average FT-IR spectra in the 1750–800 cm^{-1}

region for GCF samples at different stages of OTM were reported in Figure 16. Visual inspection of the spectra evidenced the presence of some relevant contributions. In T0 spectrum, the band at 1656 cm^{-1} is assigned to the C–O stretching of Amide I. The peak at 1598 cm^{-1} can be assigned to C=C stretching of amino acids. Other two important peaks are located at 1424 and 1039 cm^{-1} and they can be ascribed to COO- stretching of amino acids and to C–O stretching of glucose, respectively. In addition, some small contributions are positioned at 1311, 1160, and 897 cm^{-1} and they are assigned to CH_2 twist of lipids and amino acids, antisymmetric C–O stretching and COH_2 bending of lipids, and C–O stretching of glucose, respectively. Analogous contributions are also evident in the spectra of GCF samples collected in T1, T2, and T3 stages. The above-described deconvolution procedure permits to evidence other spectral features in Figure 16. This analysis for T0 spectrum shows other contributions at 1547 cm^{-1} due to the N–H bending of Amide II and at 1376 cm^{-1} due to symmetric bending of CH_3 of nucleic acids. The deconvolution procedure manifests also the presence of features located at 1253 and 1087 cm^{-1} ascribed to antisymmetric and symmetric PO_2^- stretching of nucleic acids, respectively. At 984 cm^{-1} is also present a contribution due to C–O and C=C stretching mode of amino acids. Moreover, in this region, some peaks are characterized by a wavenumber shift. For Amide I and II, these shifts are a signature of changes in the protein secondary structure. In Table 3, the spectral features present in the wavenumber regions here examined are reported for the different stages of the OTM, together with their assignments. Conformational changes and rearrangements of existing proteins, lipids, and nucleic acid structures are evidenced by the above-mentioned changes in the FT-IR spectra according to expectances because OTM induces inflammatory processes and changes in several pro-inflammatory cytokines (i.e., IL-6, IL-1, IL-1ß) enzymes (i.e., alkaline/acid phosphatase), and metabolites (i.e., prostaglandins E2) concentrations [2,40]. The results obtained by FT-IR spectroscopy agree also with the ones obtained by Raman spectroscopies [23,24,27].

4. Conclusions and Implications for Research and Practice

The vibrational spectroscopies described in this research can be considered the techniques of choice in comparison with other methodologies thanks to the ability to monitor vibrational contributions from the molecules in biofluids and fibers. Thus, it is possible to assert the innovative potential role that Raman and FT-IR spectroscopies can play in orthodontics, but more generally in dental sciences, in the evaluation and monitoring of periodontium during different clinical conditions. The analyses of GCF and PDL samples through the vibrational spectra showed similar results in terms of biochemical changes over time during the first weeks of OTM, as demonstrated by previous studies using other analytical techniques. In particular, the analysis of µ-RS directly performed on paper points impregnated of GCF, easily and quickly collected during the orthodontic appointment, is a potential appealing methodology, noticeably less expensive and less laboratory-based in comparison to other analytical techniques described in the literature.

Limitations of this study are the inclusion of a limited number of studies and a small number of patients (a total of about 63) that may be enlarged to get more evidence. Thus, the work until done in this field may be considered as a starting point for future prospective cohort studies with a wider sample using different typologies of orthodontic appliances (i.e., removable vs. fixed) assessed with vibrational spectroscopies and comparing the outcomes with other analytical methodologies and a greater interest in these optical techniques would be beneficial for dental and orthodontic research field.

This research field could be a novel step for the development, in the near future, of a vibrational spectroscopy-based non-invasive, accurate, and reliable test. Clinical implications may be found both for diagnosis and clinical purposes in specific type of patients presenting different pathological conditions (i.e., bony defects, arthritis) before starting treatment and for monitoring the status of periodontal tissues during orthodontic tooth movement by GCF collection repeated overtime. This may help the clinician in the choice of the proper type of force application on teeth individually for each patient with the final aim of improving treatment outcomes and even accelerating its overall duration.

Author Contributions: Conceptualization F.d., G.I., and M.L.; methodology, C.C., I.D., L.N., and M.P.; software, C.C., I.D., and M.L.; validation, G.I., G.M., and L.N.; investigation, C.C., I.D., I.S., and M.P.; writing—original draft preparation, F.d. and M.L.; writing—review and editing, F.d., G.I., and M.L. All authors have read and agreed to the published version of the manuscript.

Funding: This research received no external funding.

Data Availability Statement: The data presented in this study are available on request from the corresponding author.

Conflicts of Interest: The authors declare no conflict of interest.

References

1. Dolce, C.; Malone, J.S.; Wheeler, T.T. Current concepts in the biology of orthodontic tooth movement. *Semin. Orthod.* **2002**, *8*, 6–12. [CrossRef]
2. Krishnan, V.; Davidovitch, Z. Cellular, molecular, and tissue-level reactions to orthodontic force. *Am. J. Orthod. Dentofac. Orthop.* **2006**, *129*, 469.e1–469.e32. [CrossRef]
3. Proffit, W.R.; Fields, H.W., Jr.; Larso, B.; Sarver, D.M. *Contemporary Orthodontics*, 6th ed.; Elsevier Inc.: Philadelphia, PA, USA, 2018.
4. Anastasi, G.; Cordasco, G.; Matarese, G.; Rizzo, G.; Nucera, R.; Mazza, M.; Militi, A.; Portelli, M.; Cutroneo, G.; Favaloro, A. An immunohistochemical, histological, and electron-microscopic study of the human periodontal ligament during orthodontic treatment. *Int. J. Mol. Med.* **2008**, *21*, 545–554. [CrossRef] [PubMed]
5. Fleissig, O.; Reichenberg, E.; Tal, M.; Redlich, M.; Barkana, I.; Palmon, A. Morphologic and gene expression analysis of periodontal ligament fibroblasts subjected to pressure. *Am. J. Orthod. Dentofac. Orthop.* **2018**, *154*, 664–676. [CrossRef] [PubMed]
6. Li, Y.; Jacox, L.A.; Little, S.H.; Ko, C.C. Orthodontic tooth movement: The biology and clinical implications. *Kaohsiung J. Med. Sci.* **2018**, *34*, 207–214. [CrossRef] [PubMed]
7. Park, J.C.; Kim, J.M.; Jung, I.H.; Kim, J.C.; Choi, S.H.; Cho, K.S.; Kim, C.S. Isolation and characterization of human periodontal ligament (PDL) stem cells (PDLSCs) from the inflamed PDL tissue: In vitro and in vivo evaluations. *J. Clin. Periodontol.* **2011**, *38*, 721–731. [CrossRef]
8. Sugimori, T.; Yamaguchi, M.; Shimizu, M.; Kikuta, J.; Hikida, T.; Hikida, M.; Murakami, Y.; Suemitsu, M.; Kuyama, K.; Kasai, K. Micro-osteo perforations accelerate orthodontic tooth movement by stimulating periodontal ligament cell cycles. *Am. J. Orthod. Dentofac. Orthop.* **2018**, *154*, 788–796. [CrossRef] [PubMed]
9. Uhlir, R.; Mayo, V.; Lin, P.H.; Chen, S.; Lee, Y.T.; Hershey, G.; Lin, F.C.; Ko, C.C. Biomechanical characterization of the periodontal ligament: Orthodontic tooth movement. *Angle Orthod.* **2017**, *87*, 183–192. [CrossRef] [PubMed]
10. Moccia, S.; Nucci, L.; Spagnuolo, C.; d'Apuzzo, F.; Piancino, M.G.; Minervini, G. Polyphenols as potential agents in the management of temporomandibular disorders. *Appl. Sci.* **2020**, *10*, 5305. [CrossRef]
11. Gunzler, H.; Gremlich, H.U. *IR Spectroscopy: An Introduction*; Wiley-VCH: Weinheim, Germany, 2002.
12. Kong, K.; Kendall, C.; Stone, N.; Notingher, I. Raman spectroscopy for medical diagnostics. From in-vitro biofluid assays to in-vivo cancer detection. *Adv. Drug Deliv.* **2015**, *89*, 121–134. [CrossRef] [PubMed]
13. Pence, I.; Mahadevan-Jansen, A. Clinical instrumentation and applications of Raman spectroscopy. *Chem. Soc. Rev.* **2016**, *45*, 1958–1979. [CrossRef]
14. Sakudo, A. Near-infrared spectroscopy for medical applications: Current status and future perspectives. *Clin. Chim. Acta* **2016**, *455*, 181–188. [CrossRef]
15. Tsuda, H.; Arends, J. Raman spectroscopy in dental research: A short review of recent studies. *Adv. Dent. Res.* **1997**, *11*, 539–547. [CrossRef] [PubMed]
16. Baker, M.J.; Trevisan, J.; Bassan, P.; Bhargava, R.; Butler, H.J.; Dorling, K.M.; Fielden, P.R.; Fogarty, S.W.; Fullwood, N.J.; Heys, K.A.; et al. Using Fourier transform IR spectroscopy to analyze biological materials. *Nat. Protoc.* **2014**, *9*, 1771–1791. [CrossRef]
17. Lacombe, C.; Untereiner, V.; Gobinet, C.; Zater, M.; Sockalingum, G.D.; Garnotel, R. Rapid screening of classic galactosemia patients: A proof-of-concept study using high-throughput FTIR analysis of plasma. *Analyst* **2015**, *140*, 2280. [CrossRef]
18. Lovergne, L.; Clemens Lovergne, L.; Untereiner, V.; Lukaszweski, R.A.; Sockalingum, G.D.; Baker, M.J. Investigating optimum sample preparation for infrared spectroscopic serum diagnostics. *Anal. Methods* **2015**, *7*, 7140. [CrossRef]
19. Lovergne, L.; Bouzy, P.; Untereine, V.; Garnotel, R.; Baker, M.J.; Thiefin, G.; Sockalingum, G.D. Biofluid infrared spectrodiagnostics: Pre-analytical considerations for clinical applications. *Faraday Discuss.* **2016**, *187*, 521–537. [CrossRef] [PubMed]
20. Xiang, X.M.; Liu, K.Z.; Man, A.; Ghiabi, E.; Cholakis, A.; Scott, D.A. Periodontitis-specific molecular signatures in gingival crevicular fluid. *J. Period. Res.* **2010**, *45*, 345–352. [CrossRef]
21. Xiang, K.Z.; Duarte, P.M.; Lima, J.A.; Santos, V.R.; Goncxalves, T.D.; Miranda, T.S.; Liu, K.Z. Diabetes-Associated Periodontitis Molecular Features in Infrared Spectra of Gingival Crevicular Fluid. *J. Periodontol.* **2013**, *84*, 1792–1800. [CrossRef]

22. Pàscoa, R.N.M.J.; Ferreira, J.; Gomes, P.S. The diagnosis of eating disorders through mid-infrared spectroscopy of the gingival crevicular fluid: A pilot trial. *Eat. Weight Disord.* **2020**, *25*, 1111–1115. [CrossRef]
23. Camerlingo, C.; d'Apuzzo, F.; Grassia, V.; Perillo, L.; Lepore, M. Micro-Raman spectroscopy for monitoring changes in periodontal ligaments and gingival crevicular fluid. *Sensors* **2014**, *14*, 22552–22563. [CrossRef]
24. Jung, G.B.; Kim, K.A.; Han, I.; Park, Y.G.; Park, H.K. Biochemical characterization of human gingival crevicular fluid during orthodontic tooth movement using Raman spectroscopy. *Biomed. Express* **2014**, *5*, 3510–3520. [CrossRef]
25. Camerlingo, C.; d'Apuzzo, F.; Grassia, V.; Parente, G.; Perillo, L.; Lepore, M. Micro-Raman spectroscopy during orthodontic tooth movement: Follow-up of gingival status. In Proceedings of the 2015 International Conference on BioPhotonics, Florence, Italy, 20–22 May 2015.
26. d'Apuzzo, F.; Perillo, L.; Delfino, I.; Portaccio, M.; Lepore, M.; Camerlingo, C. Monitoring early phases of orthodontic treatment by means of Raman spectroscopies. *J. Biomed. Opt.* **2017**, *22*, 115001. [CrossRef] [PubMed]
27. Portaccio, M.; d'Apuzzo, F.; Perillo, L.; Grassia, V.; Errico, S.; Lepore, M. Infrared microspectroscopy characterization of gingival crevicular fluid during orthodontic treatment. *J. Mol. Struct.* **2019**, *1176*, 847–854. [CrossRef]
28. Perillo, L.; d'Apuzzo, F.; Illario, M.; Laino, L.; Di Spigna, G.; Lepore, M.; Camerlingo, C. Evaluation of biochemical and structural changes in periodontal ligament after orthodontic movement by means of micro-Raman spectroscopy. *Sensors* **2020**, *20*, 497. [CrossRef] [PubMed]
29. Camerlingo, C.; d'Apuzzo, F.; Cammarota, M.; Errico, S.; Portaccio, M.; Perillo, L.; Lepore, M. Human periodontal ligament characterization by means of vibrational spectroscopy and electron microscopy. *Eng. Proc.* **2020**, *2*, 35. [CrossRef]
30. Butler, H.J.; Ashton, L.; Bird, B.; Cinque, G.; Curtis, K.; Dorney, J.; Esmonde-White, K.; Fullwood, N.J.; Gardner, B.; Martin-Hirsch, P.L.; et al. Using Raman spectroscopy to characterize biological materials. *Nat. Protoc.* **2016**, *11*, 664–687. [CrossRef] [PubMed]
31. Le Ru, E.C.; Blackie, E.J.; Meyer, M.; Etchegoin, P.G. Surface Enhanced Raman Scattering Enhancement Factors: A Comprehensive Study. *J. Phys. Chem. C* **2007**, *111*, 13794–13803. [CrossRef]
32. Lewis, I.R.; Edwards, H.G.M. *Handbook of Raman Spectroscopy*; Marcel Dekker Inc.: New York, NY, USA, 2001.
33. Craggs, C.; Galloway, K.P.; Gardiner, D.J. Maximum entropy methods applied to simulated and observed Raman spectra. *Appl. Spectrosc.* **1996**, *50*, 43. [CrossRef]
34. Gallo, C.; Capozzi, V.; Lasalvia, M.; Perna, G. An algorithm for estimation of background signal of Raman spectra from biological cell samples using polynomial functions of different degrees. *Vibr. Spectrosc.* **2013**, *83*, 132–137. [CrossRef]
35. Greek, L.; Shane, L.; Schulze, H.G.; Blades, M.W.; Bree, A.V.; Gorzalka, B.B.; Turner, R.F.B. SNR enhancement and deconvolution of Raman spectra using a two-point entropy regularization. *Appl. Spectrosc.* **1995**, *49*, 425. [CrossRef]
36. Schulze, G.; Jirasek, A.; Yu, M.M.L.; Lim, A.; Turner, R.F.B.; Blades, M.W. Investigation of selected baseline removal techniques as candidates for automated implementation. *Appl. Spectrosc.* **2005**, *56*, 545. [CrossRef]
37. Camerlingo, C.; Zenone, F.; Gaeta, G.M.; Riccio, R.; Lepore, M. Wavelet data processing of micro-Raman spectra of biological samples. *Measur. Sci. Tech.* **2006**, *17*, 298–303. [CrossRef]
38. Thomas, G.J., Jr.; Agard, D.A. Quantitative analysis of nucleid acids, proteins, and viruses by Raman band deconvolution. *Biophys. J.* **1984**, *46*, 763–768. [CrossRef]
39. Delfino, I.; Perna, G.; Lasalvia, M.; Capozzi, V.; Manti, L.; Camerlingo, C.; Lepore, M. Visible micro-Raman spectroscopy of single human mammary epithelial cells exposed to X-ray radiation. *J. Biomed. Opt.* **2015**, *20*, 035003. [CrossRef] [PubMed]
40. Spitz, A.; Christovam, I.O.; Marañón-Vásquez, G.A.; Masterson, D.F.; Adesse, D.; Maia, L.C.; Bolognese, A.M. Global gene expression profile of periodontal ligament cells submitted to mechanical loading: A systematic review. *Arch. Oral Biol.* **2020**, *118*, 104884. [CrossRef] [PubMed]

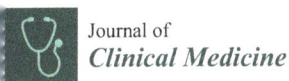

Review

The Oral Microbiota Changes in Orthodontic Patients and Effects on Oral Health: An Overview

Maria Contaldo [1,*], Alberta Lucchese [1], Carlo Lajolo [2], Cosimo Rupe [2], Dario Di Stasio [1], Antonio Romano [1], Massimo Petruzzi [3] and Rosario Serpico [1]

[1] Multidisciplinary Department of Medical-Surgical and Dental Specialties, University of Campania Luigi Vanvitelli, 80138 Naples, Italy; alberta.lucchese@unicampania.it (A.L.); dario.distasio@unicampania.it (D.D.S.); antonio.romano4@unicampania.it (A.R.); rosario.serpico@unicampania.it (R.S.)

[2] Head and Neck Department, Fondazione Policlinico Universitario A. Gemelli IRCCS, Roma Università Cattolica del Sacro Cuore, 00168 Rome, Italy; carlo.lajolo@unicatt.it (C.L.); cosimo.rupe01@icatt.it (C.R.)

[3] Interdisciplinary Department of Medicine, University of Bari "Aldo Moro", 70121 Bari, Italy; massimo.petruzzi@uniba.it

* Correspondence: Email maria.contaldo@unicampania.it; Tel.: +39-320-487-6058; Fax: +39-081-566-7674

Abstract: Nowadays, there is a considerable interest to study the biological and microbiological changes that accompany orthodontic treatment. Growing knowledge on oral microbiota allows, day after day, to identify and characterize the microbial arrangements specifically associated with oral and extra-oral conditions. The aim of the present work is to highlight any further correlations between orthodontic appliances and the qualitative and quantitative modifications of the oral microbiota, such as predisposing factors for the onset of caries, periodontal diseases, and other infections, which can impact the oral and systemic health of the orthodontic patients. When compared with subjects without orthodontic appliances, orthodontic patients reported significant qualitative and quantitative differences in supra- and subgingival plaque during the entire treatment period. Certain components of fixed appliances (mainly bonded molar brackets, ceramic brackets, and elastomeric ligatures) showed high risks of periodontal disease and tooth decay for patients. An unclear prevalence of *Candida* spp. and the paucity of studies on viruses and protozoas in the oral microbiota of orthodontic patients need to be further investigated. The evidence emerging from this study could guide clinicians in modulating the timing of controls and enhance patient motivation to prevent the formation of mature plaque, thus reducing the risks of oral-plaque-related diseases.

Keywords: orthodontics; clear aligners; brackets; microbiota; microbiome; oral health; *Candida albicans*; periodontitis; caries; dental plaque; materials; PCR

1. Introduction: Oral Dysbiosis and Related Oral Conditions in General Population

Over the years, the need and prevalence of orthodontic treatments have increased, particularly in developed countries [1], for both therapeutic and aesthetic purposes, and thanks to the development of different orthodontic devices and protocols [2–5] that meet the needs of every potential patient. Orthodontic procedures are indicated to correct dental malocclusions and craniofacial skeletal discrepancies of a genetic, family, and/or environmental nature, using fixed and/or removable orthodontic devices.

Recently, research has also investigated various biomarkers to monitor biological changes in tooth movement before and during treatment and has focused on the role and weight of numerous variables, such as oral hygiene levels and food habits related to the onset of dental and periodontal diseases during orthodontic treatment [6,7].

In general, the main plaque-related periodontal diseases are gingivitis and periodontitis. Gingivitis is a non-destructive inflammation, usually reversible after dental plaque control, while periodontitis, determined by the presence of predisposing factors—genetic and environmental—continues even after the restoration of oral hygiene [8], resulting in the irreversible loss of attachment and teeth due to a perpetuation of local inflammation, initially triggered by periodontopathogen bacteria [9].

In addition, various systematic reviews have confirmed the worsening of clinical parameters indicative of periodontal diseases, such as plaque index, bleeding on probing, attachment loss, and the onset of pockets or gingival recessions, in association with the time and type of orthodontic treatment, reporting varying degrees of reversibility after treatments.

The causes of the onset of periodontal diseases in orthodontic patients can be traced to:
- more difficult maintenance of oral hygiene,
- plaque retention to orthodontic devices,
- bone/periodontal movements and remodeling under orthodontic forces, which can favor the accumulation of subgingival plaque and enhance the periodontal pathogenic potential [10,11].

Aside from periodontal implications, plaque retention in the presence of orthodontic appliances has also been associated with increased susceptibility to caries and is influenced by transient/permanent qualitative and quantitative changes in the oral microbiota, responsible for the onset of oral infections, with systemic effects on well-being [12,13], thus predisposing orthodontic patients to suffer various pathologies more likely than non-orthodontic patients [14].

1.1. Dental Plaque Characterization

Dental plaque changes over time and depending on the location, so that early and mature plaques, supragingival and subgingival plaques, differ greatly from each other and are responsible for various and different pathologies, the most prevalent of which are caries and periodontal diseases. This is due to the fact that, by definition, dental plaque is a polymicrobial biofilm made up of various bacterial complexes, which mutually benefit from coaggregation, adhesion, and metabolic interactions [15].

Supragingival plaque is generally considered to be the main cause of caries and demineralization of enamel and dentin, as a consequence of the presence of *Streptococcus mutans* and other cariogenic bacteria, such as *Lactobacilli* and *Actinomycetes* species (spp.) as second colonizers, [14] but it also plays a key role in the late co-aggregation of periodontopathogen bacteria in the subgingival plaque, consisting mainly of gram-negative anaerobic bacteria strongly associated with periodontal diseases [16].

Thanks to culture-independent high-throughput technologies, such as reverse transcrip tase-polymerase chain reaction (RT-PCR) [17], and related, which, compared to conventional culture methods widely used in the past, allow the simultaneous evaluation of a large number of microbial species from different samples—saliva, supra-, and subgingival plaque—and from a wide range of subjects, the knowledge on the oral microbiota is enriched, day by day, allowing the characterization of the microbiota in conditions other than baseline. By definition, the oral microbiota is the collection of more than 600 microbial species—eukaryotes, archaea, bacteria, fungi, and viruses—living in specific ecological niches of the mouth [18,19], 169 of which constitute the indigenous "core oral microbiome", whose species are qualitatively and quantitatively housed in three different niches, classified as: Group 1, buccal mucosa, keratinized gingiva, and hard palate; Group 2, saliva, tongue, tonsils, and throat (back wall of oropharynx); and Group 3, sub- and supra-gingival plaque [20].

1.1.1. Subgingival Plaque and Periodontopathogen Bacteria

Subgingival plaque was first characterized in 1998, with checkerboard DNA–DNA hybridization (CDDH) when Socransky et al. analyzed the subgingival microbiota in a series of adults with and without periodontitis and grouped the forty species more frequently associated into complexes [21]. The grouping of these complexes was done on the basis of their strong or weak association with periodontitis and its clinical signs and they have been color-labeled in red, orange, yellow, green, and purple complexes; even today, this classification is used to refer to the periodontal pathogenic potential of each specific bacterium.

Periodontal damage begins thanks to the so-called "early colonizers" (the bacteria of the green and yellow complexes), which are able to adhere with their fimbriae to the dental film, thus favoring the subsequent co-adhesion and co-aggregation of the bacteria of the orange complex. The orange bacteria are the "bridge species" that connect green and red bacteria, produce toxins and enzymes responsible for the progressive loss of attachment and increase in pocket depth, thus creating a hospitable environment in the gingival sulcus/pocket for living conditions and colonization by red-complex bacteria. The latter is the "late colonizers", lodged in the deepest pockets and strongly associated with bleeding in the advanced stages of periodontitis [21].

Therefore, periodontal damage by red bacteria is the endpoint of a process during which different green/yellow and orange bacteria accumulate and co-aggregate, making the subgingival niche a hospitable habitat for the red bacteria.

1.1.2. Supragingival Plaque and Periodontopathogen Bacteria

Ten years later of their first work, Haffajee, Socransky et al. repeated a similar investigation to define relationships among bacterial species in supragingival plaque samples from a control group of periodontally healthy subjects and a test group consisting of patients who experienced attachment loss [22]. They found specific microbial complexes in the test group's supragingival plaque that were similar to those found in subgingival plaque samples, with some minor differences. Moreover, in this case, the colonization sequence of the supragingival plaque begins with the *Streptococci* (yellow complex), which are progressively replaced by the *Actinomicetes*, and then, at the bleeding sites and in the gingival pockets, they bind to the orange and red complexes, both ubiquitously present in supragingival and subgingival plaques and in inflamed and non-inflamed pockets.

1.2. The Role of Other Microscopic Agents in Gingival and Oral Health

Noteworthy, virus, fungi, and protozoa may also be involved in gingival diseases, such as linear gingival erythema associated with *Candida albicans* in children with AIDS [23] or *Entamoeba gingivalis* involved in periodontal destruction [24].

As regards *Candida* spp., they are not only responsible for a series of oral and systemic opportunistic infections [25,26], but they have also been implicated in the onset of caries as they show a synergistic relationship with *S. mutans*, with which they are frequently associated in mature plaque, mainly in children [27].

Usually, the presence of viruses in the oral microbiota (the so-called "oral virobiome") is indicative of potential infections, as the viruses are microscopic agents responsible for infection and damage to eukaryotic cells, with lifelong effects and/or recurrences [28,29]. Among the viruses commonly found at the oral sites, Epstein–Barr Virus (EBV) and Human Cytomegalovirus (CMV), as well Herpes Simplex Virus (HSV), also showed significantly higher in patients with severe periodontitis than in healthy subjects [30,31] and viral–bacterial associations in aggressive periodontitis—such as EBV/CMV with *Porphyromonas gingivalis* and *Aggregatibacter actinomycetemcomitans*—has been reported by various authors [32,33]. These viruses have been considered responsible for local immunosuppression that can favor the subgingival colonization and the multiplication of periodontal bacteria, indirectly exerting a periodontopathic effect [32,33].

1.3. Aims

On the basis of the evidence reported for the general population, the aim of the present work is to highlight any further correlations between orthodontic appliances and the related qualitative and quantitative modifications of the oral microbiota, such as predisposing factors for the onset of caries, periodontal diseases and other infections, which can impact the oral and systemic health of the orthodontic patients.

2. Microbiota Changes in Orthodontic Patients with Fixed Appliances

Several systematic reviews summarized the clinical and microbial differences found in salivary or plaque samples between orthodontic patients (case groups) and subjects not undergoing orthodontic therapies (control groups).

Pan et al. found significant differences in the number of microbial counts between 61 orthodontic and 56 non-orthodontic subjects (age range, 11–17 years) [34], reporting the highest increased in the case group three months after the placement of the orthodontic appliances and the significantly increased presence of strongly pathogenic *P. gingivalis*-specific *fimA* genotypes in the case group, defining this subtype as closely associated with orthodontic gingivitis.

The consistent quantitative and qualitative changes in the plaque one month after the start of orthodontic treatment were confirmed by a systematic review by Lucchese et al. [11]. According to it, different orthodontic appliances tended indiscriminately to alter the oral microbiota during treatment, but fixed appliances reported a greater and significant cariogenic and periodontopathogen effect than removable appliances.

2.1. Fixed Appliances and Periodontopathogen Bacteria

In 2017, Guo et al. [35] performed a meta-analysis to observe microbial changes in subgingival plaque between case/controls and before, during, and after orthodontic treatments with metal fixed appliances, focusing on the amounts of the red-complex bacteria (*P. gingivalis*, *Prevotella intermedia* and *Tannerella forsythia*, plus *A. actinomycetemcomitans*). Of these, only *T. forsythia* showed a statistically significant increase three months after orthodontic appliances, while a transient increase in all the species considered was detected six months after the start of the treatment. Furthermore, *P. intermedia* characteristically increased more significantly at the incisors than at the molars.

In 2018, Sun et al. [36] investigated microbial diversity from salivary samples from 20 healthy individuals and 30 patients with full fixed orthodontic appliances during the midterm of orthodontic treatment (10–12 months): real-time PCR analysis with gene-specific primers confirmed that the two groups expressed two distinct microbial communities with greater microbial diversity in the orthodontic group, characterized by higher amounts of *Pseudomonas* spp., *P. synxantha*, *Burkholderia* species and *Veillonella parvula*; conversely, there were no significant differences in *S. oralis* and *Neisseria lactamica* amounts.

The association between changes in clinical parameters and subgingival plaque was highlighted by Naranjo et al. in cultures from subgingival microbial specimens collected from 30 patients before and after bracket placement and 30 additional control subjects without orthodontic treatment [37]. Compared to the control group and baseline, elevated levels of *P. gingivalis*, *P. intermedia/Prevotella nigrescens*, *T. forsythia*, and *Fusobacterium* spp., were found in orthodontic patients three months after the placement of the brackets. Furthermore, a number of gram-negative superinfecting bacteria and enteric rods (*Klebsiella oxytoca, Enterobacter cloacae, Klebsiella pneumoniae, Serratia marcescens, Pseudomonas species, Enterobacter aerogenes, Enterobacter gergoviae*) were found indistinctly in all groups, without significant differences. Similarly, Kim et al. studied longitudinal changes in the subgingival microbiota by PCR before and during the first period of orthodontic treatment (up to 6 months) [38] in 30 adolescents treated with fixed appliances (conventional metal brackets with stainless steel ligatures and molar bands). From three months after placement of orthodontic appliances and thereafter, at least one periodontopathogen species—among *A. actinomycetemcomitans, T. forsythia, C. rectus, Eikenella corrodens, P. gingivalis, P. intermedia, P. nigrescens,* and *Treponema denticola*—was found in every subject. Among them, *C. rectus* and *P. nigrescens* significantly increased already after the first week of treatment, while *T. forsythia* took longer to colonize, after 3–6 months of treatment. In contrast, *A. actinomycetemcomitans* was detected at a very low level and showed no significant increase during the observation period. All frequencies of periodontopathogens were significantly higher in the molars than in the incisors. A similar decrease in *Actinomyces* spp. after 1 year of treatment was also reported by Lemos et al. in a study with CDDH on subgingival biofilm samples from

17 adults with full-fixed orthodontic appliances [39]. These authors also reported that, during treatment, *P. intermedia* and other orange complex species increased, while the proportions of the red complex species remained unchanged.

In addition to considering microbial changes *during* therapy, other authors have focused on changes that happen *after* the end of therapy, to assess whether a return to baseline occurs or if an altered microbiota remains. In their work, Guo et al. also reported a return to pretreatments levels several months after the removal of fixed appliances [35]. This was also confirmed by Choi et al. with a PCR-based study of the microbial changes occurring in subgingival plaque samples from 30 orthodontic patients three months after removal of fixed orthodontic appliances compared to 30 healthy subjects not undergoing orthodontic treatment [40]. They also reported that periodontopathogens bacteria significantly increased during orthodontic treatment (mainly *T. forsythia, C. rectus,* and *E. corrodens*) and then significantly reduced within three months of removing the appliance, eventually returning to levels similar to those reported in healthy subjects, except for *T. forsythia* and *P. nigrescens*, which persisted at even higher but not statistically significant levels compared to the control group. Similarly, Lo et al. [41] described with cultural techniques the bacterial composition before and during fixed orthodontic treatment in 10 patients (age range, 10–17 years), up to 12 weeks from appliance placement, revealing a prevalent aerobic flora (*Streptococcus* spp., *A.odontolyticus, A. israelii*) before treatment and one year from the start, and a prevalent facultative aerobic (*A. actinomycetemcomitans, Actinomyces viscosus, Capnocytophaga gingivalis*) and anaerobic species (*E.corrodens, Fusobacterium nucleatum, Micrococcus micros, Peptostreptococcus anaerobius, P. gingivalis,* and *Pseudomonas* spp.) during the first 2–4 weeks of treatment.

2.2. Fixed Appliances and Cariogenic Species

In 2016, Klaus et al. reported the results of a cross-sectional study on 75 subjects treated with fixed appliances (mean age, 14.4 ± 1.8 years) to measure the prevalence in saliva and plaque of *Candida* spp, *S. mutans,* and *Lactobacilli*, with culture methods [42]. The subjects were divided according to their oral hygiene status into three groups: good oral hygiene (GOH), poor oral hygiene (POH), and poor oral hygiene with white spots lesions (POH/WL). All patients, regardless of groups, reported a high prevalence of *Candida* spp. both in saliva (73% of cases) and plaque (61% of cases) with a significantly higher prevalence in the POH group and in the POH/WL group compared to the GOH group. *C. ulbicans* and *C. dubliniensis* were the main species identified, found in 86% and 15% of cases, respectively. With regards to bacteria, both *S. mutans* and *Lactobacilli* were found in 100% of salivary samples and in 91% of plaque samples, respectively, higher and significantly higher, in POH and POH/WL groups than in GOH group. A similar study on the cultural identification of salivary *S. mutans*, *Lactobacillus* spp. and *C. albicans* was performed by Topaloglu-Ak et al. [43] on 35 children with fixed appliances and 34 with removable devices, reporting a significant increase in *S. mutans* and *Lactobacilli* six months after insertion of fixed/removable appliances and a statistically higher presence of *C. albicans* in the fixed appliance group than in the removable appliance group.

In 2011, Andrucioli et al. [44] assessed bacterial contaminations after 30 days of permanence of premolar bands inserted after 16 months of fixed orthodontic treatment in 18 patients (age range 11–29 years), by checkerboard DNA–DNA hybridization. Among the cariogenic species, *S. mutans* and *Streptococcus sobrinus* were found in greater numbers than *Lactobacillus acidophilus* and *Lactobacillus casei*. The detection of periodontal pathogens of the orange complex was higher than that of the red complex and represented 40% of the total bacterial count.

2.3. Conventional Brackets with Elastomeric Ligatures, Steel Ligatures, Self-Ligating Brackets and Ceramic Brackets

Among fixed appliances, metal brackets with elastomeric ligatures have been shown to retain more plaque and worsen bleeding on probing and the plaque index more significantly than steel ligatures. In detail, Türkkahraman et al., after performing a split-mouth study on 21 subjects with two different archwire ligation techniques (elastomeric rings and steel ligatures), reported more bleeding at the teeth ligated with elastomeric rings than those with steel ligatures [45]. This finding was confirmed by Alves de Souza et al. which reported significantly higher amounts of *T. forsythia* and *P. nigrescens* at elastomeric ligatures, while *P. gingivalis*, *A. actinomycetemcomitans* and *P. intermedia* did not differ significantly [46].

A third type of ligature used for archwire ligation is the self-ligating bracket: this system has been variously associated with higher bleeding, worse plaque index and with an increase in gram-negative and gram-positive bacteria (mainly *Streptococci and Lactobacilli*) in several studies, despite they did not report statistically significant differences compared to conventional brackets ligated with stainless steel ligatures [47,48]. Regarding the risk of caries, Jing et al. [49] found a significant increase in *S. mutans* in patients with conventional brackets compared to those with self-ligating brackets over 18 months after starting the treatments.

In 2002, Anhoury et al. [50] compared the total bacterial counts and the levels of various cariogenic and periodontopathogen bacteria present on 24 metallic and 32 ceramic orthodontic brackets immediately after their debonding. The mean counts of *P. gingivalis* were very similar on metallic and ceramic brackets isolated from both posterior and anterior teeth, as well for amounts of *P. nigrescens*, *Actinomyces odontolyticus*, *T. forsythia*, *Actinomyces naeslundii*, *Capnocytophaga ochracea*, *Actinomyces israelii* and cariogenic bacteria such as *S. mutans* and *L. acidophilus*. In contrast, the two types of bracket exhibited statistical differences in the counts of eight periodontopathogen species: the metallic bracket showed significant increased levels of *T. denticola*, *A. actinomycetemcomitans*, *F. nucleatum ss vincentii*, *S. anginosus* and *E. nodatum*, while in ceramic ones *E. corrodens*, *Capnocytophaga showae*, *Selenomonas noxia* were the most significantly increased species. Counts of *Streptococcus sanguis*, *Actinomyces gerencseriae*, and *Streptococcus constellatus* significantly increased in anterior ceramic brackets, while *C. rectus* was higher in posterior metallic brackets.

2.4. Molar Band vs. Bonded Molar Tubes

In 2014, Ireland et al. [51] used denaturing gradient gel electrophoresis (DGGE) and 16S rDNA microarray in a cross-mouth study on 24 orthodontic patients (age range, 11–14 years) to investigate differences in clinical parameters and microbial communities in supra- and subgingival plaque from banded molar vs bonded molar, randomly assigned, during treatment and up to one year after appliance removal. In both groups, the plaque populations changed within three months of starting fixed treatment and was characterized by an increase in *T. denticola* and *P. nigrescens*, and a decrease in *A. actinomycetemcomitans*. Post-treatment plaque associated with both types of molar attachments showed increased levels of periodontal pathogens, such as *P. gingivalis*, *T. forsythia*, and *E. nodatum*, while *C. rectus*, *Parvimonas micra*, *A. odontolyticus* and *V. parvula* were peculiarly elevated only in bonded molars. One year after the cessation of treatment, the banded molar plaque returned to its baseline composition, while a new arrangement of the microbial community persisted in the bonded molars.

In 2016, Mártha et al. [52] used DNA-strip technique to assess the presence of eleven periodontopathogen bacteria in subgingival plaque of banded and bonded molars, before and during the first two months of fixed orthodontic treatment, in 25 subjects (age range, 11–17 years). The most common bacteria, regardless of groups and time, were *F. nucleatum* (92% of samples), *E. corrodens* (76% of samples), and *Capnocytophaga* spp. (*C. gingivalis*, *C. ochracea*, *C. sputigena*), while the other eight species (*A. actinomycetemcomitans*, *P. gingivalis*, *P. intermedia*, *T. forsythia*, *T. denticola*, *Parvimonas micra*, *C. rectus*, and *Eubacterium nodatum*) were found less frequently. Among them, *E. nodatum* was found only in 2 subjects with bonded molars during treatment, while *E. corrodens*, *P. micra*, *T. denticola* and *T. forsythia* were stable over time in the banded molar group but it significantly increased two months later in the bonded group, as well as *Capnocytophaga* spp.

3. Microbiota Changes in Children with Functional/Orthodontic Appliances

Various functional/orthodontic appliances are used in interceptive orthodontics, such as in those children needing rapid maxillary expansion. The microbial changes associated to these types of appliances were studied by Ortu et al. [53] who evaluated the microbial levels of *S. mutans* and *Lactobacillus* spp. in 30 children aged 6–9 years and grouped into 10 subjects treated with rapid palatal expander (RPE), 10 treated with Mc Namara expander, and 10 patients as control. These authors found a significant increase in *Streptococci and Lactobacilli* in each group but no significant differences between the groups, except the Mc Namara group that showed significantly higher amounts of *Lactobacilli* after 6 months of treatment than in control group and RPE.

4. Clear Aligners vs. Fixed Orthodontic Appliances in Adults

In 2015, Levrini et al. [54] prospectively considered 77 patients grouped in subjects with clear aligners, fixed orthodontics, and control to assess periodontal indexes and microbial composition of the plaque before and during treatments: they found better control over biofilm formations and significantly less severe periodontal indexes in the clear aligners wearers, as confirmed by the meta-analysis made by Rossini et al. on the periodontal health of patients treated with clear aligners compared to those treated with fixed appliances [55].

With regard to the characterization of the microbiota in subjects with clear aligner vs. fixed appliances, Lombardo et al. [56] recently reported a longitudinal study of the sub-gingival microbiota in these two groups, focusing on the identification and quantification of *A. actinomycetemcomitans, P. gingivalis, F. nucleatum, C. rectus, T. denticola* and *T. forsythia* by real-time PCR. They found a significantly increased total bacterial load during both treatments and a progressive increase in *C. rectus* and *F. nucleatum* in the fixed appliances group. Conversely, *A. actinomycetemcomitans* was never detected, while *P. gingivalis, T. forsythia* and *T. denticola* were rarely detected. Similar comparisons were also reported by Mummolo et al. [57], focusing on the amounts of *Streptococci and Lactobacilli* in a prospective controlled study on 80 adults—40 subjects with clear aligners and 40 with fixed orthodontic appliances—reporting a significant increase in the amounts of those cariogenic species in the saliva of subjects with fixed appliances.

The superior periodontal health in removable appliances wearers compared to fixed orthodontic appliances has recently been confirmed by two meta-analyses by Lu et al. and Wu et al. [58,59]. The authors considered randomized controlled trials (RCTs) and prospective cohort studies comparing periodontal health status in patients undergoing orthodontic treatment with fixed and removable appliances. They compared the gingival index (GI), plaque index (PI), the sulcus probing depth (SPD), and the sulcus bleeding index (SBI) from seven and thirteen eligible studies, respectively, and found that, compared to wearers of fixed appliances, wearers of clear aligners did not show significant differences in GI and SPD but reported significantly lower PI and SBI, at any time of observation.

5. Protozoas, Fungi and Other Bacterial Species in Orthodontic Patients

While a wide variety of works have focused on cariogenic and periodontopathogen bacteria in orthodontic patients, further studies focused on other pathogenic and opportunistic microorganisms responsible for various oral and systemic diseases. In 2019, Perkowski et al. performed a cultural study on periodontal swab from 25 young orthodontic patients (6–13 years old) treated with removable orthodontic appliances and 25 older patients (14–23 years) treated with fixed appliances, each compared to 50 healthy subjects in the same age ranges of the two test groups [60] to test for any clinical and microbial differences among the four groups. As expected, caries and DMFT (decay, missed, filled teeth index) [61] were significantly higher in the younger subjects, while bleeding on probing was higher in the older subjects, irrespective of case/control groups. The fixed orthodontic group showed a higher prevalence of *Enterococcus faecalis, Enterococcus faecium, Staphylococcus aureus and Escherichia coli,* and other gram-negative such as *Enterobacter* cloacae, *P. agglomerans*, and *Klebsiella* spp. plus various strains of *Candida* spp., compared to those with removable appliance or not treated. In particular, the presence of *C.albicans* was correlated with higher bleeding indices and poor oral hygiene. Furhtermore, few older subjects reported the identification of protozoas (*Trichomonas tenax* and *Entamoeba gingivalis*) regardless of the groups, while cysts of *Acanthamoeba* spp. were exclusively found in 3 patients with fixed appliances.

The higher carriage of *Candida* spp. in orthodontic patients with fixed appliance than in non-orthodontic subjects and patients with orthodontic removable appliances has been previously discussed, as reported by Topaloglu et al. [43] and other authors [62,63]. Klaus et al. also reported a significant higher prevalence of *Candida* spp. associated with poor oral hygiene [42], as confirmed by the literature [64].

In their work, Arslan et al. characterized by culture methods *Candida* species found in 58% of a group of adolescents with fixed orthodontic appliances: *C. albicans* was predominant (73.8%), followed by *C. tropicalis*, *C. krusei* and *C. kefyr* (7.14%), and *C. parapsilosis* (4.76%) [63]. Similar rates were reported by Grzegocka et al. [65] who analyzed *Candida* spp. from oral rinses and suprangingival plaque in 17 orthodontic subjects (mean age 17 ± 7 years) founding 59% of Candida carriers among them, and a strongly correlation with the massive presence of plaque.

Contrasted with these findings, Sanz-Orrio-Soler et al. [66] recently reported the results of a prospective controlled trial on oral colonization by *Candida* species in 124 orthodontic patients before, during, and after treatment with fixed appliances. Again, *Candida* spp. identification was based on culture methods and results contrasted with the previously published literature: the authors did not observe any statistically significant increase in the colonization of *C. albicans* during the orthodontic treatment despite the fact that ceramic brackets showed a higher incidence of this fungus. Similarly, Tapia et al. [67] found colonization rates of *C. albicans* and *C. tropicalis* of 6.7% in 90 orthodontic subjects (20.6 ± 7.1 years).

6. Discussion

The present work examined the scientific literature to highlight any specific microbial changes that occur during and after different types of orthodontic treatments.

When compared with subjects without orthodontic treatment, orthodontic patients reported significant qualitative and quantitative differences in the amount and microbial composition of plaque during the entire treatment period. Removable appliances were less associated with worsening of periodontal indices and caries because, despite being worn nearly 24 h a day, they can be easily removed to allow for proper oral hygiene. These results are in line with a recent meta-analysis by Jiang et al. [68], reporting that patients with clear aligners, compared with those undergoing orthodontic treatment with fixed appliances, appear to benefit from better oral health and periodontal parameters, thus recommending clear aligners as preferential therapeutic option in those patients at high risk of developing gingivitis/periodontitis, mainly adults [69]. Furthermore, subjects with fixed appliances showed a significant increase in the number of *Streptococci* and *Lactobacilli* and, therefore, a greater risk of caries than subjects with clear aligners [57].

Among the types of brackets and ligatures used in fixed orthodontic therapies, patients with conventional brackets have shown an increase in *S. mutans* and should be considered at higher risk of developing white spot lesions and caries than patients with self-ligating brackets [49], as well as elastomeric ligatures and ceramic brackets are more associated with poor oral conditions and with a greater amount of periodontopathogen and cariogenic species. Based on these findings, while self-ligating brackets are microbiologically safer, elastomeric ligatures and ceramic brackets must be considered at higher risk of periodontal diseases and caries.

In fixed appliances, the first changes already occur during the first weeks of treatment and, within the first month, *Streptococci* and *Actynomicetes* spp. predominate, as well as *C. rectus* and *P. nigrescens* (orange complex species), *A. actinomycetemcomitans*, *A. viscosus*,

Capnocytophaga gingivalis and anaerobic species (*Eikenella corrodens, F. nucleatum, Micrococcus micros, Peptostreptococcus anaerobius, P. gingivalis and Pseudomonas species*). After 3 months, the species of the orange complex increase and account for the 40% of the total bacteria counts. The red complex bacteria *P. gingivalis, P. intermedia,* and *T. forsythia*, significantly increase after 6 months, as well as *Lactobacilli*. From the end of the treatment, the literature agreed in founding a return to the original bacterial flora of the baseline, thus considering all the microbial alterations occurred during orthodontic treatment as transitory [35]. However, some authors have disproved this finding by reporting a long-term effect on periodontal health in patient with molar bonded tubes appliances compared with the classical molar bands [51]. On this basis, more rigorous follow-up should be considered after orthodontic treatment in patients treated with molar bond.

Regarding the presence of *Candida* spp. in orthodontic patients, many studies reported a high and significant prevalence of this yeast in orthodontic patients, but other studies have refuted this hypothesis. An explanation of these discordant results can be given by analyzing the reported studies: few subjects were enrolled and the methods of fungal detection were based on culture, which underestimate the presence of those yeasts that are difficult to cultivate, especially if present in low percentages. For these reasons, more extensive studies are desirable and the use of high throughput technologies should be preferred to culture methods in order to map, without risk of underestimation, the real oral mycobiome of orthodontic patients. It should be noted that *Candida* is an opportunist agent which, under physiological conditions, is present only as a carrier. However, if local or systemic alterations occur, it can virulent with repercussions of various degrees on the health of the individual [26].

In one study, the presence of protozoas was also found: *Trichomonas tenax, Entamoeba gingivalis,* and *Acanthamoeba* spp. are not a common resident of the oral cavity and their opportunistic colonization may be associated with serious systemic conditions, such as lung abscesses, granulomatous encephalitis, and keratitis, as well their proteinases activity is capable of damaging oral mucosal tissues and invading the periodontal spaces [58].

With regard to virobiome in orthodontic subjects, the scientific literature is silent and has not reported significant works on the presence of viruses associated with orthodontic treatments. However, based on the viral–bacterial interaction found in periodontitis [32], it is reasonable to hypothesize a triggering role of HSV, EBV, and CMV (viruses frequently reported in children and adolescents [70,71]) in periodontal damage if associated with significant amounts of periodontopathogen bacteria.

7. Conclusions

The qualitative and quantitative changes in the microbial plaque of orthodontic patients occur as early as one week and they become more consistent three months after the start of treatment, with stable colonization first by orange and then by red species. Especially in patients being treated with fixed devices, it is advisable to strengthen oral hygiene and clinical checks in the first months of treatment to block the progression, maturation, and arrangement of periodontopathogen and cariogenic species in plaque.

The results of the present review were in accordance with what recently reported by Müller et al., which concluded the reversibility of the periodontal changes and the permanence of enamel demineralization and white spots, thus suggesting the use of antibacterial orthodontic bonding systems as an adjunct in the maintenance of proper dental health in orthodontic patients [72].

Furthermore, this study focused on the literature related to healthy, immunocompetent subjects without other local or systemic affections. Therefore, it is foreseeable that patients with special needs, those with immunological alterations or other oral and/or systemic comorbidities, may be more affected by the cariogenic and periodontopathogen effects of mature plaque during orthodontic treatments, and a high carriage of *Candida* spp. could be responsible for fungal stomatitis and disseminated candidiasis in fragile subjects.

Since the correlations between oral dysbiosis and systemic diseases are various and reported in the more recent literature, [73,74] it is desirable to conduct targeted research on the less investigated components of the oral microbiota (fungi, viruses, and protozoan) and on fragile populations requiring orthodontic treatments, to prevent oral and extraoral complications and to guarantee each patient personalized dentistry with personalized therapies [75], which takes into account the microbiological and clinical characteristics of each individual.

Author Contributions: Conceptualization, M.C., A.L., M.P. and R.S.; writing—original draft preparation, M.C, A.R. and D.D.S.; writing—review and editing, M.C., C.L., C.R. and M.P. All authors have read and agreed to the published version of the manuscript

Funding: This research received no external funding.

Conflicts of Interest: The authors declare no conflict of interest.

References

1. Grippaudo, M.M.; Quinzi, V.; Manai, A.; Paolantonio, E.G.; Valente, F.; La Torre, G.; Marzo, G. Orthodontic treatment need and timing: Assessment of evolutive malocclusion conditions and associated risk factors. *Eur J Paediatr Dent.* **2020**, *21*, 203–208. [CrossRef]
2. Marra, P.; Nucci, L.; Abdolreza, J.; Perillo, L.; Itro, A.; Grassia, V. Odontoma in a young and anxious patient associated with unerupted permanent mandibular cuspid: A case report. *J. Int. Oral Heal.* **2020**, *12*, 182. [CrossRef]
3. Cozzani, M.; Sadri, D.; Nucci, L.; Jamilian, P.; Pirhadirad, A.P.; Jamilian, A. The effect of Alexander, Gianelly, Roth, and MBT bracket systems on anterior retraction: A 3-dimensional finite element study. *Clin. Oral Investig.* **2019**, *24*, 1351–1357. [CrossRef]
4. Grassia, V.; D'Apuzzo, F.; Ferrulli, V.E.; Matarese, G.; Femiano, F.; Perillo, L. Dento-skeletal effects of mixed palatal expansion evaluated by postero-anterior cephalometric analysis. *Eur J Paediatr Dent.* **2014**, *15*, 59–62. [PubMed]
5. Grassia, V.; d'Apuzzo, F.; Di Stasio, D.; Jamilian, A.; Lucchese, A.; Perillo, L. Upper and lower arch changes after Mixed Palatal Expansion protocol. *Eur J Paediatr Dent.* **2014**, *15*, 375–380.
6. Grassia, V.; Lombardi, A.; Kawasaki, H.; Ferri, C.; Perillo, L.; Mosca, L.; Cave, D.D.; Nucci, L.; Porcelli, M.; Caraglia, M. Salivary microRNAs as new molecular markers in cleft lip and palate: A new frontier in molecular medicine. *Oncotarget* **2018**, *9*, 18929–18938. [CrossRef]
7. Perinetti, G.; D'Apuzzo, F.; Contardo, L.; Primozic, J.; Rupel, K.; Perillo, L. Gingival crevicular fluid alkaline phosphate activity during the retention phase of maxillary expansion in prepubertal subjects: A split-mouth longitudinal study. *Am. J. Orthod. Dentofac. Orthop.* **2015**, *148*, 90–96. [CrossRef]
8. Mombelli, A. Microbial colonization of the periodontal pocket and its significance for periodontal therapy. *Periodontology 2000* **2018**, *76*, 85–96. [CrossRef] [PubMed]
9. Ballini, A.; Cantore, S.; Farronato, D.; Cirulli, N.; Inchingolo, F.; Papa, F.; Malcangi, G.; Inchingolo, A.D.; Dipalma, G.; Sardaro, N.; et al. Periodontal disease and bone pathogenesis: The crosstalk between cytokines and porphyromonas gingivalis. *J Biol Regul Homeost Agents* **2015**, *29*, 273–281.
10. Giugliano, D.; D'Apuzzo, F.; Majorana, A.; G CAMPUS; Nucci, F.; Flores-Mir, C.; Perillo, L. Influence of occlusal characteristics, food intake and oral hygiene habits on dental caries in adolescents: A cross-sectional study. *Eur J Paediatr Dent* **2018**, *19*, 95–100.
11. Lucchese, A.; Bondemark, L.; Marcolina, M.; Manuelli, M. Changes in oral microbiota due to orthodontic appliances: A systematic review. *J. Oral Microbiol.* **2018**, *10*, 1476645. [CrossRef] [PubMed]
12. Contaldo, M.; Della Vella, F.; Raimondo, E.; Minervini, G.; Buljubasic, M.; Ogodescu, A.; Sinescu, C.; Serpico, R. Early Childhood Oral Health Impact Scale (ECOHIS): Literature review and Italian validation. *Int. J. Dent. Hyg.* **2020**, *18*, 396–402. [CrossRef]
13. Zannella, C.; Shinde, S.; Vitiello, M.; Falanga, A.; Galdiero, E.; Fahmi, A.; Santella, B.; Nucci, L.; Gasparro, R.; Galdiero, M.; et al. Antibacterial Activity of Indolicidin-Coated Silver Nanoparticles in Oral Disease. *Appl. Sci.* **2020**, *10*, 1837. [CrossRef]
14. De Freitas, A.O.A.; Marquezan, M.; Nojima, M.D.C.G.; Alviano, D.S.; Maia, L.C. The influence of orthodontic fixed appliances on the oral microbiota: A systematic review. *Dent. Press J. Orthod.* **2014**, *19*, 46–55. [CrossRef]
15. Kwon, T.; Lamster, I.B.; Levin, L. Current concepts in the management of periodontitis. *Int. Dent. J.* **2020**. [CrossRef] [PubMed]
16. Tezal, M.; Scannapieco, F.A.; Wactawski-Wende, J.; Grossi, S.G.; Genco, R.J. Supragingival Plaque May Modify the Effects of Subgingival Bacteria on Attachment Loss. *J. Periodontol.* **2006**, *77*, 808–813. [CrossRef]
17. Pannone, G.; Sanguedolce, F.; De Maria, S.; Farina, E.; Muzio, L.L.; Serpico, R.; Emanuelli, M.; Rubini, C.; De Rosa, G.; Staibano, S.; et al. Cyclooxygenase Isozymes in Oral Squamous Cell Carcinoma: A Real-Time RT-PCR Study with Clinic Pathological Correlations. *Int. J. Immunopathol. Pharmacol.* **2007**, *20*, 317–324. [CrossRef]
18. Dewhirst, F.E.; Chen, T.; Izard, J.; Paster, B.J.; Tanner, A.C.R.; Yu, W.-H.; Lakshmanan, A.; Wade, W.G. The Human Oral Microbiome. *J. Bacteriol.* **2010**, *192*, 5002–5017. [CrossRef] [PubMed]

19. Segata, N.; Haake, S.K.; Mannon, P.; Lemon, K.P.; Waldron, L.; Gevers, D.; Huttenhower, C.; Izard, J. Composition of the adult digestive tract bacterial microbiome based on seven mouth surfaces, tonsils, throat and stool samples. *Genome Biol.* **2012**, *13*, R42. [CrossRef]
20. Wade, W.; Prosdocimi, E. Profiling of Oral Bacterial Communities. *J. Dent. Res.* **2020**, *99*, 621–629. [CrossRef]
21. Socransky, S.S.; Haffajee, A.D.; Cugini, M.A.; Smith, C.; Kent, R.L., Jr. Microbial complexes in subgingival plaque. *J. Clin. Periodontol.* **1998**, *25*, 134–144. [CrossRef]
22. Haffajee, A.D.; Socransky, S.S.; Patel, M.R.; Song, X. Microbial complexes in supragingival plaque. *Oral Microbiol. Immunol.* **2008**, *23*, 196–205. [CrossRef] [PubMed]
23. Velegraki, A.; Nicolatou, O.; Theodoridou, M.; Mostrou, G.; Legakis, N.J. Paediatric AIDS - related linear gingival erythema: A form of erythematous candidiasis? *J. Oral Pathol. Med.* **2007**, *28*, 178–182. [CrossRef]
24. Dubar, M.; Zaffino, M.-L.; Remen, T.; Thilly, N.; Cunat, L.; Machouart, M.-C.; Bisson, C. Protozoans in subgingival biofilm: Clinical and bacterial associated factors and impact of scaling and root planing treatment. *J. Oral Microbiol.* **2020**, *12*, 1693222. [CrossRef] [PubMed]
25. Paoletti, I.; Fusco, A.; Grimaldi, E.; Perillo, L.; Coretti, L.; Di Domenico, M.; Cozza, V.; Lucchese, A.; Contaldo, M.; Serpico, R.; et al. Assessment of Host Defence Mechanisms Induced by Candida Species. *Int. J. Immunopathol. Pharmacol.* **2013**, *26*, 663–672. [CrossRef]
26. Supplement, D.; Contaldo, M.; Romano, A.; Mascitti, M.; Fiori, F.; Della Vella, F.; Serpico, R.; Santarelli, A. Association between denture stomatitis, candida species and diabetic status. *J Biol Regul Homeost Agents* **2019**, *33*, 35–41.
27. Bachtiar, E.W.; Bachtiar, B.M. Relationship between Candida albicans and Streptococcus mutans in early child-hood caries, evaluated by quantitative PCR. *F1000Res.* **2018**, *7*, 1645. [CrossRef]
28. Pannone, G.; Santoro, A.; Carinci, F.; Bufo, P.; Papagerakis, S.M.; Rubini, C.; Campisi, G.; Giovannelli, L.; Contaldo, M.; Serpico, R.; et al. Double Demonstration of Oncogenic High Risk Human Papilloma Virus DNA and HPV-E7 Protein in Oral Cancers. *Int. J. Immunopathol. Pharmacol.* **2011**, *24*, 95–101. [CrossRef] [PubMed]
29. Donnarumma, G.; De Gregorio, V.; Fusco, A.; Farina, E.; Baroni, A.; Esposito, V.; Contaldo, M.; Petruzzi, M.; Pannone, G.; Serpico, R. Inhibition of HSV-1 Replication by Laser Diode-Irradiation: Possible Mechanism of Action. *Int. J. Immunopathol. Pharmacol.* **2010**, *23*, 1167–1176. [CrossRef]
30. Puletic, M.; Popovic, B.; Jankovic, S.; Brajovic, G. Detection rates of periodontal bacteria and herpesviruses in different forms of periodontal disease. *Microbiol. Immunol.* **2020**, *64*, 815–824. [CrossRef]
31. Khosropanah, H.; Karandish, M.; Ziaeyan, M.; Jamalidoust, M. Quantification of Epstein-Barr Virus and Human Cytomegalovirus in Chronic Periodontal Patients. *Jundishapur J. Microbiol.* **2015**, *8*, e18691. [CrossRef]
32. Sharma, S.; Tapashetti, R.P.; Patil, S.R.; Kalra, S.M.; Bhat, G.K.; Guvva, S. Revelation of Viral - Bacterial Interrelationship in Aggressive Periodontitis via Polymerase Chain Reaction: A Microbiological Study. *J Int Oral Health.* **2015**, *7*, 101–107. [PubMed]
33. Li, F.; Zhu, C.; Deng, F.-Y.; Wong, M.C.M.; Lu, H.-X.; Feng-Ying, D. Herpesviruses in etiopathogenesis of aggressive periodontitis: A meta-analysis based on case-control studies. *PLoS ONE* **2017**, *12*, e0186373. [CrossRef] [PubMed]
34. Pan, S.; Liu, Y.; Si, Y.; Zhang, Q.; Wang, L.; Liu, J.; Wang, C.; Xiao, S. Prevalence of fimA genotypes of Porphyromonas gingivalis in adolescent orthodontic patients. *PLoS ONE* **2017**, *12*, e0188420. [CrossRef] [PubMed]
35. Guo, R.; Lin, Y.; Zheng, Y.; Li, W. The microbial changes in subgingival plaques of orthodontic patients: A systematic review and meta-analysis of clinical trials. *BMC Oral Heal.* **2017**, *17*, 1–10. [CrossRef]
36. Sun, F.; Ahmed, A.; Wang, L.; Dong, M.; Niu, W. Comparison of oral microbiota in orthodontic patients and healthy individuals. *Microb. Pathog.* **2018**, *123*, 473–477. [CrossRef]
37. Naranjo, A.A.; Triviño, M.L.; Jaramillo, A.; Betancourth, M.; Botero, J.E. Changes in the subgingival microbiota and periodontal parameters before and 3 months after bracket placement. *Am. J. Orthod. Dentofac. Orthop.* **2006**, *130*, 275-e17. [CrossRef]
38. Kim, S.-H.; Choi, D.-S.; Jang, I.; Cha, B.-K.; Jost-Brinkmann, P.-G.; Song, J.-S. Microbiologic changes in subgingival plaque before and during the early period of orthodontic treatment. *Angle Orthod.* **2012**, *82*, 254–260. [CrossRef]
39. Lemos, M.M.; Cattaneo, P.M.; Melsen, B.; Faveri, M.; Feres, M.; Figueiredo, L.C. Impact of Treatment with Full-fixed Orthodontic Appliances on the Periodontium and the Composition of the Subgingival Microbiota. *J Int Acad Periodontol.* **2020**, *22*, 174–181.
40. Choi, D.-S.; Cha, B.-K.; Jost-Brinkmann, P.-G.; Lee, S.-Y.; Chang, B.-S.; Jang, I.; Song, J.-S. Microbiologic Changes in Subgingival Plaque After Removal of Fixed Orthodontic Appliances. *Angle Orthod.* **2009**, *79*, 1149–1155. [CrossRef]
41. Lo, B.A.M.; Di Marco, R.; Milazzo, I.; Nicolosi, D.; Calì, G.; Rossetti, B.; Blandino, G. Microbiological and clinical periodontal effects of fixed orthodontic appliances in pediatric patients. *New Microbiol.* **2008**, *31*, 299.
42. Klaus, K.; Eichenauer, J.; Sprenger, R.; Ruf, S. Oral microbiota carriage in patients with multibracket appliance in relation to the quality of oral hygiene. *Head Face Med.* **2016**, *12*, 1–7. [CrossRef] [PubMed]
43. Topaloglu-Ak, A.; Ertugrul, F.; Eden, E.; Ates, M.; Bulut, H. Effect of Orthodontic Appliances on Oral Microbiota—6 Month Follow-up. *J. Clin. Pediatr. Dent.* **2011**, *35*, 433–436. [CrossRef] [PubMed]
44. Andrucioli, M.C.D.; Nelson-Filho, P.; Matsumoto, M.A.N.; Saraiva, M.C.P.; Feres, M.; De Figueiredo, L.C.; Martins, L.P. Molecular detection of in-vivo microbial contamination of metallic orthodontic brackets by checkerboard DNA-DNA hybridization. *Am. J. Orthod. Dentofac. Orthop.* **2012**, *141*, 24–29. [CrossRef]
45. Türkkahraman, H.; Sayin, M.O.; Bozkurt, F.Y.; Yetkin, Z.; Kaya, S.; Onal, S. Archwire ligation techniques, microbial colonization, and periodontal status in orthodontically treated patients. *Angle Orthod.* **2005**, *75*, 231–236. [PubMed]

46. De Souza, R.A.; Magnani, M.B.B.D.A.; Nouer, D.F.; Da Silva, C.O.; Klein, M.I.; Sallum, E.A.; Gonçalves, R.B. Periodontal and microbiologic evaluation of 2 methods of archwire ligation: Ligature wires and elastomeric rings. *Am. J. Orthod. Dentofac. Orthop.* **2008**, *134*, 506–512. [CrossRef] [PubMed]
47. Baka, Z.M.; Basciftci, F.A.; Arslan, U. Effects of 2 bracket and ligation types on plaque retention: A quantitative microbiologic analysis with real-time polymerase chain reaction. *Am. J. Orthod. Dentofac. Orthop.* **2013**, *144*, 260–267. [CrossRef]
48. Uzuner, F.D.; Kaygisiz, E.; Çankaya, Z.T. Effect of the bracket types on microbial colonization and periodontal status. *Angle Orthod.* **2014**, *84*, 1062–1067. [CrossRef] [PubMed]
49. Jing, D.; Hao, J.; Shen, Y.; Tang, G.; Lei, L.; Zhao, Z. Effect of fixed orthodontic treatment on oral microbiota and salivary proteins. *Exp. Ther. Med.* **2019**, *17*, 4237–4243. [CrossRef]
50. Anhoury, P.; Nathanson, D.; Hughes, C.V.; Socransky, S.; Feres, M.; Chou, L.L. Microbial profile on metallic and ceramic bracket materials. *Angle Orthod.* **2002**, *72*, 338–343.
51. Ireland, A.J.; Soro, V.; Sprague, S.V.; Harradine, N.W.T.; Day, C.; Al-Anezi, S.; Jenkinson, H.F.; Sherriff, M.; Dymock, D.; Sandy, J.R. The effects of different orthodontic appliances upon microbial communities. *Orthod. Craniofacial Res.* **2013**, *17*, 115–123. [CrossRef]
52. Mártha, K.; Lőrinczi, L.; Bică, C.; Gyergyay, R.; Petcu, B.; Lazăr, L.; Information, R. Assessment of Periodontopathogens in Subgingival Biofilm of Banded and Bonded Molars in Early Phase of Fixed Orthodontic Treatment. *Acta Microbiol. et Immunol. Hung.* **2016**, *63*, 103–113. [CrossRef]
53. Ortu, E.; Sgolastra, F.; Barone, A.; Gatto, R.; Marzo, G.; Monaco, A. Salivary Streptococcus Mutans and Lacto-bacillus spp. levels in patients during rapid palatal expansion. *Eur J Paed Dent.* **2014**, *15*, 271–274.
54. Levrini, L.; Mangano, A.; Montanari, P.; Margherini, S.; Caprioglio, A.; Abbate, G.M. Periodontal health status in patients treated with the Invisalign®system and fixed orthodontic appliances: A 3 months clinical and microbiological evaluation. *Eur. J. Dent.* **2015**, *9*, 404–410. [CrossRef] [PubMed]
55. Rossini, G.; Parrini, S.; Castroflorio, T.; Deregibus, A.; Debernardi, C.L. Periodontal health during clear aligners treatment: A systematic review. *Eur. J. Orthod.* **2015**, *37*, 539–543. [CrossRef] [PubMed]
56. Lombardo, L.; Palone, M.; Scapoli, L.; Siciliani, G.; Carinci, F. Short-term variation in the subgingival microbiota of two groups of patients treated with clear aligners and vestibular fixed appliances: A prospective study. *Orthod. Craniofacial Res.* **2020**. [CrossRef] [PubMed]
57. Mummolo, S.; Nota, A.; Albani, F.; Marchetti, E.; Gatto, R.; Marzo, G.; Quinzi, V.; Tecco, S. Salivary levels of Streptococcus mutans and Lactobacilli and other salivary indices in patients wearing clear aligners versus fixed orthodontic appliances: An observational study. *PLoS ONE* **2020**, *15*, e0228798. [CrossRef] [PubMed]
58. Lu, H.; Tang, H.; Zhou, T.; Kang, N. Assessment of the periodontal health status in patients undergoing orthodontic treatment with fixed appliances and Invisalign system. *Med.* **2018**, *97*, e0248. [CrossRef]
59. Wu, Y.; Cao, L.; Cong, J. The periodontal status of removable appliances vs fixed appliances. *Med.* **2020**, *99*, e23165. [CrossRef] [PubMed]
60. Perkowski, K.; Baltaza, W.; Conn, D.B.; Marczyńska-Stolarek, M.; Chomicz, L. Examination of oral biofilm microbiota in patients using fixed orthodontic appliances in order to prevent risk factors for health complications. *Ann. Agric. Environ. Med.* **2019**, *26*, 231–235. [CrossRef]
61. Levine, R.S.; Pitts, N.; Nugent, Z.J. The fate of 1,587 unrestored carious deciduous teeth: A retrospective general dental practice based study from northern England. *Br. Dent. J.* **2002**, *193*, 99–103. [CrossRef]
62. Hagg, U.; Kaveewatcharanont, P.; Samaranayake, Y.H.; Samaranayake, L.P. The effect of fixed orthodontic appliances on the oral carriage of Candida species and Enterobacteriaceae. *Eur. J. Orthod.* **2004**, *26*, 623–629. [CrossRef] [PubMed]
63. Arslan, S.G.; Akpolat, N.; Kama, J.D.; Özer, T.; Hamamcı, O. One-year follow-up of the effect of fixed orthodontic treatment on colonization by oral candida. *J. Oral Pathol. Med.* **2007**, *37*, 26–29. [CrossRef]
64. Muzurovic, S.; Babajic, E.; Masic, T.; Smajic, R.; Selmanagic, A. The Relationship Between Oral Hygiene and Oral Colonisation with Candida Species. *Med Arch.* **2012**, *66*, 415–417. [CrossRef]
65. Grzegocka, K.; Krzyściak, P.; Hille-Padalis, A.; Loster, J.E.; Talaga-Ćwiertnia, K.; Loster, B.W. Candida prevalence and oral hygiene due to orthodontic therapy with conventional brackets. *BMC Oral Heal.* **2020**, *20*, 1–9. [CrossRef] [PubMed]
66. Sanz-Orrio-Soler, I.; De Luxán, S.A.; Sheth, C.C. Oral colonization by Candida species in orthodontic patients before, during and after treatment with fixed appliances: A prospective controlled trial. *J. Clin. Exp. Dent.* **2020**, *12*, e1071–e1077. [CrossRef]
67. Tapia, C.V.; Batarce, C.; Amaro, J.; Hermosilla, G.; Rodas, P.I.; Magne, F. Microbiological characterisation of the colonisation by Candida sp in patients with orthodontic fixed appliances and evaluation of host responses in saliva. *Mycoses* **2018**, *62*, 247–251. [CrossRef]
68. Jiang, Q.; Li, J.; Mei, L.; Du, J.; Levrini, L.; Abbate, G.M.; Li, H. Periodontal health during orthodontic treatment with clear aligners and fixed appliances. *J. Am. Dent. Assoc.* **2018**, *149*, 712–720. [CrossRef] [PubMed]
69. Flores-Mir, C. Clear Aligner Therapy Might Provide a Better Oral Health Environment for Orthodontic Treatment Among Patients at Increased Periodontal Risk. *J. Évid. Based Dent. Pr.* **2019**, *19*, 198–199. [CrossRef]
70. Slots, J. Periodontal herpesviruses: Prevalence, pathogenicity, systemic risk. *Periodontol. 2000* **2015**, *69*, 28–45. [CrossRef] [PubMed]

71. Hong, C.H.L.; Dean, D.R.; Hull, K.; Hu, S.J.; Sim, Y.F.; Nadeau, C.; Gonçalves, S.; Lodi, G.; Hodgson, T.A. World Workshop on Oral Medicine VII: Relative frequency of oral mucosal lesions in children, a scoping review. *Oral Dis.* **2019**, *25*, 193–203. [CrossRef] [PubMed]
72. Müller, L.K.; Jungbauer, G.; Jungbauer, R.; Wolf, M.; Deschner, J. Biofilm and Orthodontic Therapy. *Monographs in Oral Science* **2021**, *29*, 201–213. [CrossRef] [PubMed]
73. Carinci, F.; Martinelli, M.; Contaldo, M.; Santoro, R.; Pezzetti, F.; Lauritano, D.; Candotto, V.; Mucchi, D.; Palmieri, A.; Tagliabue, A.; et al. Focus on periodontal disease and development of endocarditis. *J. Boil. Regul. Homeost. agents* **2018**, *32*, 143–147.
74. Contaldo, M.; Itro, A.; Lajolo, C.; Gioco, G.; Inchingolo, F.; Serpico, R. Overview on Osteoporosis, Periodontitis and Oral Dysbiosis: The Emerging Role of Oral Microbiota. *Appl. Sci.* **2020**, *10*, 6000. [CrossRef]
75. Contaldo, M.; Di Stasio, D.; Della Vella, F.; Lauritano, D.; Serpico, R.; Santoro, R.; Lucchese, A. Real Time In Vivo Confocal Microscopic Analysis of the Enamel Remineralization by Casein Phosphopeptide-Amorphous Calcium Phosphate (CPP-ACP): A Clinical Proof-of-Concept Study. *Appl. Sci.* **2020**, *10*, 4155. [CrossRef]

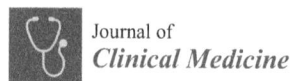

Review

Orthopedic Treatment for Class II Malocclusion with Functional Appliances and Its Effect on Upper Airways: A Systematic Review with Meta-Analysis

Darius Bidjan, Rahel Sallmann, Theodore Eliades and Spyridon N. Papageorgiou *

Clinic of Orthodontics and Pediatric Dentistry, Center of Dental Medicine, University of Zurich, 8032 Zurich, Switzerland; darius.bidjan@bluewin.ch (D.B.); rahel.sallmann@hotmail.com (R.S.); theodore.eliades@zzm.uzh.ch (T.E.)
* Correspondence: snpapage@gmail.com

Received: 26 October 2020; Accepted: 23 November 2020; Published: 25 November 2020

Abstract: Aim of this systematic review was to assess the effects of orthopedic treatment for Class II malocclusion with Functional Appliances (FAs) on the dimensions of the upper airways. Eight databases were searched up to October 2020 for randomized or nonrandomized clinical studies on FA treatment of Class II patients with untreated control groups. After duplicate study selection, data extraction, and risk of bias assessment according to Cochrane guidelines, random effects meta-analyses of mean differences (MDs) and their 95% confidence intervals (CIs) were performed, followed by subgroup/meta-regression analyses and assessment of the quality of evidence. A total of 20 nonrandomized clinical studies (4 prospective/16 retrospective) including 969 patients (47.9% male; mean age 10.9 years) were identified. Orthopedic treatment with FAs was associated with increased oropharynx volume (MD = 2356.14 mm^3; 95% CI = 1276.36 to 3435.92 mm^3; $p < 0.001$) compared to natural growth. Additionally, significant increases in nasopharynx volume, minimal constricted axial area of pharyngeal airway, and airway were seen, while removable FAs showed considerably greater effects than fixed FAs ($p = 0.04$). Finally, patient age and treatment duration had a significant influence in the effect of FAs on airways, as had baseline matching and sample size adequacy. Clinical evidence on orthopedic Class II treatment with FAs is associated with increased upper airway dimensions. However, the quality of evidence is very low due to methodological issues of existing studies, while the clinical relevance of increases in airway dimensions remains unclear.

Keywords: Class II malocclusion; mandibular retrognathism; orthopedic treatment; dentofacial orthopedics; orthodontics; functional appliances; clinical trials; systematic review; meta-analysis

1. Introduction

1.1. Background

Skeletal Class II malocclusion is the most common clinical entity the orthodontist is faced with [1] and is often due to a retrognathic mandible [2]. Among growing patients with a retrognathic mandible, orthopedic advancement of the mandible and its dentition with functional appliances is often performed with considerable success. However, functional appliances are now believed to have mostly dentoalveolar effects [3,4] and more limited effects on skeletal components [5–7].

At the same time, severe mandibular retrognathism has been linked to obstructive sleep apnea (OSA) [8] due to a retrodisplacement of the tongue and hyoid bone that may lead to a concomitant upper airway constriction [9,10]. Inversely, therapeutic advancement of the mandible with functional appliances among OSA patients has been shown to be an effective means to improve clinical OSA parameters [11]. Therefore, it might be reasonable to expect that functional appliance therapy among patients with skeletal Class II malocclusion might be associated with a beneficial effect on the patient's airways [12] and possibly breathing function [13].

A previous systematic review on the subject [14] concluded that early treatment with functional appliances had positive effects on the upper airway, especially on oropharyngeal dimensions, in growing skeletal Class II patients and might decrease potential risk of OSA for growing patients in the future. However, this review only covered literature published only up to the start of 2017, while its conclusions might be influenced by existing methodological issues like lack of an a priori protocol [15], incomplete handling of risk of bias within studies according to the latest Cochrane guidelines [16], issues with the data synthesis (double-counting of controls from multiarm studies, outdated statistical modelling, lack of sensitivity analyses) [17], and no assessment of the quality of meta-evidence [18]. Finally, that systematic review only assessed overall effects, did not associate them with differences between removable/fixed appliances [3,4] and did not assess any patient risk factors.

1.2. Objective

Therefore, the aim of this systematic review was to compare the effects of functional appliance treatment for Class II malocclusion on the upper airway dimensions with natural occurring growth in untreated Class II patients.

2. Materials and Methods

2.1. Protocol, Registration, and Review Question

This review's protocol was made a priori, registered in PROSPERO (CRD42019125897) with all post hoc changes transparently reported (Appendix A). The conduct and reporting of this review are guided by the Cochrane Handbook [19] and the PRISMA statement [20], respectively. The focused question this review tried to answer is: "Does functional appliance therapy of growing Class II patients lead to an increase in the upper airway dimensions to a degree greater than expected by natural growth alone?".

2.2. Eligibility Criteria

Based on the Participants-Intervention-Comparison-Outcome-Study design (PICOS) schema and as few randomized trials exist on this matter, included were randomized and nonrandomized clinical studies on systemically healthy growing human patients of any age (<18 years), sex, and ethnicity with Class II malocclusion with mandibular retrognathism receiving orthopedic functional appliance treatment without any limitations on language, publication year, or status. Excluded were nonclinical studies, animal studies, and case reports/series, as well as studies with obstructive sleep apnea patients, studies without functional appliance treatment, and studies without an untreated longitudinal Class II control group. The primary outcome for this review was the total volume of the upper airways or any specific airway compartment assessed with Cone Beam Computerized Tomography (CBCT). Secondary outcomes included other measures of airway dimensions in terms of linear distances or areas, measured either on lateral cephalograms or CBCTs and in either upright or supine position.

2.3. Information Sources and Search

Eight electronic databases were searched without restrictions from inception to 20 October 2020 (Table S1), while ClinicalTrials.gov Directory of Open Access Journals, Digital Dissertations, metaRegister of Controlled Trials, WHO, Google Scholar, and the reference/citation lists of included articles or existing systematic reviews were manually searched.

2.4. Study Selection

Two authors (D.B. and R.S.) screened the titles and/or abstracts of search hits to exclude obviously inappropriate studies, prior to checking their full texts. Any differences between the two reviewers were resolved by discussion with the last authors (T.E. and S.N.P.).

2.5. Data Collection Process and Items

Data from included studies was collected independently by two authors (D.B. and R.S.) with the same way to resolve discrepancies using predefined/piloted forms covering: (a) study characteristics (design, clinical setting, and country), (b) patient characteristics (age and sex), (c) eligibility criteria for patient selection, (d) treatment details (appliance and duration), and (e) outcome measurement modality.

2.6. Risk of Bias of Individual Studies

The risk of bias of included nonrandomized studies was assessed with a custom tool based on the ROBINS-I ("Risk Of Bias In Nonrandomized Studies—of Interventions") [16]. Assessment of the risk of bias was likewise independently performed by two authors (DB, RS) with the same approach being applied to resolve discrepancies.

2.7. Data Synthesis and Summary Measures

An effort was made to maximize data for the analysis; where data were missing, they were calculated by ourselves. As the outcome of upper airway dimensions is bound to be affected by patient and treatment-related characteristics (baseline dimensions, growth potential, compliance, and response to treatment), a random-effects model was a priori deemed appropriate to calculate the average distribution of true effects, based on clinical and statistical reasoning [21], and a restricted maximum likelihood variance estimator with improved performance was used according to recent guidance [22]. Mean differences (MDs) with their corresponding 95% confidence intervals (CIs) were used, while the standardized mean difference (SMD) was decided post hoc to combine similar measurements of nasopharyngeal volume (Appendix A). The extent and impact of between-study heterogeneity was assessed by inspecting the forest plots and by calculating the τ^2 (absolute heterogeneity) or the I^2 statistics (relative heterogeneity). I^2 defines the proportion of total variability in the result explained by heterogeneity, and not chance, while also considering the heterogeneity's direction (localization on the forest plot) and uncertainty around heterogeneity estimates [23]. The 95% random-effects predictive intervals were calculated to incorporate observed heterogeneity and predict expected results in a future treatment [24].

2.8. Additional Analyses and Risk of Bias across Studies

Possible sources of heterogeneity were a priori planned to be sought through random-effects subgroup analyses and meta-regressions in meta-analyses of at least five trials, according to the following factors: appliance type (removable or fixed), patient age, patient sex, and treatment duration. Reporting biases were assessed with contour-enhanced funnel plots and Egger's test [25] for meta-analyses with ≥10 studies.

The overall quality of meta-evidence (i.e., the strength of clinical recommendations) was rated using the Grades of Recommendations, Assessment, Development and Evaluation (GRADE) approach [18] following recent guidance for nonrandomized studies [26]. The produced forest plots were augmented with contours denoting the magnitude of the observed effects (Appendix A) to assess heterogeneity, clinical relevance, and imprecision [17].

Robustness of the results was checked for meta-analyses ≥ 5 studies with sensitivity analyses based on (i) the inclusion of prospective versus retrospective studies, (ii) unequal duration of treatment/observation between treated/control groups, (iii) inadequate matching (assessed with Cohen's d for baseline measurements of each outcome), and (iv) studies with inadequate versus inadequate samples, with the cut-off set at 25 patients/group. All analyses were run in Stata version 14.0 (StataCorp LP, College Station, TX, USA) by one author (S.N.P.) and the dataset was openly provided [27]. All *p* values were two sided with α = 5%, except for the test of between-studies or between-subgroups heterogeneity where α-value was set as 10% [28].

3. Results

3.1. Study Selection

A total of 2095 hits were retrieved by the literature database search and another 6 records were identified manually (Figure 1). After removing duplicates and eliminating nonrelevant reports by title/abstracts, 185 full-text papers were checked against the eligibility criteria (Table S2). In the end, 20 publications pertaining to 20 unique studies were included in this review.

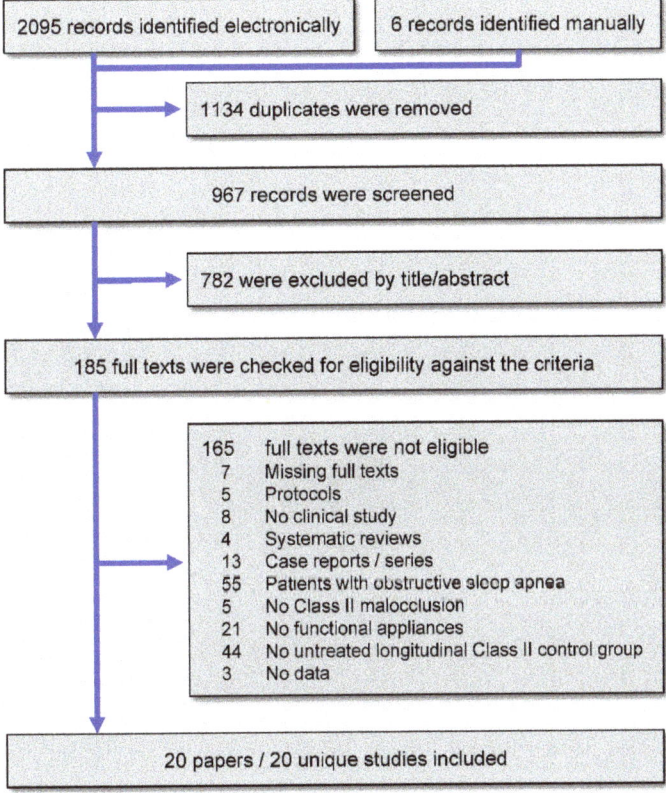

Figure 1. Preferred Reporting Items for Systematic Reviews and Meta-Analyses (PRISMA) flow diagram for the identification and selection of studies.

3.2. Study Characteristics

All 20 included studies [29–48] were nonrandomized (Table 1), with only 4 studies (20%) being prospective. All studies were conducted within a university setting (one jointly with a hospital) in 9 different countries (Brazil, Egypt, India, Italy, Pakistan, Spain, Sweden, Turkey, and the United States of America). The included studies were all published as journal papers and were in English, except from one study that was in Turkish.

Table 1. Characteristics of included studies.

Study	Design; Setting; Country *	Patients (M/F); Age †	Appliance (Active Duration)	Radio-Graph
Aksu 2017 [29]	rNRS; Uni; TR	Exp: 16 (4/12); 10.3 Control: 19 (9/10); 10.2	Exp: Activator (15.6) Control—(12.0)	Lateral ceph
Alhammadi 2019 [30]	pNRS; Uni; EG	Exp1: 23 (0/23); 11.9 Exp2: 21 (0/21); 13.5 Control: 18 (0/18); 11.3	Exp1: Twin Block (Tx end) Exp2: Forsus FRD (Tx end) Control—(as Exp1-2)	CBCT
Ali 2015 [31]	rNRS; Uni; PK	Exp: 42 (21/21); 10.4 Control ‡: 32 (16/16); 10.1	Exp: Twin Block +FA (36.4) Control—(36.0)	Lateral ceph
Atik 2017 [32]	rNRS; Uni; TR	Exp1: 15 (4/11); 8.9 Exp2: 15 (6/9); 10.6 Control: 10 (6/4); 9.3	Exp1: Fränkel-2 (14.3) Exp2: X-Bow (8.6) Control—(14.8)	Lateral ceph
Bavbek 2016 [33]	rNRS; Uni; TR	Exp: 18 (10/8); 13.6 Control: 19 (8/11); 12.7	Exp: Forsus FRD (8.7) Control—(11.9)	Lateral ceph
Cortese 2017 [34]	rNRS; Uni; IT	Exp: 10 (7/3); 10.9 Control: 10 (5/5); 10.1	Exp: Activator/Twin Block (21.6) Control—(40.8)	Lateral ceph
Drosen 2018 [35]	rNRS; Uni; SE	Exp: 13 (13/0); 12.4 Control ‡: 13 (13/0); 12.1	Exp: Herbst (21.6) Control—(25.2)	Lateral ceph
Elfeky 2015 [36]	pNRS; Uni; EG	Exp: 18 (0/18); 10.0–12.0 Control: 18 (0/18); 10.0–12.0	Exp: Twin Block (8.0) Control—(8.0)	CBCT
Entrenas 2019 [37]	pNRS; Uni; ES	Exp: 40 (20/20); 9.8 Control: 20 (10/10); 9.1	Exp: Twin Block (Tx end) Control—(12.0–24.0)	Lateral ceph
Fabiani 2017 [38]	rNRS; Uni; IT	Exp: 28 (13/15); 8.4 Control ‡: 21 (14/7); 8.5	Exp: Fränkel-2 (14.6) Control—(16.0)	Lateral ceph
Ghodke 2014 [39]	pNRS; Uni; IN	Exp: 20 (11/9); 8.0–13.0 Control: 18 (9/9); 8.0–14.0	Exp: Twin Block (6.0) Control: ± sectionals (6.0)	Lateral ceph
Goymen 2019 [40]	rNRS; Uni; TR	Exp1: 15 (7/8); 12.1 Exp2: 15 (7/8); 14.5 Control ‡: 10 (NR); 13.0	Exp1: Twin Block (Tx end) Exp2: Forsus FRD (Tx end) Control—(6.0)	Lateral ceph
Jena 2013 [41]	rNRS; Uni; IN	Exp: 16 (9/7); 12.8 Exp2: 21 (11/10); 11.4 Control 16 (9/7); 10.6	Exp1: MAPA4 (6.2) Exp2: Twin Block (9.4) Control: ± sectionals (9.9)	Lateral ceph
Kilinc 2018 [42]	uNRS; Uni; TR	Exp: 19 (11/8); NR Control: 19 (7/12); NR	Exp: Activator (11.5) Control—(11.3)	Lateral ceph
Oliveira 2020 [43]	rNRS; Uni; BR	Exp: 24 (15/9); NR Control: 18 (10/8); NR	Exp: Herbst (8.0) Control: Pre-Tx (10.4)	CBCT
Ozbek 1998 [44]	rNRS; Uni; TR	Exp: 26 (11/15) 11.5 Control: 15 (7/8) 11.3	Exp: Activator±headgear (17.4) Control—(23.0)	Lateral ceph
Pavoni 2017 [45]	uNRS; Uni; IT	Exp: 51 (27/24); 9.9 Control: 31 (15/16); 10.1	Exp: Activator (21.6) Control—(22.8)	Lateral ceph
Rizk 2016 [46]	rNRS; Uni; US	Exp: 20 (7/13); 11.7 Control: 73 (NR); NR	Exp: MARA+FA (27.4) Control—(NR)	CBCT
Rongo 2020 [47]	rNRS; Hosp/Uni; IT	Exp: 34 (21/13); 11.1 Control: 34 (25/9); 10.4	Exp: Sander (14.8) Control—(13.9)	Lateral ceph
Ulusoy 2014 [48]	rNRS; Uni; TR	Exp: 16 (8/8); 11.4 Control: 19 (8/11); 12.1	Exp: Activator (11.0) Control—(11.4)	Lateral ceph

* given with the country's ISO 3166 alpha-2 code, † given as mean (one value) or if mean not reported, given as range (two values), ‡ historical control from growth study or archive. CBCT, cone beam computerized tomography; ceph, cephalogram; Exp, experimental group; FA, fixed appliance (braces); FRD, fatigue-resistant device; MAPA4, Mandibular Protraction Appliance-IV; MARA, Mandibular Anterior Repositioning Appliance; pNRS, prospective nonrandomized study; Pract, private practice; rNRS, retrospective nonrandomized study; Tx, treatment; Uni, university clinic; uNRS, nonrandomized study with unclear design.

The eligible studies included a total of 969 patients (536 treated/433 untreated), to a median sample size of 40.5 patients/study (range: 20–93 patients/study). Among the 20 studies reporting the patients' gender, 47.9% of the patients were male (424 of the total 886), while from the 16 studies reporting mean age, the average across studies was 10.9 years (range of average age/study 8.4–14.5 years). The identified studies used dental Class II molar relationship, cephalometric skeletal anteroposterior jaw relationship, overjet, or vertical jaw configuration as eligibility criteria to include patients, while 5 studies (25%) also included explicit reporting of no respiratory problems (Table S3). Removable functional appliances (Activator, Fränkel-2, Twin Block, or Sander appliance) were used in 16 studies, while fixed functional appliances (Herbst, Forsus Fatigue Resistant Device, Mandibular Protraction Appliance-IV, Mandibular Anterior Repositioning Appliance, or X-Bow appliance) were used in 8 studies (with 4 studies using both removable and fixed appliances). One study [32] also included a prefabricated myofunctional appliance (Trainer 4 Kids), but this was omitted from the review, due to the different modus operandi [49]. One study [44] incorporated headgear to the Activator for anchorage reinforcement, while another study [31] also included a second phase treatment with braces after a first phase with Twin Block. Airway dimensions were assessed by lateral cephalograms in 16 (80%) of the studies and by CBCT in the remaining 4 (20%)—all of them made in an upright position. All studies reported outcome results before and after treatment with functional appliances, while only one study [35] reported long-term follow-up after treatment (6 years).

3.3. Risk of Bias within Studies

The risk of bias of included nonrandomized studies is summarized in Table 2 and given in detail in Table S4. For most studies, inclusion of patients in the study was not based on any factor that could influence treatment outcome (85%), and the treatment/control groups were clearly defined (95%). Treated/untreated patients were explicitly reported to be selected from the same source and time in only half (50%) of the studies, while the rate of adequate matching at baseline for potential confounders (age, sex, malocclusion, airway dimensions, and treatment/observation duration) between treated/control patients ranged from 35% to 65%. Finally, no study blinded the person measuring the cephalometric/CBCT variables, while the sample size was deemed to be adequate (≥50 patients) in 4 (20%) studies. All included studies were judged to be in critical risk of bias, as issues existed for at least three domains per study.

Table 2. Risk of bias summary of included nonrandomized studies.

Question	Yes/Probably Yes	No/Probably No	No Information
Was the study prospective?	5 (25%)	15 (75%)	–
Was selection of patients based on any factor that could influence the outcome (malocclusion, airways, compliance, missed appointments, breakages)?	3 (15%)	17 (85%)	–
Were FA/CTR groups clearly defined?	19 (95%)	1 (5%)	–
Were FA/CTR patients treated/observed at the same place/time?	10 (50%)	4 (20%)	6 (30%)
Were FA/CTR patients matched for baseline age?	11 (55%)	5 (25%)	4 (20%)
Were FA/CTR patients matched for baseline sex?	13 (65%)	5 (25%)	2 (10%)
Were FA/CTR patients matched for baseline malocclusion?	12 (60%)	5 (25%)	3 (15%)
Were FA/CTR patients matched for baseline airway measurements?	7 (35%)	13 (65%)	–
Was the use of other appliances the same among FA/CTR patients?	14 (70%)	6 (30%)	–
Was the observation period similar for FA/CTR patients?	9 (45%)	7 (35%)	4 (20%)
Were FA/CTR patients measured exactly the same way?	20 (100%)	–	–
Were FA/CTR patients measured blindly?	–	20 (100%)	–
Was the adequate sample? (25 patients per group)	4 (20%)	16 (80%)	–

CTR, untreated control group; FA, functional appliance group.

3.4. Results of Individual Studies and Data Synthesis

The results of studies not included in any meta-analyses are given in Table S5. Functional appliances were associated with a statistically significant but clinically irrelevant reduction in hypopharynx dimensions compared to untreated controls. Additionally, functional appliances were associated with statistically significant increases in nasopharynx dimensions, oropharynx cross-section, and pharynx height—with the increase in nasopharynx being also clinically relevant.

Meta-analyses of the effects of functional appliances on upper airway dimensions are given in Table 3. Orthopedic therapy with functional appliances was associated with statistically significant increases in the volume of both the nasopharynx (3 studies; SMD = 0.95; 95% CI = 0.36 to 1.54; $p = 0.002$) and the oropharynx (4 studies; MD = 2356.14 mm^3; 95% CI = 1276.36 to 3435.92 mm^3; $p < 0.001$; Figure 2) compared to natural growth.

Moderate heterogeneity existed among studies (I^2 60% and 69%, respectively), which, however, influenced only the precise quantification of the improvement seen through treatment (as all included studies were on the same side of the forest plot).

Furthermore, functional appliance therapy was associated with statistically significant increases in (i) the minimal constricted axial area of pharyngeal airway (2 studies; MD = 59.91 mm^2); (ii) superoposterior airway space (8 studies; MD = 1.63 mm); (iii) middle airway space (11 studies; MD = 1.25 mm); (iv) inferior airway space (10 studies; MD = 1.32 mm); (v) McNamara's lower pharynx dimension (3 studies; MD = 2.31 mm); (vi) lower adenoid thickness (2 studies; MD = 1.16 mm); and (vii) pharyngeal dimension at the epiglottal base (4 studies; MD = 0.70 mm). Heterogeneity was relatively moderate, except from the meta-analyses of middle and inferior airway space, where considerable heterogeneity was seen ($I^2 > 75\%$).

3.5. Subgroup and Meta-Regression Analyses

Differences in the effects of removable and fixed functional appliances were assessed in Table 4 and tested formally with subgroup interaction for meta-analyses of at least 5 studies. For most outcomes, removable functional appliances showed considerable greater benefits in terms of airway dimensions than fixed appliances, like nasopharynx volume (SMDs of 1.64 and 0.73, respectively), superoposterior airway space (MDs of 1.41 and 1.08 mm, respectively), middle airway space (MDs of 1.37 and 1.02 mm, respectively), and inferior airway space (MDs of 1.52 and 0.79 mm, respectively). Additionally, increases in McNamara's lower pharynx and sagittal depth of the nasopharynx were seen only with removable functional appliances and had no significant effect with fixed functional appliances. Furthermore, an effect reversal was seen for the minimal constricted axial area of pharyngeal airway, where an increase was seen with removable appliances and a reduction was seen with fixed appliances. However, all these differences were not confirmed by formal subgroup interaction—possibly due to low statistical power. The only exception was for the primary outcome of oropharynx volume, where removable appliances induced a statistically significantly greater increase than fixed appliances (MDs of 2595.56 and 2303.57 mm^3; $p = 0.04$).

Table 3. Random-effects meta-analyses for the effect of any functional appliance versus untreated controls on airways.

Outcome	Studies	MD (95% CI)	p	I^2 (95% CI)	tau^2 (95% CI)	95% Prediction
Superoposterior airway space (mm)	8	1.63 (1.03, 2.23)	<0.001	68% (28%, 92%)	0.42 (0.08, 2.15)	−0.13, 3.39
Posterior airway space (mm)	8	0.52 (−0.20, 1.24)	0.15	47% (0%, 87%)	0.44 (0, 3.44)	−1.34, 2.38
Middle airway space (mm)	11	1.25 (0.53, 1.98)	0.001	81% (58%, 93%)	1.09 (0.36, 3.69)	−1.25, 3.76
Inferior airway space (mm)	10	1.32 (0.34, 2.31)	0.009	90% (76%, 97%)	1.97 (0.75, 6.47)	−2.12, 4.76
McNamara's upper pharynx (mm)	3	1.35 (−0.57, 3.27)	0.17	87% (45%, 99%)	2.45 (0.31, 48.50)	−22.12, 24.82
McNamara's lower pharynx (mm)	3	2.31 (0.79, 3.82)	0.003	70% (0%, 99%)	1.18 (0, 41.05)	−14.64, 19.25
Upper adenoid thickness (AD2-H; mm)	2	0.24 (−2.10, 2.58)	0.84	93% (NE)	2.65 (NE)	NE
Lower adenoid thickness (AD1-Ba; mm)	2	1.16 (0.46, 1.86)	0.001	0% (NE)	0 (NE)	NE
Upper airway thickness (PNS-AD2; mm)	5	0.38 (−0.18, 0.94)	0.19	13% (0%, 89%)	0.06 (0, 3.00)	−0.81, 1.57
Nasopharynx height (PNS-BaN; mm)	2	0.13 (−0.77, 1.02)	0.78	51% (NE)	0.21 (NE)	NE
Upper pharyngeal airway passage (Ptm-UPW; mm)	2	−0.37 (−1.73, 0.99)	0.60	0% (NE)	0 (NE)	NE
Base of epiglottis-posterior pharyngeal wall (V-LPW; mm)	4	0.70 (0.11, 1.29)	0.02	14% (0%, 93%)	0.05 (0, 4.46)	−0.93, 2.33
Sagittal depth of bony nasopharynx (Ba-PNS; mm)	2	1.25 (0.06, 2.43)	0.04	21% (NE)	0.18 (NE)	NE
Minimum axial area (mm²)	2	59.91 (41.46, 78.35)	<0.001	0% (NE)	0 (NE)	NE
Oropharynx sagittal dimension (mm)	2	1.20 (−2.12, 4.52)	0.48	97% (80%, 100%)	5.58 (0.68, 721.82)	NE
Oropharynx area (units)	2 *	556.10 (−279.88, 1392.08)	0.19	0% (NE)	0 (NE)	NE
Nasopharynx volume (mm³)	3	0.95 † (0.36, 1.54)	0.002	60% (0%, 98%)	0.16 (0, 5.02)	−5.44, 7.34
Oropharynx volume (mm³)	4	2356.14 (1276.36, 3435.92)	<0.001	69% (0%, 98%)	>100 (0, >100)	−1931.83, 6644.10

CI, confidence interval; MD, mean difference; NE, not estimable. * Study of Ozbek 1998 omitted due to different measurement method. † SMD used instead of MD due to big differences in the control group baseline measurements.

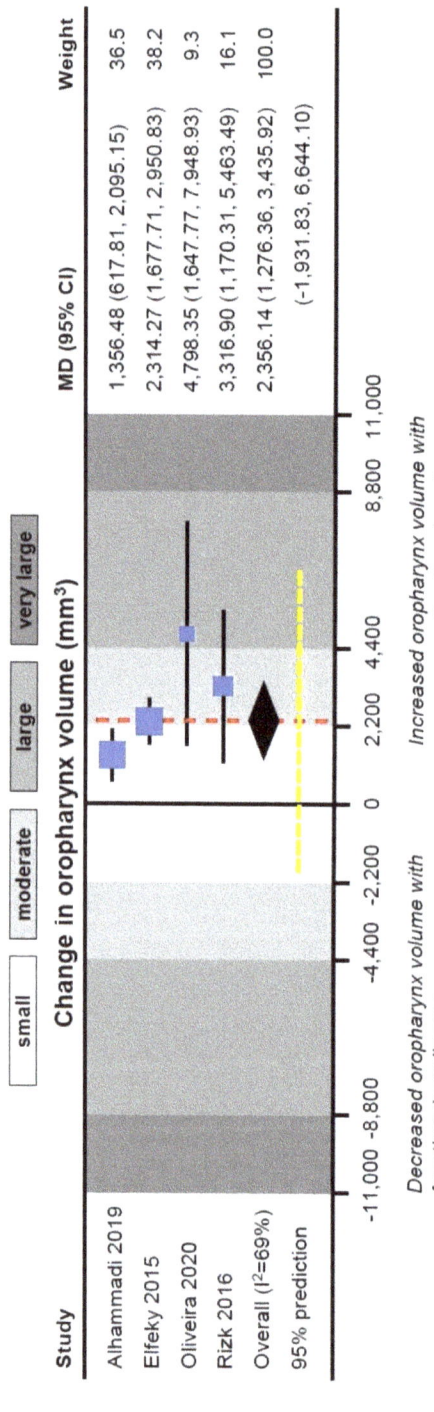

Figure 2. Contour-enhanced forest plot for the effect of functional appliances on oropharynx volume.

Table 4. Subgroup analyses for the effect of removable or fixed functional appliances analyses versus untreated controls on airways.

Outcome	All Appliances MD (95% CI)	p	Removable Appliances MD (95% CI)	p	Fixed Appliances MD (95% CI)	p	P$_{SG}$
Superoposterior airway space (mm)	$n = 8$ 1.63 (1.03, 2.23)	<0.001	$n = 7$ 1.41 (0.65, 2.17)	<0.001	$n = 2$ 1.08 (0.35, 1.82)	0.004	0.20
Posterior airway space (mm)	$n = 8$ 0.52 (−0.20, 1.24)	0.15	$n = 6$ 0.83 (−0.18, 1.84)	0.11	$n = 2$ 0.14 (−0.77, 1.06)	0.76	0.35
Middle airway space (mm)	$n = 11$ 1.25 0.53, 1.98)	0.001	$n = 9$ 1.37 (0.47, 2.26)	0.003	$n = 3$ 1.02 (0.29, 1.75)	0.006	0.26
Inferior airway space (mm)	$n = 10$ 1.32 (0.34, 2.31)	0.009	$n = 8$ 1.52 (0.32, 2.72)	0.01	$n = 2$ 0.79 (0.03, 1.54)	0.04	0.15
McNamara's upper pharynx (mm)	$n = 4$ 1.35 (−0.57, 3.27)	0.17	$n = 3$ 2.05 (−0.04, 4.14)	0.06	$n = 1$ −0.20 (−1.81, 1.41)	0.81	NT
McNamara's lower pharynx (mm)	$n = 3$ 2.31 (0.79, 3.82)	0.003	$n = 2$ 2.95 (2.13, 3.78)	<0.001	$n = 1$ 0 (−2.67, 2.67)	1.00	NT
Upper adenoid thickness (AD2-H; mm)	$n = 2$ 0.24 (−2.10, 2.58)	0.84	$n = 2$ 0.24 (−2.10, 2.58)	0.84	–		NT
Lower adenoid thickness (AD1-Ba; mm)	$n = 5$ 1.16 (0.46, 1.86)	0.001	$n = 4$ 1.16 (0.46, 1.86)	0.001	$n = 1$		NT
Upper airway thickness (PNS-AD2; mm)	$n = 2$ 0.38 (−0.18, 0.94)	0.19	$n = 2$ 0.13 (−0.51, 0.78)	0.69	$n = 1$ 0.61 (−1.90, 3.12)	0.63	0.73
Nasopharynx height (PNS-BaN; mm)	$n = 2$ 0.13 (−0.77, 1.02)	0.78	$n = 2$ 0.27 (−1.01, 1.56)	0.68	$n = 1$ 0.02 (−0.88, 0.92)	0.97	NT
Upper pharyngeal airway passage (Ptm-UPW; mm)	$n = 2$ −0.37 (−1.73, 0.99)	0.60	$n = 2$ −0.04 (−1.52, 1.44)	0.96	$n = 1$ −1.12 (−3.06, 0.82)	0.26	NT
Base of epiglottis-posterior pharyngeal wall (V-LFW; mm)	$n = 4$ 0.70 (0.11, 1.29)	0.02	$n = 3$ 0.65 (−0.33, 1.62)	0.19	$n = 2$ 0.51 (−0.46, 1.48)	0.30	NT
Sagittal depth of bony nasopharynx (Ba-PNS; mm)	$n = 2$ 1.25 (0.06, 2.43)	0.04	$n = 2$ 1.62 (0.57, 2.68)	0.003	$n = 1$ −0.71 (−2.91, 1.49)	0.53	NT
Minimum axial area (mm^2)	$n = 2$ 59.91(41.46, 78.35)	<0.001	$n = 2$ 91.60 (19.14, 197.56)	0.01	$n = 1$ −26.97 (−44.18, −9.76)	0.002	NT
Oropharynx sagittal dimension (mm)	$n = 2$ 1.20 (−2.12, 4.52)	0.48	$n = 1$ −0.65 (−0.89, −0.42)	<0.001	$n = 2$ 1.30 (−1.83, 4.42)	0.42	NT
Oropharynx area (units)	$n = 2$ * 556.10 (−279.88, 1392.08)	0.19	$n = 2$ 114.35 (98.61, 130.09)	<0.001	$n = 1$ 607.00 (−452.17, 1666.17)	0.26	NT
Nasopharynx volume (mm^3)	$n = 3$ 0.95 † (0.36, 1.54)	0.002	$n = 1$ 1.64 † (0.88, 2.40)	<0.001	$n = 1$ 0.73 † (0.10, 1.36)	0.02	NT
Oropharynx volume (mm^3)	$n = 4$ 2356.14 (1276.36, 3435.92)	<0.001	$n = 2$ 2595.56 (2013.07, 3178.05)	<0.001	$n = 3$ 2303.57 (−808.11, 5415.25)	0.15	0.04

CI, confidence interval; MD, mean difference; NT, not tested; P$_{SG}$, p value for subgroup differences. * Study of Ozbek 1998 omitted due to different measurement method. † SMD used instead of MD due to big differences in the control group baseline measurements.

Meta-regression analyses indicated that patient age had a significant influence on the effects of functional appliances (Table 5), as treatment-induced increase in posterior airway space was reduced on average by −0.36 mm (95% CI = −0.75 to 0.03 mm) for each additional year of age. Additionally, a dose-response relationship was seen between increases in airway and treatment duration, as for each additional treatment month, additional increases in superoposterior airway space (coefficient = 0.12 mm; 95% CI = −0.02 to 0.26 mm) and inferior airway space (coefficient = 0.29 mm; 95% CI = 0.12 to 0.45 mm) were seen. Limiting the meta-regressions to only removable functional appliances revealed a greater influence of patient's age on increases in posterior airway space (coefficient = −0.99 mm; 95% CI = −1.91 to −0.08 mm) and of treatment duration on inferior airway space (coefficient = 0.41 mm; 95% CI = 0.26 to 0.56 mm), which might be anticipated, due to the greater treatment effects of removable appliances on the airways.

Table 5. Meta-regression analysis on the effect of functional appliances on airways.

Outcome	Any Functional Appliance (Removable/Fixed)			Only Removable Appliances		
	Patient Age (Per Year)	Male % in Sample (Per %)	Treatment Duration (Per Month)	Patient Age (Per Year)	Male % in Sample (Per %)	Treatment Duration (Per Month)
Upper airway thickness (PNS-AD2; mm)	b = −0.55, p = 0.30	b = −4.03, p = 0.43	b = 0.03, p = 0.26	NT	b = −4.71, p = 0.46	NT
Superoposterior airway space (mm)	b = 0.11, p = 0.69	b = 1.99, p = 0.47	b = 0.12, p = 0.09	b = 0.41, p = 0.41	b = 2.13, p = 0.49	b = 0.17, p = 0.12
Posterior airway space (mm)	b = −0.36, p = 0.06	b = −6.00, p = 0.15	b = 0.07, p = 0.45	b = −0.99, p = 0.04	b = −6.15, p = 0.24	b = 0.07, p = 0.70
Middle airway space (mm)	b = 0.03, p = 0.91	b = −2.59, p = 0.41	b = 0.09, p = 0.28	b = 0.10, p = 0.84	b = −3.40, p = 0.37	b = 0.09, p = 0.48
Inferior airway space (mm)	b = −0.13, p = 0.78	b = 1.56, p = 0.71	b = 0.29, p = 0.003	b = 0.02, p = 0.98	b = 1.61, p = 0.73	b = 0.41, p < 0.001
Base of epiglottis-posterior pharyngeal wall (V-LPW; mm)	b = 0.29, p = 0.46	b = −12.09, p = 0.41	b = −0.13, p = 0.38	NT	b = −13.62, p = 0.55	NT
Oropharynx volume (mm^3)	b = −1256.28, p = 0.17	b = 5027.43, p = 0.23	b = 13.37, p = 0.92	NT	NT	NT

b, meta-regression coefficient; NT, not tested (as less than 5 studies contributed to the analysis).

3.6. Reporting Biases and Sensitivity Analyses

Reporting biases (including the possibility for publication bias) could be assessed only for the meta-analyses of middle and inferior airway space that included at least 10 studies. The funnel plots (Figure S1) indicated asymmetry, which was confirmed by Egger's test in both instances ($p = 0.07$ and $p = 0.006$, respectively). However, this was interpreted as small-study effects, with smaller/more imprecise studies reporting greater treatment effects than larger studies.

Sensitivity analyses according to methodological issues of existing studies are seen in Table 6. No significant differences in the meta-analyses were seen between prospective versus retrospective studies nor according to the difference between treatment and observation durations. However, adequate baseline matching had a significant effect on the reported treatment effects of functional appliances. Studies with greater baseline differences between treated/untreated patients (i.e., without adequate matching) reported significantly greater increases in middle (coefficient = 0.93 mm) and posterior airway space (coefficient = 1.86 mm). Furthermore, studies with adequate sample size (≥50 patients) reported significantly higher increases of inferior airway space (coefficient = 2.05 mm) compared to smaller studies. Therefore, future clinical recommendations should be based on studies with adequate baseline matching (preferably through randomization) and with adequate sample size.

Table 6. Sensitivity analyses on the effect of methodological characteristics on the effect of functional appliances on airways.

Outcome	Prospective Vs Retrospective (Ref)	Tx-Ctr Difference in Duration (Per Month)	Tx-Ctr Difference in Baseline Outcome (In Absolute Cohen's d)	Adequate Sample (≥ 50) vs. Inadequate (Ref)
Upper airway thickness (PNS-AD2; mm)	NE	b = 0.05 p = 0.82	b = 0.38 p = 0.26	b = 0.39 p = 0.59
Superoposterior airway space (mm)	NE	b = −0.07 p = 0.32	b = 0.82 p = 0.15	b = 0.91 p = 0.36
Posterior airway space (mm)	NE	b = 0.04 p = 0.83	b = 1.86 p = 0.08	b = −0.46 p = 0.65
Middle airway space (mm)	b = −0.65 p = 0.62	b = 0.01 p = 0.91	b = 0.93 p = 0.04	b = −1.56 p = 0.27
Inferior airway space (mm)	NE	b = −0.03 p = 0.79	b = 0.51 p = 0.64	b = 2.05 p = 0.09
Base of epiglottis-posterior pharyngeal wall (V-LPW; mm)	b = 0.95 p = 0.26	b = 0.03 p = 0.90	b = −0.48 p = 0.60	b = −1.45 p = 0.29
Oropharynx volume (mm^3)	b = −2334.16 p = 0.27	NE	b = −3586.53 p = 0.36	b = −1406.38 p = 0.51

b, meta-regression coefficient; Ctr, control; NE, not estimable; Ref, reference; Tx, treatment.

3.7. Quality of Evidence

The quality of evidence according to GRADE was very low in all instances (downgraded by two points), due to the lack of randomization and the many methodological issues from the identified retrospective studies that might introduce bias. Therefore, our confidence in current estimates is very low and future studies might change current recommendations.

4. Discussion

4.1. Evidence in Context

The present systematic review summarizes clinical evidence from existing studies assessing the effects of Class II orthopedic treatment with functional appliances on airway dimensions to untreated Class II controls. A total of 20 studies including 536 treated and 433 untreated Class II patients were finally included in the meta-analyses.

Mandibular advancement with removable or fixed functional appliances was associated with statistically significant increases in airway dimensions directly after treatment compared to what could be expected by Class II growth alone. Specifically, benefits were seen for volume of the naso- and oropharynx, the minimal constricted axial area of pharyngeal airway, and many sagittal measurements of the oropharynx (Table 3). However, many of these changes, especially at the upper pharynx, were small to moderate in magnitude, which means that they might have little clinical relevance. On the contrary, greater effects were seen at the lower part of the pharynx and this indicates that any clinically relevant benefits in airway dimensions or breathing might be attributed in this compartment. There is some evidence indicating that normal patients and patients with sleep-disordered breathing have significant differences in the dimensions of the pharyngeal airway or the thickness of the pharyngeal wall [50], and the lower retropalatal/retroglossal areas are mostly affected [51]. This area has also emerged as a sensitive parameter enabling to consistently assess the patient's respiratory conditions [52]. However, even though increases in airway volume or cross-section might be indicative of improved breathing, functional confirmation through improved nasal airflow resistance, nasal pressure, and patient-relevant outcomes is needed. Some data indicate that treatment with Herbst appliance improved nocturnal breathing in adolescents [53], but the evidence is weak due to the lack of a control group and further studies are needed.

The exact mechanism with which these changes on the upper airway occur is currently unknown, but it might be that the mesial displacement of the lower dentition and the labial flaring of the lower incisors, might cause anterior traction on the tongue and hyoid bone [48], thereby causing adaptive changes of the soft palate and leading to an increase in pharyngeal airway dimensions [33]. This is also compatible with the observation that the soft palate is anteriorly repositioned after functional appliance treatment of Class II [39,41] as the tongue moves away from the palate. However, confirmatory studies are needed.

The effects of orthopedic mandibular advancement on the airways were highly variable among the included studies, which was reflected in between-study heterogeneity. Part of this heterogeneity was explained by several patient- or treatment-related characteristics including patient age, appliance design, and treatment duration (Tables 4 and 5). Removable functional appliances were shown to exert greater changes in the upper airway dimensions than fixed appliances for most of the analyzed variables. This might be due to different skeletal/dentoalveolar effects of removable/fixed appliances that have been previously reported [4]. On the other hand, this might be due to the fact that fixed functional appliances are usually placed on older patients after most deciduous teeth have been shed, whereas removable functional appliances are often placed in the mixed dentition (an age difference also seen among the included studies). This might act as a confounding factor at least to some part, since patient age was consistently associated with the observed airway benefits, both for the whole set of included studies and, specifically, for the subset of removable appliances (Table 5). It is generally believed that, moreover, skeletal effects of functional appliances are more pronounced in patients treated before or during the growth peak [54].

Existing clinical studies only demonstrated the short-term beneficial effect of functional appliances on the upper airways. However, it remains to be seen whether such benefits remain stable in the long term. The sole included study assessing long-term status of treated Class II patients [35] indicated that not only were the benefits of functional appliance treatment retained 6 years afterwards, but a significantly greater post-treatment increase was seen. This is also consistent with previous evidence on the long-term stability of increased airway dimensions among patients with skeletal Class III treated orthopedically with maxillary protraction [55].

4.2. Strengths and Limitations

Among the strengths of the current review can be counted it is a priori registration [15], the extensive searching of the literature, the inclusion of untreated Class II controls, the use of contemporary statistical methods [22], the gauging of the quality of meta-evidence according to GRADE [18], and the transparent open provision of the dataset [56].

On the other hand, some limitations also exist, like the inclusion of weak study designs like retrospective nonrandomized studies [57] with historical controls [58], which might introduce bias. Additionally, most studies had small sample sizes and this can affect the precision of the estimated effects [59]. Moreover, many included studies were inadequately matched in terms of similar baseline airway dimensions, and baseline dissimilarities were associated with inflated treatment effects (Table 6), which is in agreement with previous meta-epidemiological evidence [60,61]. Furthermore, airways before and after treatment were assessed with radiographs done in the upright position and not in a supine position, since most studies were retrospective with nonapneic patients that received functional appliance treatment for their underlying malocclusion and airways were only secondarily assessed. However, changes between supine or upright posture can influence airways measurements [62–64], even though oropharyngeal area measurement from lateral cephalograms can be used as an initial screening measurement to predict the upright upper airway 3D volume [64]. Finally, the small number and the limited reporting of existing studies did not enable extensive subgroup and meta-regression analyses to identify and account for sources of confounding, like patient age, sex, growth pattern, and presence/size of tonsils or adenoid, which might influence the observed results. Further prospective, ideally randomized, studies with open provision of their full dataset [56] will help in shedding on the pure airway effects of orthopedic treatment for Class II malocclusion.

5. Conclusions

Current evidence indicates that orthopedic treatment with functional appliances for Class II malocclusion might be associated with increased volume and dimensions of the upper airways, which are dependent on patient- and treatment-related factors. However, our confidence in these data is very low due to the poor quality of existing studies and their small number. It is crucial that the clinical relevance of such anatomical changes is confirmed by functional analyses of breathing ability before concrete recommendations can be formulated.

Supplementary Materials: The following are available online at http://www.mdpi.com/2077-0383/9/12/3806/s1, Figure S1: Contour-enhanced funnel plots for assessing reporting biases and publication bias; Table S1: Literature searches with resulting hits (last search date: 20 October 2020); Table S2: List of studies identified from the literature search and their inclusion/exclusion status, with reasons; Table S3: Malocclusion characteristics of the patients within the included studies; Table S4: Detailed risk of bias of included nonrandomized studies; Table S5: Results of individual studies not included in meta-analyses.

Author Contributions: D.B., T.E. and S.N.P. developed the research protocol. D.B. and R.S. independently performed study selection in duplicate, data extraction, and risk of bias assessment. Disagreements were resolved with the last authors (T.E. and S.N.P.). Literature searches analysis were performed by the first author (D.B.) and data analysis was performed by the last author (S.N.P.). All authors (D.B., R.S., T.E. and S.N.P.) read and approved the final manuscript. All authors have read and agreed to the published version of the manuscript.

Funding: This research received no external funding.

Conflicts of Interest: The authors declare no conflict of interest.

Appendix A

Additional details of methods and deviations from protocol.

Additional method details:

- When before-and-after treatment values were provided, these were converted to treatment-induced increments (post minus pre) according to Cochrane guidelines assuming a pre/post correlation of 0.75 [19].
- The produced forest plots were augmented with contours denoting the magnitude of expected effects: small (up to half a Standard Deviation [SD]), moderate (half to one SD), large (one to two SDs) and very large (more than 2 SDs). The SD for each outcome's forest plot was based on the average pre-treatment SD of the response variable across all eligible studies for each meta-analysis (rounded up to 2 decimals).

Post hoc changes:

- The standardized mean difference was chosen over the mean difference for the meta-analysis of nasopharynx volume since considerable differences were seen among the measurements of the included studies (one study reporting baseline volume in the control group being twice as large as the volume in the other two studies).

References

1. Josefsson, E.; Bjerklin, K.; Lindsten, R. Malocclusion frequency in Swedish and immigrant adolescents—Influence of origin on orthodontic treatment need. *Eur. J. Orthod.* **2007**, *29*, 79–87. [CrossRef] [PubMed]
2. McNamara, J.A., Jr. Components of class II malocclusion in children 8–10 years of age. *Angle Orthod.* **1981**, *51*, 177–202. [CrossRef] [PubMed]
3. Koretsi, V.; Zymperdikas, V.F.; Papageorgiou, S.N.; Papadopoulos, M.A. Treatment effects of removable functional appliances in patients with Class II malocclusion: A systematic review and meta-analysis. *Eur. J. Orthod.* **2015**, *37*, 418–434. [CrossRef] [PubMed]
4. Zymperdikas, V.F.; Koretsi, V.; Papageorgiou, S.N.; Papadopoulos, M.A. Treatment effects of fixed functional appliances in patients with Class II malocclusion: A systematic review and meta-analysis. *Eur. J. Orthod.* **2016**, *38*, 113–126. [CrossRef]

5. Franchi, L.; Pavoni, C.; Faltin, K., Jr.; McNamara, J.A., Jr.; Cozza, P. Long-term skeletal and dental effects and treatment timing for functional appliances in Class II malocclusion. *Angle Orthod.* **2013**, *83*, 334–340. [CrossRef]
6. Batista, K.B.; Thiruvenkatachari, B.; Harrison, J.E.; O'Brien, K.D. Orthodontic treatment for prominent upper front teeth (Class II malocclusion) in children and adolescents. *Cochrane Database Syst. Rev.* **2018**, *3*, CD003452. [CrossRef]
7. Kyburz, K.S.; Eliades, T.; Papageorgiou, S.N. What effect does functional appliance treatment have on the temporomandibular joint? A systematic review with meta-analysis. *Prog. Orthod.* **2019**, *20*, 32. [CrossRef]
8. Arens, R.; Marcus, C.L. Pathophysiology of upper airway obstruction: A developmental perspective. *Sleep* **2004**, *27*, 997–1019. [CrossRef]
9. Schellenberg, J.B.; Maislin, G.; Schwab, R.J. Physical findings and the risk for obstructive sleep apnea. The importance of oropharyngeal structures. *Am. J. Respir. Crit. Care Med.* **2000**, *162*, 740–748. [CrossRef]
10. Claudino, L.V.; Mattos, C.T.; Ruellas, A.C.; Sant' Anna, E.F. Pharyngeal airway characterization in adolescents related to facial skeletal pattern: A preliminary study. *Am. J. Orthod. Dentofac. Orthop.* **2013**, *143*, 799–809. [CrossRef]
11. Koretsi, V.; Eliades, T.; Papageorgiou, S.N. Oral Interventions for Obstructive Sleep Apnea. *Dtsch. Arztebl. Int.* **2018**, *115*, 200–207. [CrossRef] [PubMed]
12. Lanteri, V.; Farronato, M.; Ugolini, A.; Cossellu, G.; Gaffuri, F.; Parisi, F.M.R.; Cavagnetto, D.; Abate, A.; Maspero, C. Volumetric Changes in the Upper Airways after Rapid and Slow Maxillary Expansion in Growing Patients: A Case-Control Study. *Materials* **2020**, *13*, 2239. [CrossRef] [PubMed]
13. Shete, C.S.; Bhad, W.A. Three-dimensional upper airway changes with mandibular advancement device in patients with obstructive sleep apnea. *Am. J. Orthod. Dentofac. Orthop.* **2017**, *151*, 941–948. [CrossRef] [PubMed]
14. Xiang, M.; Hu, B.; Liu, Y.; Sun, J.; Song, J. Changes in airway dimensions following functional appliances in growing patients with skeletal class II malocclusion: A systematic review and meta-analysis. *Int. J. Pediatr. Otorhinolaryngol.* **2017**, *97*, 170–180. [CrossRef]
15. Sideri, S.; Papageorgiou, S.N.; Eliades, T. Registration in the international prospective register of systematic reviews (PROSPERO) of systematic review protocols was associated with increased review quality. *J. Clin. Epidemiol.* **2018**, *100*, 103–110. [CrossRef]
16. Sterne, J.A.; Hernán, M.A.; Reeves, B.C.; Savović, J.; Berkman, N.D.; Viswanathan, M.; Henry, D.; Altman, D.G.; Ansari, M.T.; Boutron, I.; et al. ROBINS-I: A tool for assessing risk of bias in non-randomised studies of interventions. *BMJ* **2016**, *355*, i4919. [CrossRef]
17. Papageorgiou, S.N. Meta-analysis for orthodontists: Part II—Is all that glitters gold? *J. Orthod.* **2014**, *41*, 327–336. [CrossRef]
18. Guyatt, G.H.; Oxman, A.D.; Schünemann, H.J.; Tugwell, P.; Knottnerus, A. GRADE guidelines: A new series of articles in the Journal of Clinical Epidemiology. *J. Clin. Epidemiol.* **2011**, *64*, 380–382. [CrossRef]
19. Higgins, J.P.T.; Green, S. *Cochrane Handbook for Systematic Reviews of Interventions Version 5.1.0*; The Cochrane Collaboration: London, UK, 2011.
20. Liberati, A.; Altman, D.G.; Tetzlaff, J.; Mulrow, C.; Gøtzsche, P.C.; Ioannidis, J.P.A.; Clarke, M.; Devereaux, P.J.; Kleijnen, J.; Moher, D. The PRISMA statement for reporting systematic reviews and meta-analyses of studies that evaluate health care interventions: Explanation and elaboration. *J. Clin. Epidemiol.* **2009**, *62*, e1–e34. [CrossRef]
21. Papageorgiou, S.N. Meta-analysis for orthodontists: Part I—How to choose effect measure and statistical model. *J. Orthod.* **2014**, *41*, 317–326. [CrossRef]
22. Langan, D.; Higgins, J.P.T.; Jackson, D.; Bowden, J.; Veroniki, A.A.; Kontopantelis, E.; Viechtbauer, W.; Simmonds, M. A comparison of heterogeneity variance estimators in simulated random-effects meta-analyses. *Res. Synth. Methods* **2019**, *10*, 83–98. [CrossRef] [PubMed]
23. Higgins, J.P.T.; Thompson, S.G.; Deeks, J.J.; Altman, D.G. Measuring inconsistency in meta-analyses. *BMJ* **2003**, *327*, 557–560. [CrossRef] [PubMed]

24. IntHout, J.; Ioannidis, J.P.A.; Rovers, M.M.; Goeman, J.J. Plea for routinely presenting prediction intervals in meta-analysis. *BMJ Open* **2016**, *6*, e010247. [CrossRef]
25. Egger, M.; Davey Smith, G.; Schneider, M.; Minder, C. Bias in meta-analysis detected by a simple, graphical test. *BMJ* **1997**, *315*, 629–634. [CrossRef] [PubMed]
26. Schünemann, H.J.; Cuello, C.; Akl, E.A.; Mustafa, R.A.; Meerpohl, J.J.; Thayer, K.; Morgan, R.L.; Gartlehner, G.; Kunz, R.; Katikireddi, S.V.; et al. GRADE guidelines: 18. How ROBINS-I and other tools to assess risk of bias in nonrandomized studies should be used to rate the certainty of a body of evidence. *J. Clin. Epidemiol.* **2019**, *111*, 105–114. [CrossRef] [PubMed]
27. Bidjan, D.; Sallmann, R.; Eliades, T.; Papageorgiou, S.N. Orthopedic treatment for Class II malocclusion with functional appliances and its effect on upper airways: A systematic review with meta-analysis [dataset]. *Zenodo* **2020**. [CrossRef]
28. Ioannidis, J.P.A. Interpretation of tests of heterogeneity and bias in meta-analysis. *J. Eval. Clin. Pract.* **2008**, *14*, 951–957. [CrossRef]
29. Aksu, M.; Gorucu-Coskuner, H.; Taner, T. Assessment of upper airway size after orthopedic treatment for maxillary protrusion or mandibular retrusion. *Am. J. Orthod. Dentofac. Orthop.* **2017**, *152*, 364–370. [CrossRef]
30. Alhammadi, M.S.; Elfeky, H.Y.; Fayed, M.S.; Ishaq, R.A.R.; Halboub, E.; Al-Mashraqi, A.A. Three-dimensional skeletal and pharyngeal airway changes following therapy with functional appliances in growing skeletal Class II malocclusion patients: A controlled clinical trial. *J. Orofac. Orthop.* **2019**, *80*, 254–265. [CrossRef]
31. Ali, B.; Shaikh, A.; Fida, M. Effect of Clark's twin-block appliance (CTB) and non-extraction fixed mechano-therapy on the pharyngeal dimensions of growing children. *Dent. Press J. Orthod.* **2015**, *20*, 82–88. [CrossRef]
32. Atik, E.; Gorucu-Coskuner, H.; Kocadereli, I. Dentoskeletal and airway effects of the X-Bow appliance versus removable functional appliances (Frankel-2 and Trainer) in prepubertal Class II division 1 malocclusion patients. *Aust. Orthod. J.* **2017**, *33*, 3–13.
33. Bavbek, N.C.; Tuncer, B.B.; Turkoz, C.; Ulusoy, C.; Tuncer, C. Changes in airway dimensions and hyoid bone position following class II correction with forsus fatigue resistant device. *Clin. Oral Investig.* **2016**, *20*, 1747–1755. [CrossRef] [PubMed]
34. Cortese, M.; Pigato, G.; Casiraghi, G.; Ferrari, M.; Bianco, E.; Maddalone, M. Evaluation of the Oropharyngeal Airway Space in Class II Malocclusion Treated with Mandibular Activator: A Retrospective Study. *J. Contemp. Dent. Pract.* **2020**, *21*, 666–672. [PubMed]
35. Drosen, C.; Bock, N.C.; von Bremen, J.; Pancherz, H.; Ruf, S. Long-term effects of Class II Herbst treatment on the pharyngeal airway width. *Eur. J. Orthod.* **2018**, *40*, 82–89. [CrossRef] [PubMed]
36. Elfeky, H.Y.; Fayed, M.M.S. Three-dimensional effects of twin block therapy on pharyngeal airway parameters in Class II malocclusion patients. *J. World Fed. Orthod.* **2015**, *4*, 114–119. [CrossRef]
37. Entrenas, I.; González-Chamorro, E.; Álvarez-Abad, C.; Muriel, J.; Menéndez-Díaz, I.; Cobo, T. Evaluation of changes in the upper airway after Twin Block treatment in patients with Class II malocclusion. *Clin. Exp. Dent. Res.* **2019**, *5*, 259–268. [CrossRef] [PubMed]
38. Fabiani, G.; Galván Galván, J.; Raucci, G.; Elyasi, M.; Pachêco-Pereira, C.; Flores-Mir, C.; Perillo, L. Pharyngeal airway changes in pre-pubertal children with Class II malocclusion after Frankel-2 treatment. *Eur. J. Paediatr. Dent.* **2017**, *18*, 291–295. [CrossRef] [PubMed]
39. Ghodke, S.; Utreja, A.K.; Singh, S.P.; Jena, A.K. Effects of twin-block appliance on the anatomy of pharyngeal airway passage (PAP) in class II malocclusion subjects. *Prog. Orthod.* **2014**, *15*, 68. [CrossRef]
40. Göymen, M.; Mourad, D.; Güleç, A. Evaluation of Airway Measurements in Class II Patients Following Functional Treatment. *Turk. J. Orthod.* **2019**, *32*, 6–10. [CrossRef]
41. Jena, A.K.; Singh, S.P.; Utreja, A.K. Effectiveness of twin-block and Mandibular Protraction Appliance-IV in the improvement of pharyngeal airway passage dimensions in Class II malocclusion subjects with a retrognathic mandible. *Angle Orthod.* **2013**, *83*, 728–734. [CrossRef]
42. Kilinc, D.D.; Sayar, G. Pharyngeal airway changes of patients after Class II activator treatment. *Selcuk Dent. J.* **2018**, *5*, 8–12. [CrossRef]

43. Oliveira, P.M.; Cheib-Vilefort, P.L.; de Pársia Gontijo, H.; Melgaço, C.A.; Franchi, L.; McNamara, J.A., Jr.; Souki, B.Q. Three-dimensional changes of the upper airway in patients with Class II malocclusion treated with the Herbst appliance: A cone-beam computed tomography study. *Am. J. Orthod. Dentofac. Orthop.* **2020**, *157*, 205–211. [CrossRef]
44. Ozbek, M.M.; Memikoglu, T.U.; Gogen, H.; Lowe, A.A.; Baspinar, E. Oropharyngeal airway dimensions and functional-orthopedic treatment in skeletal Class II cases. *Angle Orthod.* **1998**, *68*, 327–336. [CrossRef] [PubMed]
45. Pavoni, C.; Cretella Lombardo, E.; Franchi, L.; Lione, R.; Cozza, P. Treatment and post-treatment effects of functional therapy on the sagittal pharyngeal dimensions in Class II subjects. *Int. J. Pediatr. Otorhinolaryngol.* **2017**, *101*, 47–50. [CrossRef] [PubMed]
46. Rizk, S.; Kulbersh, V.P.; Al-Qawasmi, R. Changes in the oropharyngeal airway of Class II patients treated with the mandibular anterior repositioning appliance. *Angle Orthod.* **2016**, *86*, 955–961. [CrossRef] [PubMed]
47. Rongo, R.; Martina, S.; Bucci, R.; Festa, P.; Galeotti, A.; Alessandri Bonetti, G.; Michelotti, A.; D'Antò, V. Short-term effects of the Sander bite-jumping appliance on the pharyngeal airways in subjects with skeletal Class II malocclusion: A retrospective case-control study. *J. Oral Rehabil.* **2020**. [CrossRef] [PubMed]
48. Ulusoy, C.; Canigur Bavbek, N.; Tuncer, B.B.; Tuncer, C.; Turkoz, C.; Gencturk, Z. Evaluation of airway dimensions and changes in hyoid bone position following class II functional therapy with activator. *Acta Odontol. Scand.* **2014**, *72*, 917–925. [CrossRef] [PubMed]
49. Papageorgiou, S.N.; Koletsi, D.; Eliades, T. What evidence exists for myofunctional therapy with prefabricated appliances? A systematic review with meta-analyses of randomised trials. *J. Orthod.* **2019**, *46*, 297–310. [CrossRef]
50. Schwab, R.J.; Gupta, K.B.; Gefter, W.B.; Metzger, L.J.; Hoffman, E.A.; Pack, A.I. Upper airway and soft tissue anatomy in normal subjects and patients with sleep-disordered breathing. Significance of the lateral pharyngeal walls. *Am. J. Respir. Crit. Care Med.* **1995**, *152*, 1673–1689. [CrossRef]
51. Schwab, R.J.; Gefter, W.B.; Hoffman, E.A.; Gupta, K.B.; Pack, A.I. Dynamic upper airway imaging during awake respiration in normal subjects and patients with sleep disordered breathing. *Am. Rev. Respir. Dis.* **1993**, *148*, 1385–1400. [CrossRef]
52. Poole, M.N.; Engel, G.A.; Chaconas, S.J. Nasopharyngeal cephalometrics. *Oral Surg. Oral Med. Oral Pathol.* **1980**, *49*, 266–271. [CrossRef]
53. Schütz, T.C.; Dominguez, G.C.; Hallinan, M.P.; Cunha, T.C.; Tufik, S. Class II correction improves nocturnal breathing in adolescents. *Angle Orthod.* **2011**, *81*, 222–228. [CrossRef] [PubMed]
54. Cozza, P.; Baccetti, T.; Franchi, L.; De Toffol, L.; McNamara, J.A., Jr. Mandibular changes produced by functional appliances in Class II malocclusion: A systematic review. *Am. J. Orthod. Dentofac. Orthop.* **2006**, *129*, 599.e1–599.e12. [CrossRef] [PubMed]
55. Havakeshian, G.; Koretsi, V.; Eliades, T.; Papageorgiou, S.N. Effect of Orthopedic Treatment for Class III Malocclusion on Upper Airways: A Systematic Review and Meta-Analysis. *J. Clin. Med.* **2020**, *9*, 3015. [CrossRef]
56. Papageorgiou, S.N.; Cobourne, M.T. Data sharing in orthodontic research. *J. Orthod.* **2018**, *45*, 1–3. [CrossRef]
57. Papageorgiou, S.N.; Xavier, G.M.; Cobourne, M.T. Basic study design influences the results of orthodontic clinical investigations. *J. Clin. Epidemiol.* **2015**, *68*, 1512–1522. [CrossRef]
58. Papageorgiou, S.N.; Koretsi, V.; Jäger, A. Bias from historical control groups used in orthodontic research: A meta-epidemiological study. *Eur. J. Orthod.* **2016**, *39*, 98–105. [CrossRef]
59. Cappelleri, J.C.; Ioannidis, J.P.A.; Schmid, C.H.; De Ferranti, S.D.; Aubert, M.; Chalmers, T.C.; Lau, J. Large Trials vs. Meta-analysis of Smaller Trials. *JAMA* **1996**, *276*, 1332–1338. [CrossRef]
60. Papageorgiou, S.N.; Höchli, D.; Eliades, T. Outcomes of comprehensive fixed appliance orthodontic treatment: A systematic review with meta-analysis and methodological overview. *Korean J. Orthod.* **2017**, *47*, 401–413. [CrossRef]
61. Konstantonis, D.; Vasileiou, D.; Papageorgiou, S.N.; Eliades, T. Soft tissue changes following extraction vs. nonextraction orthodontic fixed appliance treatment: A systematic review and meta-analysis. *Eur. J. Oral Sci.* **2018**, *126*, 167–179. [CrossRef]
62. Battagel, J.M.; Johal, A.; Smith, A.M.; Kotecha, B. Postural variation in oropharyngeal dimensions in subjects with sleep disordered breathing: A cephalometric study. *Eur. J. Orthod.* **2002**, *24*, 263–276. [CrossRef] [PubMed]

63. Hsu, W.E.; Wu, T.Y. Comparison of upper airway measurement by lateral cephalogram in upright position and CBCT in supine position. *J. Dent. Sci.* **2019**, *14*, 185–191. [CrossRef] [PubMed]
64. Eslami, E.; Katz, E.S.; Baghdady, M.; Abramovitch, K.; Masoud, M.I. Are three-dimensional airway evaluations obtained through computed and cone-beam computed tomography scans predictable from lateral cephalograms? A systematic review of evidence. *Angle Orthod.* **2017**, *87*, 159–167. [CrossRef] [PubMed]

Publisher's Note: MDPI stays neutral with regard to jurisdictional claims in published maps and institutional affiliations.

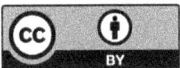

© 2020 by the authors. Licensee MDPI, Basel, Switzerland. This article is an open access article distributed under the terms and conditions of the Creative Commons Attribution (CC BY) license (http://creativecommons.org/licenses/by/4.0/).

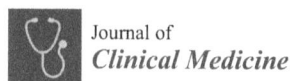

Review

Combined Surgical and Orthodontic Treatments in Children with OSA: A Systematic Review

Laura Templier [1,2], Cecilia Rossi [1,2], Manuel Miguez [3], Javier De la Cruz Pérez [1], Adrián Curto [2], Alberto Albaladejo [2] and Manuel Lagravère Vich [4,*]

[1] Division of Orthodontics, School of Dentistry, University of Alfonso X el Sabio, 28016 Madrid, Spain; Faculty of Medicine; lauratemplier@hotmail.fr (L.T.); cecilia.rossi.uni@hotmail.it (C.R.); jdela@uax.es (J.D.l.C.P.)
[2] Faculty of Medicine, University of Salamanca, 37007 Salamanca, Spain; adrian_odonto@usal.es (A.C.); albertoalbaladejo@hotmail.com (A.A.)
[3] Sleep Dental Medicine Spanish Society (SEMDeS), Dental Sleep Medicine Program, Catholic University of Murcia UCAM, 30107 Murcia, Spain; miguez@infomed.es
[4] Division of Orthodontics, School of Dentistry, Faculty of Medicine and Dentistry, University of Alberta, Edmonton, AB T6G 2R3, Canada
* Correspondence: mlagravere@ualberta.ca

Received: 30 May 2020; Accepted: 23 July 2020; Published: 26 July 2020

Abstract: Obstructive sleep apnea (OSA) is a sleeping breathing disorder. In children, adenotonsillar hypertrophy remains the main anatomical risk factor of OSA. The aim of this study was to assess the current scientific data and to systematically summarize the evidence for the efficiency of adenotonsillectomy (AT) and orthodontic treatment (i.e., rapid maxillary expansion (RME) and mandibular advancement (MA)) in the treatment of pediatric OSA. A literature search was conducted in several databases, including PubMed, Embase, Medline, Cochrane and LILACS up to 5th April 2020. The initial search yielded 509 articles, with 10 articles being identified as eligible after screening. AT and orthodontic treatment were more effective together than separately to cure OSA in pediatric patients. There was a greater decrease in apnea hypoapnea index (AHI) and respiratory disturbance index (RDI), and a major increase in the lowest oxygen saturation and the oxygen desaturation index (ODI) after undergoing both treatments. Nevertheless, the reappearance of OSA could occur several years after reporting adequate treatment. In order to avoid recurrence, myofunctional therapy (MT) could be recommended as a follow-up. However, further studies with good clinical evidence are required to confirm this finding.

Keywords: surgical; orthodontic treatments; apnea

1. Introduction

Obstructive sleep apnea (OSA) is described as a sleeping breathing disorder, characterized by prolonged partial upper airway obstruction and/or intermittent complete obstruction [1]. This syndrome is commonly correlated with intermittent hypoxemia and sleep fragmentation [2]. The prevalence of OSA has been estimated, in a general orthodontic population, by questionnaires and it was found to be 10.8%, which is more than double that reported by similar methods in a healthy pediatric population [3].

OSA has also been associated with frequent snoring, disturbed sleep, daytime neurobehavioral problems, neurocognitive impairments, academic underperformance, hypertension, cardiac dysfunction and systemic inflammation. Daytime sleepiness may occur but is uncommon in young children [4]. Etiological factors include any condition that reduces the caliber of the upper airways, such as craniofacial dysmorphism, hypertrophy of lymphoid tissues, obesity, hypotonic neuromuscular diseases and neuromotor control alterations during sleep. However, adenotonsillar hypertrophy remains the main anatomical risk factor [4–7].

Therefore, adenotonsillectomy (AT) is the recommended first-line treatment for pediatric OSA in children with adenotonsillar hypertrophy [4,8–10]. It has been demonstrated that AT reduced the severity of OSA in most children, and reduced symptoms and improved behavior, quality of life and polysomnographic findings [9]. However, a significant number of patients with pediatric OSA undergoing AT exhibit residual persistent post-surgery OSA [10].

Moreover, it was proven that children with OSA and large tonsils had some craniofacial morphology characteristics like a narrow and long face, a narrow upper airway, maxillary constriction and/or some degree of mandibular retrusion [11–16]. Hence, AT was not always successful in controlling OSA in children, and orthodontic treatments such as rapid maxillary expansion (RME) or mandibular advancement (MA) could be a helpful complement. Nowadays, there are a lot of systematic reviews and meta-analyses about OSA treatments but none has compared the different treatments together and the information about both treatments in concurrence is very limited.

The aim of this systematic review was to assess the current scientific data and to summarize, in a systematic manner, evidence for the efficiency of a combination of surgery (e.g., AT) and orthodontic treatment (i.e., RME and MA) in the treatment of pediatric OSA.

2. Materials and Methods

A Preferred Reporting Items for Reporting Systematic reviews and Meta-Analyses (PRISMA) protocol was followed for reporting this systematic review [17].

2.1. Protocol and Registration

Protocol registration was not available.

2.2. Eligibility Criteria

The Population, Intervention, Comparison, Outcomes and Study design (PICOS) process was used to select abstracts and potential articles retrieved from the databases. The inclusion criteria were:

- Population: children diagnosed with OSA by polysomnography (PSG) or by a home sleep study.
- Intervention: subjects who underwent surgery such as AT and orthodontic treatment (i.e., RME, MA). RME and MA were searched for individually since the focus was on orthodontic treatment (either RME or MA or both together with surgery (tonsillectomy or adenoidectomy)).
- Comparison: a combination of clinical assessments to evaluate the efficiency of surgery and orthodontic treatment to resolve OSA.
- Outcomes: three main outcomes were evaluated: severity of OSA, oxygen saturation and recurrence of OSA after treatment.
- Study design: randomized, non-randomized trials, cohort and case-control studies, case series and case reports were included.

The exclusion criteria were syndromic patients, animal studies, book or conference abstracts, systematic reviews and meta-analyses. Studies comparing AT and expansion independently as treatments were also excluded. There were no restrictions on language, year or status of publication for inclusion.

2.3. Information Sources

A literature search was conducted online in several databases, including PubMed, Embase, Medline, Cochrane and LILACS up to 5 April 2020.

2.4. Search Strategy

The search was performed using keywords, combinations of keywords with truncations, medical subject headings (Mesh) and Boolean logical operators such as "OR" to be more sensitive. The search strategy is presented in Table A1.

Additional potentially relevant articles were identified by performing a manual search via Google, looking for reference lists of retrieved articles.

2.5. Study Selection

The selection of the studies consisted of two phases. During the first phase, two reviewers (L.T. and C.R.) independently identified and checked the titles and abstracts of all records. Those references that met the eligibility criteria were included. Full texts of references containing insufficient information in the title and/or abstract for a decision on inclusion or exclusion were retrieved for evaluation in phase two. In the second phase of article selection, the same two reviewers evaluated the full texts of the remaining articles. Those studies that met the eligibility criteria were included. In cases of disagreement, in both phases, a third reviewer (M.L.V.) settled by consensus.

2.6. Data Collection Process

Two authors (L.T. and C.R.) independently extracted and reviewed data from the included studies. Any disagreement was discussed between them.

2.7. Data Items

From the included studies, various data were collected, such as authors, year, sample size, age, gender, body mass index (BMI), types of screening used to diagnose OSA and types of treatments. They are summarized in Table 1.

2.8. Risk of Bias in Individual Studies

To assess the methodological quality/risk of bias in trials and case–control studies, the first and second authors independently used the checklist by Downs and Black [28], consisting of 26 items categorized in five subgroups: Reporting (nine items), External validity (three items), Bias (seven items), Confounding (six items) and Power (one item). For each item, one point was scored when the respective question was answered "yes" except as described in the original paper for question 5 (Reporting subscale) which can be scored 0, 1 or 2 and question 27 (Power subscale) which can be scored 0, 1, 2, 3, 4 or 5. However, as a study either has or does not have sufficient power to detect a clinically important effect, question 27 was scored, in the present study, 0 or 1. A score of 26 to 28 was considered excellent, 20 to 25 good, 15 to 19 fair and 14 or below was considered to have a poor clinical importance effect. The risk of bias in individual studies is shown in Table A2.

Moreover, the same authors evaluated case reports with the CAse REport (CARE) checklist. It is composed of 13 items: Title, Keywords, Abstract, Introduction, Patient information, Clinical findings, Timeline, Diagnostic assessments, Therapeutic intervention, Follow-up and outcomes, Discussion, Patient perspective and Informed consent. Items are divided by subscale. Each question is answered with "yes" or "no" [29]. To evaluate the different case reports, we gave 1 for the answer: "yes" and 0 for "no" and made the sum to compare them. The accuracy and transparency of the case reports are reported in Table A3.

2.9. Summary Measures

The main outcomes assessed were: apnea hypoapnea index (AHI), respiratory disturbance index (RDI), mean of the lowest oxygen saturation, nadir oxygen saturation, average oxygen saturation and the ODI (oxygen desaturation index) at different times: before both treatments (initial), after the first treatment of surgery or orthodontic treatment (intermediate) and after both treatments (final). These outcomes are presented in Tables 2 and 3.

Table 1. Study characteristics.

Year—Principal Author	Type of Study	Type of Treatment	Type of Screening	Sample Size	Age of Participants (Year) Mean + SD	Sex	BMI (kg/m^2) Mean + SD
2019 Alexander et al. [18]	Case report	RME followed by AT	HST	2	9	F	/
2019 Bignotti et al. [19]	Case report	AT followed by twin block	PSG	1	12	M	22.2
2019 Nauert [20]	Case report	AT followed by Bionator	PSG	1	3	F	/
2018 Gracco et al. [21]	Case report	At the same time: RME + epiglottoplasty + reduction of the tongue base	PSG	1	8	F	/
2014 Villa et al. [22]	NRCT	Group 1: AT: 25 Group 2: RME: 22 Group 3: AT + RME: 5	PSG	52	Group 1: 3.7 ± 0.92 * Group 2: 6.58 ± 1.83 * Group 3: 4.6 ± 3.2	Group 1 and 2: 34M/13F Group 3: 3M/2F	Group 1: 15.75 ± 1.82 * Group 2: 18.82 ± 3.44 * Group 3: 16.65 ± 3.65
2014 Kim [23]	Case report	AT followed by RME F: Final treatment FU: Follow-up 2–5 years after treatment	PSG	1	11	M	22.4
2013 Guilleminault et al. [24]	Case–Control	AT followed by RME, Follow-up: MT or WMT	PSG	24 †; Group MT: 11 Group WMT: 13	I: 5.5 ± 1.2 F: 7.3 ± 1.5 FU: 11.6 ± 1.2	14M/10F	/
2013 Guilleminault et al. [25]	Case–Control	Follow-up study of OSA in teenagers after AT + RME treated in their childhood	PSG	29	I: 7.6 ± 1.7 F: 8.6 ± 2.8 FU: 14.4 ± 0.9	20M/9F	NR: 15.9 ± 1.9 R: 15.7 ± 2.1
2012 Pirelli et al. [26]	NRCT	Group 1: RME: 40 Group 2: AT: 40 Group 3: Residual OSA RME + AT and AT + RME 42	HST	Group 1 and 2: 80 Group 3: 42	7.3	43M/37F	<24
2011 Guilleminault et al. [27]	RCT	Group 1: AT followed by RME, Group 2: RME followed by AT	PSG	31: Group 1: 16 Group 2: 15 †	6.5 ± 0.2	14M/17F	/

RCT—randomized controlled trial; NRCT—non-randomized controlled trial; OSA—obstructive sleep apnea; AT—adenotonsillectomy; RME—rapid maxillary expansion; MT—myofunctional therapy; WMT—without myofunctional therapy; PSG—polysomnography; HST—home sleep study; I—before treatment; F—final treatment; FU—follow-up; R—patients without relapse; NR—patients with relapse; M—male; F—female; * $p < 0.05$; † One patient did not have AT.

Table 2. Summary of severity of OSA.

Year—Principal Author	Type of Treatment	AHI Initial (Events/h) Mean + SD	AHI Intermediate (Events/h) Mean + SD	AHI Final (Events/h) Mean + SD	RDI Initial (Events/h) Mean + SD	RDI Intermediate (Events/h) Mean + SD	RDI Final (Events/h) Mean + SD
2019 Alexander et al. [18]	RME followed by AT	Patient A: 74 Patient B: 16	Post RME: Patient A: 11 Patient B: 4	Patient A: 0.9 Patient B: 1.6	/	/	/
2019 Bignotti et al. [19]	AT followed by twin block	25.5	Post AT: 3.4	0.7	/	/	/
2019 Nauert [20]	AT followed by Bionator	/	Post AT: 10.2	5-year follow-up: normal cognitive development and any evidence of OSA	/	/	/
2018 Gracco et al. [21]	At the same time: RME + epiglottoplasty + reduction of the tongue base	21.8		0.6	/	/	/
2014 Villa et al. [22]	Group 1: AT: 25 Group 2: RME: 22 Group 3: AT + RME: 5	Group 1: 17.25 ± 13.94 * Group 2: 5.81 ± 6.05 * Group 3: 10.14 ± 7.25	/	Group 1: 1.79 ± 1.82 * Group 2: 2.64 ± 3.11 * Group 3: 0.88 ± 0.95	/	/	/
2014 Kim et al. [23]	AT followed by RME F: Final treatment FU: Follow-up 2–5 years after treatment	/	18.9	F: 4.4 FU: 1	/	19.8	F and FU: 5.9
2013 Guilleminault et al. [24]	AT followed by RME, Follow-up: MT or WMT	10.5 ± 2.6	Post AT†: 4.3 ± 1.6	F: 0.4 ± 0.3 MT: 0.5 ± 0.4 * WMT: 5.3 ± 1.5	/	/	/
2013 Guilleminault et al. [25]	Follow-up study of OSA in teenagers after AT + RME treated in their childhood	9 ± 5	Post AT: 3 ± 4	F: 0.4 ± 0.4 NR: 0.5 ± 0.2 * R: 3.1 ± 1 *	15 ± 6.4	Post AT: 7 ± 6	F: 0.6 ± 0.5 NR: 1.5 ± 1.2 * R: 7 ± 1.2
2012 Pirelli et al. [26]	Group 1: RME: 40; Group 2: AT: 40; Group 3: Residual OSA: RME + AT and AT + RME: 42	Group 1 and 2: 12.8	Group 3: RME + AT: 13 ± 3.5 AT + RME: 15 ± 2.9	Group 1 (6/40) and G2 (15/40): 6.5 ± 3.1 Group 3: 39/42 patients were cured	/	/	
2011 Guilleminault et al. [27]	Group 1: AT followed by RME, Group 2: RME followed by AT	Group 1: 12.5 ± 0.8 Group 2: 11.1 ± 0.7	Group 1: 4.9 ± 0.6 Group 2: 5.4 ± 0.6	Group 1: 0.9 ± 0.3 Group 2: 0.9 ± 0.3	Group 1: 21.3 ± 1.0 Group 2: 19.5 ± 1.0	Group 1: 8.0 ± 0.7 Group 2: 7.9 ± 0.5	Group 1: 1.6 ± 0.6 Group 2: 1.7 ± 0.8

OSA—obstructive sleep apnea; AT—adenotonsillectomy; RME—rapid maxillary expansion; MT—myofunctional therapy; WMT—without myofunctional therapy; F—final treatment; FU—follow-up; R—patients with relapse; NR—patients without relapse; * $p < 0.05$; † One patient did not have AT.

Table 3. Summary of oxygen saturation.

Year—Principal Author	Lowest SaO$_2$ Initial (%) Mean + SD	Lowest SaO$_2$ Intermediate (%) Mean + SD	Lowest SaO$_2$ Final (%) Mean + SD	Average SaO$_2$ Initial (%) Mean + SD	Average SaO$_2$ Intermediate (%) Mean + SD	Average SaO$_2$ Final (%) Mean + SD	ODI Initial (Events/Hour)	ODI Intermediate (Events/h)	ODI Final (Events/h)
2019 Alexander et al. [18]	/	/	/	/	/	/	/	/	/
2019 Bignotti et al. [19]	Nadir: 89	Nadir: 93	Nadir: 50	97.3	96.0	96.0	22.0	0.7	3.2
2019 Nauert [20]	/	/	/	/	/	/	/	/	/
2018 Gracco et al. [21]	/	/	/	96.5%	/	98.1	23.4	/	1
2014 Villa et al. [22]	/	/	/	Group 1: 96.11 ± 2.7 * Group 2: 96.56 ± 1.47 * Group 3: 97.85 ± 1.28	/	Group 1: 97.50 ± 1.14 * Group 2: 97.42 ± 1.84 * Group 3: 97.42 ± 2.06	/	/	/
2014 Kim e al. [23]	/	Nadir: 60	Nadir FT: 85 Nadir FU: 94	/	/	/	/	/	/
2013 Guilleminault et al. [24]	90 ±1.5	Post AT†: 92 ± 1	F: 95 ± 1 MT: 96 ± 1 * WMT: 91 ± 1.8	/	/	/	/	/	/
2013 Guilleminault et al. [25]	91 ± 2.5	Post AT: 94 ± 3	F: 98 ± 1.5 NR: 97 ± 1 * R: 92.5 ± 1.5 *	/	/	/	/	/	/
2012 Pirelli et al. [26]	/	/	/	/	/	/	/	/	/
2011 Guilleminault et al. [27]	Group 1: 92.1 ± 0.5 Group 2: 92.5 ± 0.4	Group 1: 95.2 ± 0.3 Group 2: 95.9 ± 0.3	Group 1: 98.0 ± 0.2 * Group 2: 97.6 ± 0.3 *	/	/	/	/	/	/

AT—adenotonsillectomy; MT—myofunctional therapy; WMT—without myofunctional therapy; F—final treatment; FU—follow-up; R—patients with relapse; NR—patients without relapse; SaO$_2$—oxygen saturation; ODI—oxygen desaturation index; * $p < 0.05$; † One patient did not have AT.

3. Results

3.1. Selection of Studies

The information flow of the search and selection of studies is shown in Figure 1. Following the electronic database searches, 505 articles were identified and screened for retrieval and four additional records were identified through other sources. Among the initially identified articles, 259 studies were retrieved after the removal of duplicates. Thus, in the first selection phase, a total of 244 articles were excluded on the basis of title and abstract. In the second phase, on the examination of their full texts, five articles were eliminated and the reasons for exclusion were: overview article ($n = 2$), not related to OSA ($n = 1$), patients who did not receive both treatments, i.e., surgical and orthodontic treatment ($n = 1$) and retracted article ($n = 1$). Therefore, ten studies met all the inclusion criteria and remained for quantitative synthesis.

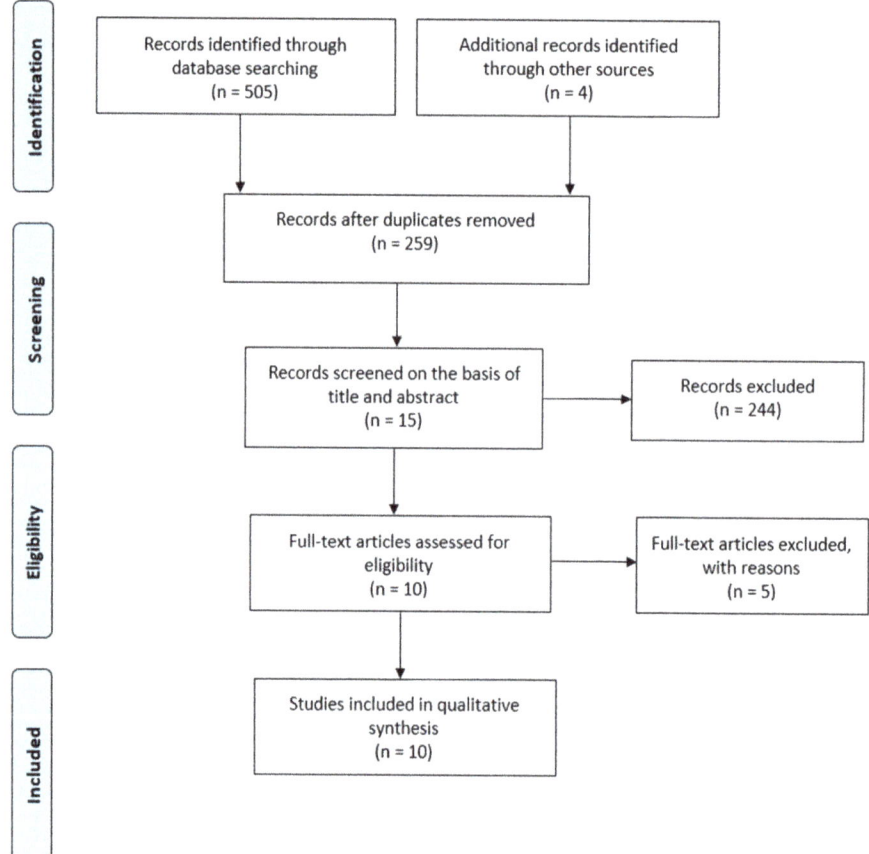

Figure 1. Flow chart of selection process.

3.2. Study Characteristics

The included studies were categorized into one randomized controlled trial (RCT) [27], two non-randomized controlled trials (NRCTs) [22,26], two observational case–control studies [24,25] and five case reports [18–21,23]. The sample sizes ranged from one to 80 subjects. The mean age of participants before starting treatment ranged from 3 to 12 years. In three case reports [19,23,25], the participants were female. In the other studies, males made up a higher proportion than females. The mean

BMI varied between 15.75 and 22.4, however, only five studies reported the BMI [19,22,23,25,26]. To diagnose and evaluate the severity of OSA, eight studies [19–25,27] employed PSG and two [18,26] used home sleep studies (HSTs). All study participants received surgery and orthodontic treatment. Among the surgical treatments, AT was the most commonly used, but there was also one case report [21] which performed other types of surgery: epiglottoplasty and a reduction of the tongue base. Two types of orthodontic treatment were carried out: RME or MA. However, only two case reports used MA as an orthodontic treatment [19,20]. Concerning the order of treatment, five studies [19,20,23–25] performed AT before orthodontic treatment, one case report [21] performed both treatments at the same time, one study [18] completed the orthodontic treatment before AT and three trials [22,26,27] compared both in different groups: AT followed by RME and RME followed by AT.

3.3. Risk of Bias Within Studies

The level of evidence in the trials and case–control studies was assessed by the Downs and Black checklist questionnaire. Two studies [22,26] had a low level of evidence and were evaluated as poor. One case–control study was qualified as fair [24]. An RCT trial [27] and a case-control study [25] were estimated as good. The main reasons for downgrading the quality of evidence pertained to the inclusion of case reports and non-randomized studies with critical methodological issues that most probably introduced bias. Villa et al. [22] compared three groups: one group was treated by AT, the second one by RME and the last one was treated by both. In comparison to the other two groups, the third one had a small numbers of subjects. Therefore, there was a large age difference between each group. The mean age for groups 1, 2 and 3 were 3.7 ± 0.92, 6.58 ± 1.83 and 4.6 ± 3.2, respectively. In the same way, in the trial of Pirelli et al. [26], there were discrepancies among the distribution of characteristics of patients in each group: subjects with indicators of chronic adenotonsillar inflammatory problems were placed in the group to be initially treated with AT, while those not clearly presenting this problem were placed in the initial orthodontic treatment group.

As case reports are considered weak evidence in the hierarchy of research evidence, all of them were classified as having a low level of evidence. However, to evaluate their accuracy and transparency, the CARE checklist was applied. Among the five case reports, Gracco et al.'s had the best rating [21]. The worst score was given to Nauert et al.'s case report [20].

3.4. Results of Individual Studies

In these studies, three main outcomes were assessed: the severity of OSA, oxygen saturation and the recurrence of OSA after surgical and orthodontic treatment.

3.4.1. Severity of OSA

The severity of OSA was evaluated by different measures, such as AHI or RDI. The AHI is the number of apneas or hypopneas recorded during the study per hour of sleep, whereas the RDI means the average number of episodes of apnea, hypopnea and respiratory event-related arousals per hour of sleep. Unlike the AHI, the RDI counts not only respiratory events during sleep, but it also takes into consideration respiratory effort-related arousals which can be defined as arousals from sleep [30].

To evaluate the effectiveness of treatment, most of the studies reported and compared the initial and final AHI. Eight papers [18–20,23–27] also described the intermediate AHI, that is, after patients underwent the first treatment. Only three studies [23,25,27] assessed the RDI.

All studies reported a higher decrease in the AHI or RDI after both treatments (surgery and orthodontic treatment) [18–27]. According to Guilleminault et al. [27], there was no significant difference between the group beginning with orthodontic treatment and the one beginning with surgical treatment after the first phase of treatment. The means of the intermediate AHI were 5.4 ± 0.6 and 4.9 ± 0.6, respectively.

On the other hand, Pirelli et al. [26] reported a greater effectiveness of RME as an initial treatment parameter. In the RME group, 15 subjects (37.5%) had a normal clinical evaluation and a normal polygraphy at the initial post-treatment evaluation, four months after the completion of treatment; 17 presented a significant improvement (AHI 6.5 ± 3.1) and eight had minimal or no improvement (AHI 13 ± 3.5). However, in the AT group, only six patients (15%) presented total remission, 18 presented an improvement in OSA (AHI 6 ± 3.1) and 16 had minimal or no improvement (AHI 15 ± 2.9).

In the same way, two case reports [20,23] appeared not to respond to AT and showed an improvement in the symptoms of pediatric OSA after undergoing orthodontic treatment. Kim et al. [23] described a pre-RME AHI, final AHI and a two-and-a-half-year follow-up AHI of 18.9, 4.4 and 1, respectively.

Furthermore, Villa et al. [22] evaluated and compared the persistence of OSA in children who only underwent AT or RME and in children who received both. They described how in approximately 40% of the children who underwent the surgical procedure, there was a complete resolution of OSA. One year after treatment, subjects who underwent RME treatment were found to have a higher post-treatment AHI than those who underwent AT even though they had a mild form of the disease prior to treatment. The one-year post-RME AHI and the one-year post-surgery AHI were 2.64 ± 3.11 and 1.79 ± 1.82, respectively, and these results were significant. In the group treated by AT and RME, there was a significant decrease in AHI from the beginning (AHI initial: 10.14 ± 7.25) to one year after the end of treatment (AHI final: 0.88 ± 0.95).

3.4.2. Oxygen Saturation

To measure the oxygen saturation, various outcomes were assessed: the mean of the lowest oxygen saturation, the nadir oxygen saturation, the average oxygen saturation and the ODI.

Oxygen saturation is the fraction of oxygen-saturated hemoglobin relative to total hemoglobin (unsaturated + saturated) in the blood. Many patients suffering from OSA have intermittent oxygen desaturation associated with periods of apnea or hypopnea [31]. The nadir oxygen saturation may refer to the lowest point of oxygen saturation, whereas the ODI is the number of times that the blood oxygen level drops by a certain degree from the baseline per hour of sleep.

Three trials [24,25,27] measured the mean of the lowest oxygen saturation before, after the first phase of treatment and at the end of both treatments. All these experimental studies found a significant increase in the lowest oxygen saturation, and it was higher after both treatments (surgery and orthodontic treatment) but not after the first phase of treatment.

Two case reports [19,23] described the nadir oxygen saturation. Kim et al. [23] reported an increase from 60% to 94% of the nadir oxygen saturation compared to before RME and two and a half years after orthodontic treatment, in a child who did not respond to AT. Bignotti et al. [19] illustrated an increase in nadir oxygen saturation after AT from 89% to 93% but a decrease from 93% to 50% after twin block treatment.

Three articles [19,21,22] reported the average of oxygen saturation. Bignotti et al. [19] have shown a lower level of oxygen saturation in patients who have undergone both treatments (AT and twin block), as opposed to Gracco et al. [21], who described a higher level of oxygen saturation after surgery and RME. Similarly, the third study [22] reported a significant increment in the average oxygen saturation one year after surgical treatment or RME therapy. However, they did not find any differences in mean overnight oxygen saturation in the group treated by RME and AT before and one year after treatment (97.85 ± 1.28% vs. 97.42 ± 2.06%).

ODI was assessed by two case reports at the beginning, after surgery treatment and at the end of both treatments. In these articles, ODI decreased by a higher amount after both treatments than after only surgical treatment [19,21].

3.4.3. Recurrence

Two case–control studies [24,25] had a large follow-up of their patients and reported the recurrence of OSA in patients who were treated by AT followed by RME. Guilleminault et al. [25] evaluated and monitored a group of 29 teenagers considered cured of OSA (AHI 0.4 ± 0.4) and with no clinical complaints after undergoing an AT and RME in early childhood. After several years, 20 of the 29 subjects presented with clinical complaints and a mean AHI of 3.1 ± 1.0, whereas nine patients did not report clinical complaints and had a mean AHI of 0.5 ± 0.2. Likewise, Guilleminault et al. [24] evaluated 24 subjects treated with AT followed by RME, with or without follow-up myofunctional re-education. Thirteen of the 24 subjects who did not undergo myofunctional re-education developed the recurrence of symptoms with a mean AHI of 5.3 ± 1.5 and a mean minimum oxygen saturation of 91 ± 1.8%. All the 11 subjects who completed myofunctional re-education for 24 months revealed healthy results (AHI 0.5 ± 0.4).

4. Discussion

4.1. Summary of Evidence

4.1.1. Severity of OSA

All the included studies [18–27] highlighted a major decrease in polysomnographic indexes (AHI or RDI) after undergoing surgical and orthodontic treatments. Most children needed both treatments to have complete resolution of their symptoms and a normalization of PSG [22,27].

These results were independent of the different types of treatment used. However, most studies performed the same types of treatment: RME as an orthodontic treatment and AT as a surgical treatment. Only two case reports [19,20] performed MA as an orthodontic treatment and one case report [21] described an epiglottoplasty and a reduction of the tongue base as surgical treatments. Therefore, the type of surgical treatment should be determined depending on the obstruction site. Hence, in patients with residual OSA after undergoing AT and RME, additional sites of obstruction during sleep could be considered, such as epiglottis collapse [32], supraglottic collapse or tongue base collapse [33].

Besides, except in two trials classified as having a high risk of bias [22,26], there were no differences observed between the various first treatment approaches, that is to say, between subjects who began with orthodontic treatment or with surgical treatment. Pirelli et al. [26] reported a greater effectiveness of RME as an initial treatment parameter, however, it was not a randomized trial and the selection of patients which had AT was not adequate. Conversely, Villa et al. [22] highlighted a higher post-treatment AHI in the group who underwent RME than those who underwent AT. However, in this study, there was an important difference between the mean age in the group treated by AT and the group treated by RME.

4.1.2. Oxygen Saturation

Two trials with a low risk of bias and one with a moderate risk of bias found a significant increase in the mean of the lowest oxygen saturation, and it was higher after receiving both surgery and orthodontic treatment than after the first phase of treatment [24,25,27]. Concerning the nadir oxygen saturation, the results were heterogeneous and had a high risk of bias [19,23].

Among the studies which evaluated the average oxygen saturation, there were a lot of discrepancies between the results and a lack of strong evidence. After undergoing both treatments, the mean level of oxygen saturation was lower according to Bignotti et al. [19], higher as reported by Gracco et al. [21] and did not change according to Villa et al. [22].

In the same way, two case reports of poor clinical relevance described a higher ODI reduction in patients who were subjected to both treatments than those undergoing only surgical treatment [19,21].

4.1.3. Recurrence

The recurrence of OSA after AT and RME were reported in two retrospective case–control studies [24,25]. In the first one [25], characterized to be of good clinical relevance, Guilleminault et al. highlighted a reoccurrence of OSA in 20 of the 29 patients treated in their childhood by AT and

RME. Thus, they suggested that the reappearance of OSA could occur several years after reporting an adequate treatment, following adequate surgical and orthodontic treatment.

Interestingly, they assessed that 12 of the 20 teenagers with sleep-related complaints had the same Friedman scale score of 4, and 16 of the 20 children with OSA recurrence had "high and narrow hard palates" and 14 of the 20 children had "an overjet of more than 2.5 mm", suggesting that these patients presented skeletal relapse despite prior maxillary expansion.

In the same way, the second case–control study [24], which related the recurrence of OSA, was evaluated as having a moderate risk of bias. It showed the follow-up of 24 children with ($n = 11$) or without MT ($n = 13$). All the children were cured (AHI 0.4 ± 0.3) by the combination of AT and palatal expansion.

The children who received MT over the long term remained cured of OSA compared to children who were never trained to perform these exercises and they subsequently had a recurrence of OSA. Similar results were reported by Villa et al. [34] in post-adenotonsillectomy patients who were randomized to either receive MT or not.

Thus, as various studies reported the benefits of the combination of orthodontic or surgical treatment with myofunctional re-education on breathing, speech, swallowing, orofacial growth and the elimination of abnormal head–neck posture, MT could be considered effective as a follow-up therapy to avoid the recurrence of OSA in children treated by adenotonsillectomy and orthodontic treatment.

4.2. Importance of Pediatric Treatment

Sleep disorders in children occur during the critical period of brain development. The consequences of not treating them can be of high relevance, leading to the following health conditions: stunted growth, cognitive and behavioral abnormalities such as hyperactivity, poor school performance, cardiovascular and endothelial dysfunction and an overall reduced quality of life. That is why it is deemed important to treat pediatric patients with OSA [9,35].

4.2.1. Multidisciplinary Approaches

As OSA is a multifactorial syndrome [36], a multidisciplinary approach should be taken to treat OSA in children. That is why, when combined soft tissue surgery, orthodontic treatment and myofunctional therapy worked more effectively together, reducing the AHI [18–27], which was irrespective of the order in which the treatments were performed [27].

In the same way, AT and RME treatments affect the growth patterns of patients with OSA in a positive way. One non-randomized trial assessed the craniofacial changes after AT and RME in mouth-breathing children. Nevertheless, this article was excluded from our quantitative analysis because it did not tie together AT and RME with OSA. This study compared children with oral breathing treated ($n = 33$) or not ($n = 20$) by AT. In the group of children subjected to AT, 17 of the 33 underwent RME. The authors found that AT controlled the facial vertical growth but not maxillomandibular sagittal growth. However, in children subjected to surgery and RME, they noticed that the vertical growth pattern was controlled, and the maxillomandibular sagittal measurements were significantly changed, with a consequent improvement in facial profile. Furthermore, in the frontal view, the group treated by AT and RME showed a significant cross-sectional gain in maxillary width and nasal width measures [37].

4.2.2. Optimal Age

Any child aged 1 to 18 years old could be a candidate for tonsillectomy [38]. The most common late complications of AT were dehydration or secondary post-tonsillectomy hemorrhage (PTH) [39]. In the retrospective study of Lindquist et al. [40], 5225 patients under the age of eighteen years were identified, with an overall late complication rate of 12.8%. Patients younger than three years of age were more likely to present dehydration. This was most significant for children under 2 years of age. However, PTH was more common in older children.

RME has to be performed before the fusion of maxillary sutures, which is completed at the age of 14–15 in females and 15–16 in males [41]. According to Melsen et al. [42], in the early stage (up to 10 years old), the suture was smooth and broad. In the juvenile stage (from 10 to 13 years old), it started to have overlapping sections. Finally, during the adolescent stage (13 and 14 years of age), the suture was wavier with increased interdigitations. In patients with an advanced stage of skeletal maturation, orthopedic maxillary expansion was not possible.

Hence, for the treatment of skeletal class II malocclusion with functional appliance, it has been shown that the functional treatment was efficient when it was performed during the pubertal growth spurt [43–45]. However, if it is performed before the pubertal growth spurt, class II functional appliance will not have clinically relevant effects to correct the skeletal relationship. Nonetheless, there was a dentoalveolar correction, effective in reducing overjet and severity of malocclusion [46]. In one case report [20], after an AT treatment failure, a patient of three years old received a functional therapy of class II. However, in early cases with class II malocclusion it is recommended that only the transversal deficiency of the maxilla is treated [47].

4.3. Limitations

At the systematic methodological review level, no reportable limitations exist, as the PRISMA guidelines were followed, and two reviewers independently selected articles, extracted data and evaluated the clinical relevance to reduce selection bias.

At the study level, the most important limitation was that most of the articles retrieved displayed limited to poor clinical evidence and this was the reason why it was not possible to assess a meta-analysis.

One notable weakness that impacted the methodological quality/risk of retrieved articles was that, in most of studies, the number of subjects undergoing surgical and orthodontic treatment was too low.

One of the limitations in our review was that, in most studies, treatments were only applied in young children. Before undergoing treatment, only two case reports [19,23] had patients older than ten years and the oldest participant was twelve years old [19].

Another important limitation was that various studies did not report the BMI of their population. However, OSA syndrome is considered as one of the adverse consequences of childhood obesity. Narang et al. [48] reported that OSA occurred in up to 60% of obese children. In the same way, Mitchell et al. [49] showed that obese children are more likely to have a higher level of pre- and post-adenotonsillectomy OSA when compared with children of normal weight.

5. Conclusions

A limitation present in this review was the availability of few studies and most of them were considered to have a high risk of bias. Nevertheless, considering the available information, AT and orthodontic treatment were more effective together rather than separately to cure OSA in pediatric patients. There was a greater decrease in AHI and RDI, a major increase in the mean of the lowest oxygen saturation and the ODI in patients after undergoing both treatments. The reappearance of OSA could occur several years after reporting adequate treatment. In order to avoid recurrence, MT could be recommended as a follow-up. Further research with good clinical evidence is required to confirm this finding.

Author Contributions: Conceptualization, L.T., C.R., M.M., M.L.V., J.D.l.C.P., A.C., and A.A.; Methodology, L.T., C.R., M.M., M.L.V., J.D.l.C.P., A.C., and A.A.; Formal Analysis, L.T., C.R., M.M., M.L.V., J.D.l.C.P., A.C., and A.A.; Writing—Original Draft Preparation, L.T., C.R., M.M., M.L.V., J.C.l.C.P., A.C., and A.A.; Writing—Review and Editing, L.T., M.M., and M.L.V.; Supervision, M.M., M.L.V., J.C.l.C.P., A.C., and A.A.; Project Administration, M.M., M.L.V., J.C.l.C.P., A.C., and A.A. All authors have read and agreed to the published version of the manuscript.

Funding: This research received no external funding.

Conflicts of Interest: The authors declare no conflict of interest.

Abbreviations

AHI	Apnea hypoapnea index
AT	Adenotonsillectomy
BMI	Body mass index
HST	Home sleep study
MA	Mandibular advancement
MT	Myofunctional therapy
NRCT	Non-randomized controlled trial
ODI	Oxygen desaturation index
OSA	Obstructive sleep apnea
PSG	Polysomnography
RCT	Randomized controlled trial
RDI	Respiratory disturbance index
RME	Rapid maxillary expansion
PTH	Post-tonsillectomy hemorrhage

Appendix A

Table A1. Search strategy.

Source	Query			Hits
MedLine (N = 129) (Ovid) http://ovidsp.tx.ovid.com	Database: Ovid MEDLINE(R) ALL <1946 to 1 April 2020> Search Strategy: 1) apnea.mp. or exp Apnea/ 2) expansion.mp. 3) extraction.mp. 4) orthodon *.mp. 5) 2 or 3 or 4 6) tonsil *.mp. 7) adenoid *.mp. 8) 6 or 7 9) 1 and 5 and 8			55,675 167,509 275,062 57,238 491,026 36,364 17,236 47,732 129
Embase (N = 194) (Ovid) http://ovidsp.tx.ovid.com	Database: Embase <1974 to 1 April 2020> Search Strategy: 1) exp apnea/or apnea.mp. 2) expansion.mp. 3) exp extraction/or extraction.mp. 4) orthodon *.mp. 5) 2 or 3 or 4 (704,171) 6) tonsil *.mp. (42,139) 7) adenoid *.mp. 8) 6 or 7 9) 1 and 5 and 8			92,729 215,648 443,345 54,485 704,171 −42,139 18,653 55,708 194
PubMed (N = 136) http://www.ncbi.nln.nih.gov/pubmed	#12	Add	Search (#1 and #6 and #10) Filters: Humans	136
	#11	Add	Search (#1 and #6 and #10)	156
	#10	Add	Search (#8 or #9)	47,643
	#9	Add	Search adenoid *	17,210
	#8	Add	Search tonsil *	36,293
	#6	Add	Search (#2 or #3 or #5)	504,872
	#5	Add	Search orthodon *	73,679
	#3	Add	Search extraction	274,317
	#2	Add	Search expansion	166,756
	#1	Add	Search apnea	58,662
Cochrane (N = 38)	ID	Search	Hits	
	#1	apnea		9046
	#2	Expansion		5534
	#3	Extraction		21,029
	#4	Orthodon *		4587
	#5	#2 or #3 or #4		29,693
	#6	Tonsil *		3659
	#7	Adenoid *		1189
	#8	#6 or #7		4129
	#9	#1 and #5 and #8		38
LILACS (N = 8)	Apnea, orthodon *, extraction, expansion, tonsil *, adenoid *			

Table A2. Quality index.

		2014 Villa et al. [22]	2013 Guilleminault et al. [24]	2013 Guilleminault et al. [25]	2012 Pirelli al. [26]	2011 Guilleminault et al. [27]
Question 1	0 no, 1 yes	1	1	1	1	0
Question 2	0 no, 1 yes	1	1	1	1	1
Question 3	0 no, 1 yes	1	1	1	1	1
Question 4	0 no, 1 yes	1	1	1	1	1
Question 5	0 no, 1 partially, 2 yes	1	0	2	0	1
Question 6	0 no, 1 yes	1	1	1	0	1
Question 7	0 no, 1 yes	0	1	1	0	1
Question 8	0 no, 1 yes	0	0	0	0	0
Question 9	0 no, 1 yes	1	1	1	0	1
Question 10	0 no, 1 yes	1	1	0	0	1
Question 11	0 no, 1 yes	0	1	1	1	1
Question 12	0 no, 1 yes	0	0	1	1	1
Question 13	0 no, 1 yes	0	1	1	1	1
Question 14	0 no, 1 yes	0	0	0	0	0
Question 15	0 no, 1 yes	0	0	0	0	0
Question 16	0 no, 1 yes	0	1	1	1	1
Question 17	0 no, 1 yes	1	1	1	1	1
Question 18	0 no, 1 yes	1	1	1	1	1
Question 19	0 no, 1 yes	1	0	1	1	0
Question 20	0 no, 1 yes	1	1	1	0	1
Question 21	0 no, 1 yes	0	0	0	1	1
Question 22	0 no, 1 yes	1	0	1	1	1
Question 23	0 no, 1 yes	0	0	0	0	1
Question 24	0 no, 1 yes	0	0	0	0	0
Question 25	0 no, 1 yes	0	0	1	0	1
Question 26	0 no, 1 yes	1	1	1	0	1
Question 27	0, 1, 2, 3, 4, 5	0	0	0	0	0
Total score		14	15	20	13	20
Quality		Poor	Fair	Good	Poor	Good

Good = 2, Fair = 1, Poor = 2.

Table A3. CAse REport (CARE) checklist.

Topic	Item	2014 Kim et al. [23]	2019 Alexander et al. [18]	2019 Bignotti et al. [19]	2019 Nauert et al. [20]	2018 Gracco et al. [21]
Title	1	0	0	1	1	1
Key Words	2	0	0	0	0	0
Abstract	3a	0	1	0	0	1
	3b	0	1	1	1	1
	3c	1	1	1	1	1
	3d	1	1	1	1	1
Introduction	4	0	0	0	0	1
Patient Information	5a	1	1	1	1	1
	5b	1	1	1	1	1
	5c	1	1	1	1	1
	5d	1	0	1	1	1
Clinical Findings	6	1	1	1	1	1
Timeline	7	1	1	1	1	1
Diagnostic Assessment	8a	1	1	1	1	1
	8b	0	0	0	0	0
	8c	0	0	0	0	1
	8d	0	0	0	0	0
Therapeutic Intervention	9a	1	1	1	1	1
	9b	1	1	1	1	1
	9c	1	1	1	1	1
Follow-up and Outcomes	10a	1	1	1	1	1
	10b	1	1	1	0	1
	10c	0	0	1	1	1
	10d	0	0	0	0	0
Discussion	11a	1	1	0	0	0
	11b	1	1	1	0	1
	11c	1	1	1	0	1
	11d	1	1	1	0	1
Patient Perspective	12	0	0	0	0	0
Informed Consent	13	0	0	0	0	0
Total		18	19	20	16	23

Yes = 1, No = 0.

References

1. Loughlin, G.M.; Brouillette, R.T.; Brooke, L.J.; Carroll, J.L.; Chipps, B.E.; England, S.J.; Ferber, P.; Ferraro, N.F.; Gaultier, C.; Givan, D.C.; et al. Standards and indications for cardiopulmonary sleep studies in children. *Am. J. Respir. Crit. Care Med.* **1996**, *153*, 866–878.
2. Marcus, C.L.; Annett, R.D.; Brooks, L.J.; Brouillette, R.T.; Carroll, J.L.; Givan, D.; Gozal, D.; Kiley, J.; Redline, S.; Rosen, C.L.; et al. Cardiorespiratory sleep studies in children. Establishment of normative data and polysomnographic predictors of morbidity. *Am. J. Respir. Crit. Care Med.* **1999**, *160*, 1381–1387. [CrossRef]
3. Abtahi, S.; Witmans, M.; Alsufyani, N.A.; Major, M.P.; Major, P.W. Pediatric sleep-disordered breathing in the orthodontic population: Prevalence of positive risk and associations. *Am. J. Orthod. Dentofac. Orthop.* **2020**, *157*, 466–473. [CrossRef] [PubMed]
4. Marcus, C.L.; Brooks, L.J.; Draper, K.A.; Gozal, D.; Halbower, A.C.; Jones, J.; Schechter, M.S.; Sheldon, S.H.; Spruyt, K.; Ward, S.D.; et al. Diagnosis and management of childhood obstructive sleep apnea syndrome. *Pediatrics* **2012**, *130*, 576–584. [CrossRef] [PubMed]
5. Marcus, C.L.; McColley, S.A.; Carroll, J.L.; Loughlin, G.M.; Smith, P.L.; Schwartz, A.R. Upper airway collapsibility in children with obstructive sleep-apnea syndrome. *J. Appl. Physiol.* **1994**, *77*, 918–924. [CrossRef] [PubMed]
6. Arens, R.; Marcus, C.L. Pathophysiology of upper airway obstruction: A developmental perspective. *Sleep* **2004**, *27*, 997–1019. [CrossRef]
7. Redline, S.; Amin, R.; Beebe, D.; Chervin, R.D.; Garetz, S.L.; Giordani, B.; Marcus, C.L.; Moore, R.H.; Rosen, C.L.; Arens, R.; et al. The childhood adenotonsillectomy trial (CHAT): Rationale, design, and challenges of a randomized controlled trial evaluating a standard surgical procedure in a pediatric population. *Sleep* **2011**, *34*, 1509–1517. [CrossRef]
8. Schechter, M.S. Technical report: Diagnosis and management of childhood obstructive sleep apnea syndrome. *Pediatrics* **2002**, *109*, e69. [CrossRef]
9. Marcus, C.L.; Moore, R.H.; Rosen, C.L.; Giordani, B.; Garetz, S.L.; Taylor, H.G.; Mitchell, R.B.; Amin, R.; Katz, E.S.; Arens, R.; et al. A randomized trial of adenotonsillectomy for childhood sleep apnea. *N. Engl. J. Med.* **2013**, *368*, 2366–2376. [CrossRef]
10. Tan, H.L.; Kheirandish-Gozal, L.; Gozal, D. Obstructive sleep apnea in children: Update on the recognition, treatment and management of persistent disease. *Expert. Rev. Respir. Med.* **2016**, *10*, 431–439. [CrossRef]
11. Pirilä-Parkkinen, K.; Pirttiniemi, P.; Nieminen, P.; Tolonen, U.; Pelttari, U.; Löppönen, H. Dental arch morphology in children with sleep-disordered breathing. *Eur. J. Orthod.* **2009**, *31*, 160–167. [CrossRef] [PubMed]
12. Guilleminault, C.; Partinen, M.; Praud, J.P.; Quera-Ssalva, M.A.; Powell, N.; Riley, R. Morphometric facial changes and obstructive sleep-apnea in adolescents. *J. Pediatr.* **1989**, *114*, 997–999. [CrossRef]
13. Guilleminault, C.; Li, K.K.; Khramtsov, A.; Pelayo, R.; Martinez, S. Sleep disordered breathing: Surgical outcomes in prepubertal children. *Laryngoscope* **2004**, *114*, 132–137. [CrossRef] [PubMed]
14. Tasker, C.; Crosby, J.H.; Stradling, J.R. Evidence for persistence of upper airway narrowing during sleep, 12 years after adenotonsillectomy. *Arch. Dis. Child.* **2002**, *86*, 34–37. [CrossRef] [PubMed]
15. Mitchell, R.B.; Kelly, J. Outcome of adenotonsillectomy for severe obstructive sleep apnea in children. *Int. J. Pediatr. Otorhinolaryngol.* **2004**, *68*, 1375–1379. [CrossRef]
16. Souki, B.Q.; Pimenta, G.B.; Souki, M.Q.; Franco, L.P.; Becker, H.M.G.; Pinto, J.A. Prevalence of malocclusion among mouth breathing children: Do expectations meet reality? *Int. J. Pediatr. Otorhinolaryngol.* **2009**, *73*, 767–773. [CrossRef]
17. Moher, D.; Liberati, A.; Tetzlaff, J.; Altman, D.G.; PRISMA Group. Preferred reporting items for systematic reviews and meta-analyses: The PRISMA statement. *PLoS Med.* **2009**, *6*, e1000097. [CrossRef]
18. Alexander, N.; Boota, A.; Hooks, K.; White, J.R. Rapid maxillary expansion and adenotonsillectomy in 9-year-old twins with pediatric obstructive sleep apnea syndrome: An interdisciplinary effort. *J. Am. Osteopath. Assoc.* **2019**, *119*, 126–134. [CrossRef]
19. Bignotti, D.; De Stefani, A.; Mezzofranco, L.; Bruno, G.; Gracco, A. Multidisciplinary approach in a 12-year-old patient affected by severe obstructive sleep apnea: A case-report. *Sleep Med. Res.* **2019**, *10*, 103–107. [CrossRef]
20. Nauert, K. Kieferorthopädische Behandlung der obstruktiven Schlafapnoe im Kindesalter—Ein Fallbericht. *Atemwegs Lungenkrankh.* **2019**, *45*, 46–48. [CrossRef]

21. Gracco, A.; Bruno, G.; de Stefani, A.; Ragona, R.M.; Mazzoleni, S.; Stellini, E. Combined orthodontic and surgical treatment in a 8-years-old patient affected by severe obstructive sleep apnea: A case-report. *J. Clin. Pediatr. Dent.* **2018**, *42*, 79–84. [CrossRef] [PubMed]
22. Villa, M.P.; Castaldo, R.; Miano, S.; Paolini, M.C.; Vitelli, O.; Tabarrini, A.; Mazzotta, A.R.; Cecili, M.; Barreto, M. Adenotonsillectomy and orthodontic therapy in pediatric obstructive sleep apnea. *Sleep Breath* **2014**, *18*, 533–539. [CrossRef] [PubMed]
23. Kim, M. Orthodontic treatment with rapid maxillary expansion for treating a boy with severe obstructive sleep apnea. *Sleep Med. Res.* **2014**, *5*, 33–36. [CrossRef]
24. Guilleminault, C.; Huang, Y.S.; Monteyrol, P.J.; Sato, R.; Quo, S.; Lin, C.H. Critical role of myofascial reeducation in pediatric sleep-disordered breathing. *Sleep Med.* **2013**, *14*, 518–525. [CrossRef]
25. Guilleminault, C.; Huang, Y.-S.; Quo, S.; Monteyrol, P.-J.; Lin, C.-H.; , C-H. Teenage sleep-disordered breathing: Recurrence of syndrome. *Sleep Med.* **2013**, *14*, 37–44. [CrossRef] [PubMed]
26. Pirelli, P.; Saponara, M.; Guilleminault, C. Rapid maxillary expansion before and after adenotonsillectomy in children with obstructive sleep apnea. *Somnologie Schlafforschung Schlafmed.* **2012**, *16*, 125–132. [CrossRef]
27. Guilleminault, C.; Monteyrol, P.-J.; Huynh, N.T.; Pirelli, P.; Quo, S.; Li, K. Adeno-tonsillectomy and rapid maxillary distraction in pre-pubertal children, a pilot study. *Sleep Breath* **2011**, *15*, 173–177. [CrossRef]
28. Downs, S.H.; Black, N. The feasibility of creating a checklist for the assessment of the methodological quality both of randomised and non-randomised studies of health care interventions. *J. Epidemiol. Community Health* **1998**, *52*, 377–384. [CrossRef]
29. Riley, D.S.; Barber, M.S.; Kienle, G.S.; Aronson, J.K.; von Schoen-Angerer, T.; Tugwell, P.; Kiene, H.; Helfand, M.; Altman, D.G.; Sox, H.; et al. CARE guidelines for case reports: Explanation and elaboration document. *J. Clin. Epidemiol.* **2017**, *89*, 218–235. [CrossRef]
30. Goyal, M.; Johnson, J. Obstructive sleep apnea diagnosis and management. *Mo. Med.* **2017**, *114*, 120–124.
31. Landsberg, R.; Friedman, M.; Ascher-Landsberg, J. Treatment of hypoxemia in obstructive sleep apnea. *Am. J. Rhinol.* **2001**, *15*, 311–313. [PubMed]
32. Torre, C.; Camacho, M.; Liu, S.Y.; Huon, L.K.; Capasso, R. Epiglottis collapse in adult obstructive sleep apnea: A systematic review. *Laryngoscope* **2016**, *126*, 515–523. [CrossRef] [PubMed]
33. Camacho, M.; Dunn, B.; Torre, C.; Sasaki, J.; Gonzales, R.; Liu, S.-C.; Chan, D.K.; Certal, V.; Cable, B.B. Supraglottoplasty for laryngomalacia with obstructive sleep apnea: A systematic review and meta-analysis. *Laryngoscope* **2016**, *126*, 1246–1255. [CrossRef] [PubMed]
34. Villa, M.P.; Brasili, L.; Ferretti, A.; Vitelli, O.; Rabasco, J.; Mazzotta, A.R.; Pietropaoli, N.; Martella, S. Oropharyngeal exercises to reduce symptoms of OSA after AT. *Sleep Breath* **2015**, *19*, 281–289. [CrossRef] [PubMed]
35. Luz Alonso-Álvarez, M.; Canet, T.; Cubell-Alarco, M.; Estivill, E.; Fernández-Julián, E.; Gozal, D.; Jurado-Luque, M.J.; Lluch-Roselló, M.A.; Martínez-Pérez, F.; Merino-Andreu, M.; et al. Consensus document on sleep apnea-hypopnea syndrome in children (full version). Sociedad Española de Sueño. El Área de Sueño de la Sociedad Española de Neumología y Cirugía Torácica(SEPAR). *Arch. Bronconeumol.* **2011**, *47*, 2–18. [CrossRef]
36. Behrents, R.G.; Shelgikar, A.V.; Conley, R.S.; Flores-Mir, C.; Hans, M.; Levine, M.; McNamara, J.A.; Palomo, J.M.; Pliska, B.; Stockstill, J.W.; et al. Obstructive sleep apnea and orthodontics: An American Association of Orthodontists White Paper. *Am. J. Orthod. Dentofac. Orthop.* **2019**, *156*, 13–28. [CrossRef]
37. Pereira, S.R.A.; Weckx, L.L.M.; Ortolani, C.L.F.; Bakor, S.F. Estudo das alterações craniofaciais e da importância da expansão rápida da maxila após adenotonsilectomia. *Braz. J. Otorhinolaryngol.* **2012**, *78*, 111–117. [CrossRef]
38. Mitchell, R.B.; Archer, S.M.; Ishman, S.L.; Rosenfeld, R.M.; Coles, S.; Finestone, S.A.; Friedman, N.R.; Giordano, T.; Hildrew, D.M.; Kim, T.W.; et al. Clinical Practice Guideline: Tonsillectomy in Children (Update)-Executive Summary. *Otolaryngol. Head Neck Surg.* **2019**, *160*, 187–205. [CrossRef]
39. Belyea, J.; Chang, Y.; Rigby, M.H.; Corsten, G.; Hong, P. Post-tonsillectomy complications in children less than three years of age: A case-control study. *Int. J. Pediatr. Otorhinolaryngol.* **2014**, *78*, 871–874. [CrossRef]
40. Lindquist, N.R.; Feng, Z.; Patro, A.; Mukerji, S.S. Age-related causes of emergency department visits after pediatric adenotonsillectomy at a tertiary pediatric referral center. *Int. J. Pediatr. Otorhinolaryngol.* **2019**, *127*, 109668. [CrossRef] [PubMed]

41. Haas, A.J. Long-term posttreatment evaluation of rapid palatal expansion. *Angle Orthod.* **1980**, *50*, 189–217. [PubMed]
42. Melsen, B.; Melsen, F. The postnatal development of the palatomaxillary region studied on human autopsy material. *Am. J. Orthod.* **1982**, *82*, 329–342. [CrossRef]
43. Baccetti, T.; Franchi, L.; Stahl, F. Comparison of 2 comprehensive Class II treatment protocols including the bonded Herbst and headgear appliances: A double-blind study of consecutively treated patients at puberty. *Am. J. Orthod. Dentofac. Orthop.* **2009**, *135*, 1–10. [CrossRef] [PubMed]
44. Baccetti, T.; Franchi, L.; Toth, L.R.; McNamara, J.A., Jr. Treatment timing for Twin-block therapy. *Am. J. Orthod. Dentofac. Orthop.* **2000**, *118*, 159–170. [CrossRef] [PubMed]
45. Martina, R.; Cioffi, I.; Galeotti, A.; Tagliaferri, R.; Cimino, R.; Michelotti, A.; Valletta, R.; Farella, M.; Paduano, S. Efficacy of the Sander bite-jumping appliance in growing patients with mandibular retrusion: A randomized controlled trial. *Orthod. Craniofac. Res.* **2013**, *16*, 116–126. [CrossRef]
46. O'Brien, K.; Wright, J.; Conboy, F.; Sanjie, Y.; Mandall, N.; Chadwick, S.; Connolly, I.; Cook, P.; Birnie, D.; Hammond, M.; et al. Effectiveness of early orthodontic treatment with the Twin-block appliance: A multicenter, randomized, controlled trial. Part 1: Dental and skeletal effects. *Am. J. Orthod. Dentofac. Orthop.* **2003**, *124*, 234–243.
47. Baccetti, T. El tiempo: La cuarta dimensión en el plan de tratamiento de la maloclusión de Clase II. *Rev. Esp. Ortod.* **2011**, *41*, 199–204.
48. Narang, I.; Mathew, J.L. Childhood obesity and obstructive sleep apnea. *J. Nutr. Metab.* **2012**, *2012*, 134202. [CrossRef]
49. Mitchell, R.B.; Boss, E.F. Pediatric obstructive sleep apnea in obese and normal-weight children: Impact of adenotonsillectomy on quality-of-life and behavior. *Dev. Neuropsychol.* **2009**, *34*, 650–661. [CrossRef]

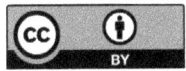

© 2020 by the authors. Licensee MDPI, Basel, Switzerland. This article is an open access article distributed under the terms and conditions of the Creative Commons Attribution (CC BY) license (http://creativecommons.org/licenses/by/4.0/).

MDPI
St. Alban-Anlage 66
4052 Basel
Switzerland
www.mdpi.com

Journal of Clinical Medicine Editorial Office
E-mail: jcm@mdpi.com
www.mdpi.com/journal/jcm

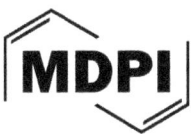

Disclaimer/Publisher's Note: The statements, opinions and data contained in all publications are solely those of the individual author(s) and contributor(s) and not of MDPI and/or the editor(s). MDPI and/or the editor(s) disclaim responsibility for any injury to people or property resulting from any ideas, methods, instructions or products referred to in the content.

www.ingramcontent.com/pod-product-compliance
Lightning Source LLC
LaVergne TN
LVHW070510100526
838202LV00014B/1825